EAST ASIA

HISTORY, POLITICS, SOCIOLOGY, CULTURE

Edited by
Edward Beauchamp
University of Hawaii

A ROUTLEDGE SERIES

East Asia: History, Politics, Sociology, Culture

Edward Beauchamp, *General Editor*

ACCOMMODATING THE CHINESE
THE AMERICAN HOSPITAL IN CHINA,
1880–1920

Michelle Renshaw

Routledge
New York & London

Published in 2005 by
Routledge
Taylor & Francis Group
711 Third Avenue
New York, NY 10017

First issued in paperback 2013

Published in Great Britain by
Routledge
Taylor & Francis Group
2 Park Square
Milton Park, Abingdon
Oxon, OX14 4RN

International Standard Book Number-10: 0-415-97285-X (Hardcover)
International Standard Book Number-13: 978-0-415-97285-7 (Hardcover)
International Standard Book Number-13: 978-0-415-64562-1 (Paperback)
Library of Congress Card Number 2004026222

Library of Congress Cataloging-In-Publication Data

Renshaw, Michelle.
  Accommodating the Chinese : the American hospital in China, 1880–1920 / Michelle Renshaw.
     p. cm.
  Includes bibliographical references and index.
  ISBN: 0-415-97285-X
  1. Hospitals--China--History--19th century.   2. Hospitals--China--History--20th century.
  3. Missions, Medical--China--History--19th century.   I. Title.

RA990.C5R46 2005
362.11'0951--dc22   2004026222

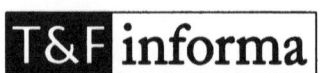

Taylor & Francis Group
is the Academic Division of T&F Informa plc.

Visit the Taylor & Francis Web site at
http://www.taylorandfrancis.com

and the Routledge Web site at
http://www.routledge-ny.com

Contents

List of Figures

List of Illustrations

A complete set of photographs, plans, and charts referred to in the text, including the Chronology, are available at www.michellerenshaw.com

Abbreviations

ABCFM	American Board of Commissioners for Foreign Missions
ABFMS	American Baptist Foreign Missionary Society
ACM	American Church Mission (Domestic and Foreign Missionary Society of the Protestant Episcopal Church in the U.S.A.)
APM (N)	American Presbyterian Mission (North)
APM (S)	American Presbyterian Mission (South)
CCC	China Continuation Committee of the National Missionary Conference
CIM	China Inland Mission
CMMA	China Medical Missionary Society
CMB	China Medical Board of the Rockefeller Foundation
CMJ	*China Medical Journal, The* (from 1907)
CMMJ	*China Medical Missionary Journal, The* (1887–1907)
CMS	Church Missionary Society
EBM	English Baptist Mission
FCMS	Foreign Christian Missionary Society
LMS	London Missionary Society
MEM	Methodist Episcopal Mission
MEM(S)	Methodist Episcopal Mission (South)
PUMC	Peking Union Medical College
RAC	Rockefeller Archive Center
SOAS	School of Oriental and African Studies, University of London
SPG	Society for the Propagation of the Gospel in Foreign Parts
WUMS	Women's Union Missionary Society
WMMS	Wesleyan Methodist Missionary Society

Glossary

Other than when citing or directly quoting from primary sources, I have used the Pinyin system in the text. The terms in parenthesis are the various spellings used in primary sources.

Aiyutang (Oi Yuk Tong)	爱育堂
anji fang	安济坊
anle fang	安乐坊
Baoli yiyuan (Pau li)	保黎医院
Cixi baoli yihui	慈溪保黎医会
baoyi (pau i)	包医
beitian fang (Peit'ien fang)	背田坊
beitian yuan (Peit'ien yuan)	背田院
bie fang	别坊
Cixi baoli yihui	慈溪保黎医会
dili	地理
Fangbiansuo (Fong Pin Sho)	方便所
fengrenyuan	疯人院
fengshui (fengshuy)	风水
futian yuan	幅田院
gang (kang)	缸
Guangdong shanhou zongju (Kwong Tung Shin Hau Tsung Kuk)	广东善后总局
Guandong zhi	广东志
Guangren hui	广仁会
Guangren yiyuan	广仁医院
Houmen (Ho Men)	后门
Hua Mei (Hwa Mei)	华美
huimin yaoju	惠民药局
jian (chien)	间

juyang fa	居养法
kang (k'ang)	炕
Laoren yuan	老人院
Liubing guan	六病馆
Mafeng yuan	麻风院
matouqiang	马头墙
mingyi	名医
Minzhengbu (Minchengbu)	民政部
neicheng guan yiyuan	内城官医院
Neiwubu	内务部
Puji yuan	普济院
qi	气
qiaojiao	翘角
ruyi	儒医
shiyi	时医
Shiyi gongu	施医公局
Tongren yuan	同仁堂院
Tongshan hui	同善会
waicheng guan yiyuan	外城官医院
waike	外科
Wai Yuan	外院
Weisheng si	卫生司
wuxing	五行
Yiyi (Hsi yi)	西医
xiandai xiyi yiyuan	现代西医医院
yamen	衙们
yinyang	阴阳
Yanghang huiguan	洋行会馆
yangzi yuan	养子院
Zhong xi yiyuan (Chung Si Yi Yuan)	中西医院
Zhongyi (Chung Yi)	中医
zuchuan shiyi	祖传世医

PLACE NAMES[1]   PROVINCE

Anhui (Anhuei, Anwei)	安徽	
Anking (Anqing)	安庆	Anhui

1. Sources used: Index of Geographical Names in K C. Wong and Wu Lien-teh, *History of Chinese Medicine: Being a Chronicle of Medical Happenings in China from Ancient Times to the Present Period*, 2nd. ed. (Shanghai: National Quarantine Service, 1936), pp. 860–64;

PLACE NAMES   PROVINCE

Baodingfu (Paotingfu)	保定府	Hebei
Baofushan (Ponasang)	保福山	Fujian
Cangzhou (T'sang-chow, Ts'angchou)	滄州	Hebei
Changan	长安	Shaanxi
Changde (Changteh)	常德	Hunan
Changsha	长沙	Hunan
Changzhou (Chenchow)	长州	Hunan
Chengdu (Chengtu, Chen-tu)	成都	Sichuan
Chizhou (Chi-chou)	祁州	Shanxi
Chongqing (Chungking)	重庆	Sichuan
Chuzhou (Chuchow)	滁州	Anhui
Cixi (Tzeki, Tzu-chi)	慈溪	Zhejiang
Dalian (Dairen)	大连	Liaoning
Daye (Taye, Tayyeh)	大冶	Hubei
Dongwan (Tungkun)	东莞	Guangdong
Foshan (Fatshan)	佛山	Guangzhou
Fujian (Fukien, Fuhkien)	福建	
Funing (Fuh-ning)	福甯	Fujian
Fuzhou (Foochow)	福州	Fujian
Guangdong (Kwangtung, Kuangtung)	广东	
Guangxi (Kwangsi)	廣西	
Guangzhou (Canton)	广州	Guangdong
Hangzho (Hangchow)	杭州	Zhejiang
Hankou (Hankow)	汉口	Hubei
Hanyang	汉阳	Hubei
Hebei (Hopei)	河北	
Hengzhoufu (Yungchowfu, Hengchowfu)	衡州府	Hunan
Haikou (Hoihow)	海口	Guangdong
Huaiyuan (Hwai-yuen)	怀远	Anhui
Huangxian (Hwang-hien, Hwanghsien)	黄县	Shandong
Hubei (Hupeh, Hupei)	湖北	
Hunan	湖南	
Jiangbei (Kiang-peh)	江北	Sichuan
Jiangsu (Kiangsu)	江苏	
Jiangxi (Kiangsi)	江西	

"Alphabetical List of the Provinces, Departments, and Districts in China, with Their Latitudes and Longitudes," Chinese Repository 13, no. 6, 7, 8, 9, 10 (1844) and Samuel Couling, The Encyclopaedia Sinica (Shanghai: Literature House, Ltd., 1917; reprint, 1964).

PLACE NAMES   PROVINCE

Jieyang (Kieh-yang, Kit-yang)	揭扬	Guangdong
Jinan (Tsinan)	济南	Shandong
Jinzhou (Chinchow)	锦州	Liaoning
Jiujiang (Kiukiang, Chiu-chiang)	九江	Jiangxi
Leling (Laoling)	乐陵	Shandong
Linqing (Linch'ing)	临清	Hebei
Lianzhou (Lien-chow)	廉州	Guangdong
Linqingzhou (Lintsingchow, Linch'ing chow)	臨清州	Hebei
Luzhoufu (Lu-cheo fu, Luchowfu)	盧州府	Anhui
Nanjing (Nanking)	南京	Jiangsu
Ningbo (Ningpo)	宁波	Zhejiang
Pangjiazhuang (Pangjiachwang, P'ang Chuang)	庞家庄	Shandong
Pingyin (Ping-yin, P'ing Yin)	平阴	Shandong
Qingdao (Tsingdao, Tsingtau)	青岛	Shandong
Qingjiangpu (Tsingjkiangpu)	清江浦	Jiangsu
Qingzhoufu (Ch'ingchoufu)	青州府	Shandong
Qizhou (Chi-chou, Chichow)	祁州	Anhui
Quanzhoufu (Chuanchowfu, Chinchewfu)	泉州府	Fujian
Shanghai	上海	Zhejiang
Shaowu	邵武	Fujian
Shaoxing (Shaohsing)	绍兴	Zhejiang
Suidingfu (Sui-ting-fu)	绥定府	Sichuan
Suzhou (Soochow)	苏州	Jiangsu
Tianjin (Tientsin)	天津	Shandong
Tongchuanfu (T'ungch'uang fu)	潼川府	Sichuan
Tongzhou (Tungchow)	通州	Hebei
Wanxian (Wanhsien)	万县	Sichuan
Weixian (Weihsien)	卫县	Shandong
Wenzhou (Wenchow)	温州	Zhejiang
Wuchang	武昌	Hubei
Wuzhou (Wuchow)	梧州	Guangxi
Wuhu	芜湖	Anhui
Wuxi (Wusih, Wusieh)	无锡	Jiangsu
Xiamen (Amoy)	厦门	Fujian
Xianyou (Sing-iu, Sienyu)	仙游	Fujian
Xiaogan (Hiau-kan)	孝感	Hubei
Xinghua (Hinghwa)	兴化	Fujian
Yangzhou (Yangchow)	扬州	Jiangsu

PLACE NAMES

		PROVINCE
Yanping (Yen-ping)	延平	Fujian
Yantai (Chefoo)	烟台	Shandong
Yichang (Ichang)	宜昌	Hubei
Yizhoufu (I-chow-fu)	沂州府	Shandong
Yongchun (Engch'un, Engchhun)	永春	Fujian
Zhangpu (Chang-poo)	漳浦	Fujian
Zhenjiang (Chinkiang)	镇江	Jiangsu

PEOPLE

Chen Xiating	陈夏堂
Hu Jinying (Hü King-eng)	胡金英
Huizong	徽宗
Jin Yunmei (Kin Yamei)	金韵梅
Kang Aide (Ida Kahn, Kang Cheng)	康爱德
Li Deyu	李德裕
Lin Wenqing	林文庆
Qianlong	乾隆
Shi Meiyu (Shih Ma-yu, Mary Stone)	石美玉
Song Jing (Sung Ching)	宋景
Su Shi	苏轼
Tang Jian	唐坚
Wu Weiyu	吴为雨
Wu Lianting	吴莲艇
Xie Kangyou	谢康尤
Yongzheng	雍正
You Jingsen	游敬森
Zhu Xianhua	朱先华
Zuo Runqing	奏润卿

著手成春

友如吳秋□圖

Woman Physician, Li Ying, at work in the *Hongkou Tongren Yiyuan*, 1884

Source: Dianshizhai Huabao 1 (1884): 81

Once upon a time, there was a woman doctor from one of the Western countries whose name was Li Ying. In the beginning, she was living here temporarily. Her major is gynecology but she has knowledge of surgery as well. A beautiful woman had a very big tumor. She went to the *Hongkou Tongren* Hospital (in a suburb of Shanghai). The Western woman doctor checked and said this tumor could be cured. The she cut the tumor off with a sharp knife, and put some medicine on the cuts. The woman has fully recovered after one month. The tumor was very big—about one fourth of the human body. Where would this patient be if she had not met this Western doctor? And who would know of the wonderful skill of the doctor if she had not met this patient? It might be fate that brought them together.

Translation, courtesy of Zheng Jianping

Acknowledgments

This book has been a long time coming and the debts I have accumulated over the years are manifold. Firstly, I wish to thank Dr. Judith Raftery for her friendship and unflagging support, good humor, availability, attention to detail, and willingness to enter into debate with me. Dr. Carney Fisher's encouragement, guidance and friendship over the past eight years have also been invaluable.

I am grateful to the Barr Smith Library at the University of Adelaide for acquiring microfilm reproductions of primary sources for this study, the *Chinese Medical Missionary Journal* (1887–1921) and the *Customs Gazette, Medical Reports,* (1871–1900), and to the staff for their unfailing helpfulness. Other libraries and their staffs who gave welcome assistance included the Australian National Library, Australian National University Library, Flinders University Library, State Library of South Australia, New York Public Library and, in particular, the East Asian Librarian at the Melbourne University Library, Bick-har Yeung.

I wish to acknowledge Thomas Rosenbaum and the staff at the Rockefeller Archive Center and the staff of School of Oriental and African Studies Library for providing me with access to their collections, professional assistance, and permission to reproduce photographs they hold. Sarah Myers, the Director, and Claire McCurdy the Archivist and Head of Special Collections at the Burke Library of the Union Theological College in New York came to the rescue magnificently when there was a danger that this project would be still-born.

Many individuals have assisted me in a number of ways. They include Yi-Li Wu who read my dissertation and offered "frank and fearless" advice for which I will be forever grateful. My friend Zheng Jianping kindly translated the text which accompanies the line drawings from the *Dianshizhai Huabao* reproduced here. Thanks are due, too, to those who have read parts of the manuscript at its various stages and encouraged me to persist.

They include Colin Grant, Steven Grieve, Edward Halloran, Jo Melling, Tina Phillips, Jonathan Reinarz, and Ann Rudkin. To the members of the "chimed" internet list—Bridie Andrews, Paul Buell, Tina Phillips, Reiko Shinno, Nathan Sivin, and Wang Hsui-Yun—who were so willing to answer my various queries, I wish to express my gratitude. I also wish to thank the various authors who entered into a dialogue with an anonymous email correspondent and gave of themselves so generously: Eugene Anderson, Jeffrey Cody, Asaf Goldschmidt, Ronald Knapp, Frederick Lisowski, Guenter Risse and Richard Smith.

I am grateful to participants in a number of seminars conducted in the course of researching and writing this book in the Adelaide University departments of Public Health, History, and Asian Studies and, in particular, to my colleagues Nona Verco, Gerald Donaghy, and Andrew Ratledge. I was also fortunate to be able to attend and present papers at two significant international social history of medicine conferences—at Manchester University in 2003 and Oxford University in 2004—where I met many scholars who encouraged me in the project and offered valuable suggestions.

I could not have traveled to England without the generous support of the department of Public Health at Adelaide University and the Wellcome Unit for the History of Medicine at the University of Oxford. The University of Adelaide, through the Research Abroad Research Scholarship and the departments of Asian Studies and Public Health also assisted my travel to Britain and America to undertake the initial research. A big debt is owed to the internet for lessening the distance between Australia and the rest of the world.

To Professor Edward Beauchamp for recommending the manuscript to Routledge and Kimberly Guinta and Benjamin Holtzman for being such responsive and helpful editors, I express my thanks. I could never have completed the book without the encouragement of my family and my son Tom, whose expertise kept my computer running. Lastly, I have valued the proofreading, constructive criticism, support and, indeed, urging of Peter Horne whose belief in the project sustained me.

Introduction

Prior to the introduction of modern medicine [by missionaries] into China there was nothing in the whole country that was at all analogous to the western hospital. . . . There was no Chinese institution that undertook to receive and treat the sick poor.

—Harold Balme 1921

When I first came across this statement by a medical missionary to China, Harold Balme, I wondered if it could possibly be true.[1] I had not expected that the "modern" hospital would have arisen in China but, in the West, the modern hospital has a long and continuous history, beginning with institutions where medicine was not necessarily paramount. Could it be that nowhere in China's history were the sick cared for in institutions? I discovered the view Balme expressed—that the hospital, as a concomitant element of Western medicine, was introduced into China by Protestant missionaries in the 19th century—was commonly held.[2] The implication is that the transfer was one-way, complete, and into virgin soil. Were this so, one would expect a number of consequences to be evident in the historical record. If the introduction had been a straightforward transfer from the West, then one might suppose that hospitals the Chinese subsequently established would be closely modeled on the Western example. When I subsequently found a reproduction of a rough sketch-plan and brief description of a hospital established by the Chinese government in 1906 I realized that this might not have happened. The hospital in question, the *Minzhengbu yiyuan* 民政部医院, bore little resemblance physically to hospitals in the Protestant missionaries' home countries. Although I did not find plans of any other government hospitals, it seems that this one is representative. Firstly, according to a member of the medical staff of the Methodist Episcopal Mission (MEM) hospital at Beijing, John Mullowney (who described this hospital for the benefit of his missionary colleagues in 1912), the *Minzhengbu* (or Ministry of Civil Affairs) operated hospitals in several of China's largest cities and,

1

although they may "differ a little, in a general way they are practically laid out on the same plan."[3] And secondly, Ronald Knapp, an expert in vernacular Chinese architecture, finds the plan to be what he "would have expected. It looks like the general plan of complexes all over China in the 19th and 20th century, even to the present."[4] It would seem that the plan and design were indigenous to China. (see Plate 1)

One of the most striking features of the layout was the style of patient accommodation—I was reminded of a plan I had seen of a Roman infirmary excavated at Inchtuthil in Perthshire, Scotland. This Roman building, in the form of an open courtyard surrounded on all sides by a double row of individual cubicles separated by a corridor, was apparently typical of a *valetudinarium* (hospital for soldiers) in a legionary fortress.[5] Rather than in communal wards, as one might have expected if it had been based on an American or British model, Chinese patients in the *Minzhengbu* hospital lived in small, one or two-bed, rooms arranged around a central courtyard. I imagined that this hospital might have looked like a present-day small hospital, with which I was familiar, in the grounds of the *Wai Yuan* 外院 (Foreign Languages Institute) in Xian 西安 (Shaanxi), the layout of which shares features with this early-twentieth-century institution. (see Plate 2)

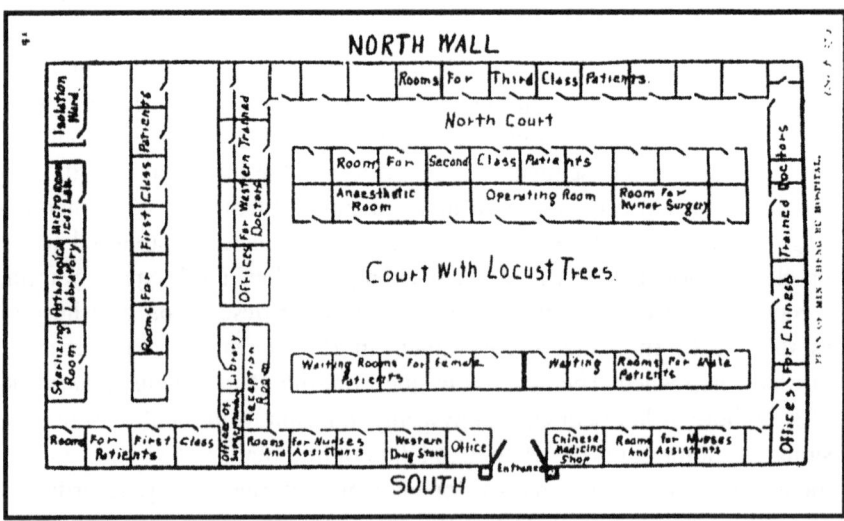

Plate 1. Plan of the *Mingzhenbu Yiyuan*, Beijing, 1912

Source: John J. Mullowney, "Modern Hospitals for Chinese by Chinese." *CMJ* 26, no.1 (1912): opp.36

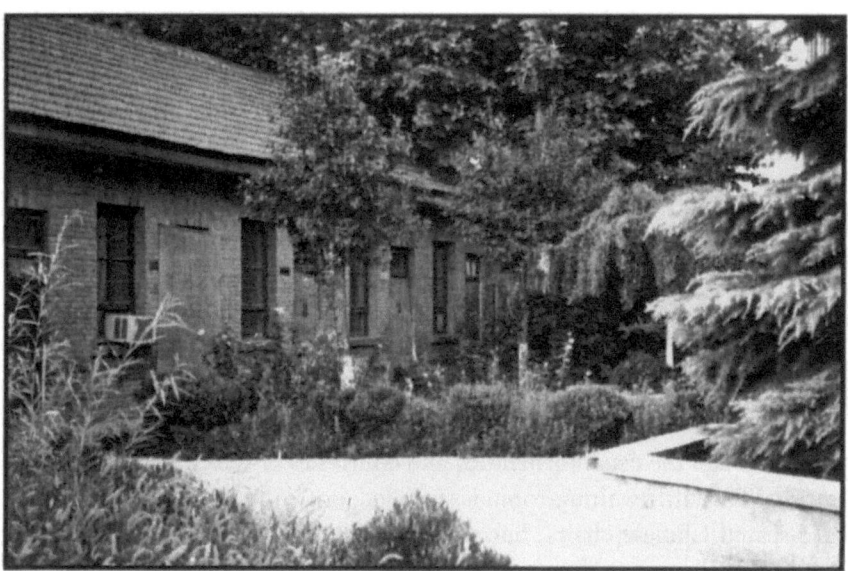

Plate 2. Small wards facing into courtyard of *Waiyuan Yiyuan,* Xian, Shaanxi, 2001

In terms of organization, it seemed this hospital was also distinctive in that patients were not only divided along the anticipated lines of gender and class but were further divided according to which type of medicine they preferred: traditional Chinese or Western. Outpatients entered the hospital compound through a southern gate set between long, low buildings to the right and left. The first room of the building on the left side was the "little office, where the patients must tell whether they wish to see the *Chung Yi* 中 医, the Chinese trained doctor, or the *Hsi Yi* 西医, the Western-trained doctor."[6] The distinction between the two schools of medicine was expressed physically: Western medicine on the western side and Chinese on the eastern. As Mullowney put it, "[t]he enclosure forms a rectangle; the entrance divides this into two parts, one of which is given over to the adherents of the Old School, and one to the disciples of the Western Sciences."

Mullowney was impressed with many aspects of the hospital plan, construction, and operation but the feature that he found most interesting was the way in which the two systems of medicine were integrated. In his opinion, rather than being a case of the Chinese emulating the mission example, it was a Chinese attempt to not only preserve what was useful in Chinese traditional medicine but also to introduce the people to Western medicine. He commended the Chinese government's approach, describing it thus: "instead of antagonizing and embittering the old by the new, they have given each a chance to work out its own salvation. And the natural law will work out here as elsewhere, it will be 'the survival of the fittest.'"[7] Provision had been made for all aspects of both systems of medicine including, for example, separate drug stores: "a finely-equipped modern drug-store, where all the important Western remedies are found ... [and] a fine large room containing, not the bottles, beakers, mortars and paraphernalia of a Western drug-store, but all sorts of herbs, leaves, barks, and other substances in the neatly labelled drawers and jars, large and small, of the old-type Chinese medicine shop."[8]

There were separate waiting rooms for men and women as well as a reception room for those first class patients who chose Western medicine. Furnished in Western style, "the visitor is invited after passing in his card and going through the usual formalities and courtesies of which the Chinese are masters. This little waiting-room is supplied, not with the old straight-back, hard-seated Chinese chairs, but with the fine upholstered European kind, and in it is a large table covered with a spotless white table-cloth, a fine side-board, a coat and hat rack and a wash-stand with towels. The walls are made cheery by a few artistic pictures and an enlarged photograph of Prince Su, who, as the head of the Board of Interior, is the titular chief of this system of Min Cheng Bu Hospitals."[9]

The hospital appeared to be relatively well endowed so far as physicians were concerned. When Mullowney visited in 1911, he noted that under the supervision of the "Chief of the Sanitary Department of the Board of the Interior," who had studied in England and Germany, there were seven Western-trained physicians. One had been trained in France, two in Japan, three at the government medical school in Tianjin, "where the teachers are Frenchmen," and one at the St John's Medical School at Shanghai. The three "doctors of the old school" had trained at "the old-fashioned medical school, outside the Ho Men in Peking."[10] A photograph of hospital staff sitting against one of the buildings accompanied Mullowney's article. (see Plate 3) Although he does not identify the members of staff, the group aptly reflects the hospital's policy and management. Standing at the back, a guard wearing a police uniform represents the department under whose auspices the hospital was run. The Chinese doctor, wearing Western coat, collar and tie, and holding a straw hat, was presumably one of those trained in Western medicine whereas those on either side of him, in Chinese dress, represent traditional Chinese medicine.

For me, this hospital raised further questions. Firstly, if this late Qing hospital was indeed modeled on the hospital introduced into China, what was the nature of the template hospital? In what ways, if any, did it differ

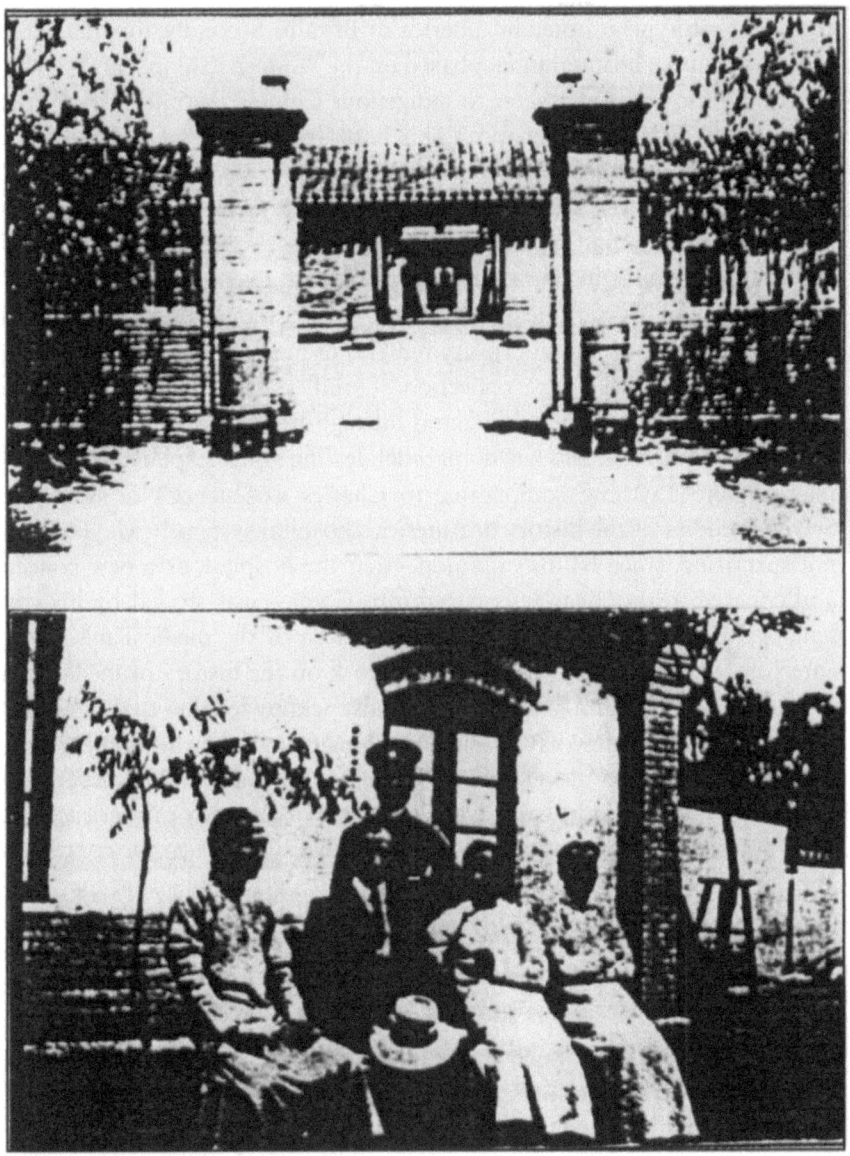

Plate 3. **Entrance and staff of the *Minzhengbu Yiyuan*, Beijing, 1912**

Source: John J. Mullowney, "Modern Hospitals for Chinese by Chinese." *CMJ* 26, no. 1 (1912): opp.36

from its prototype at home in America or Britain? Secondly, to what extent was this Chinese hospital in fact based on the Western example and to what extent did it owe its character to indigenous Chinese institutions? In other words, what was *its* provenance? This book is the result of my attempt to answer these questions.

Neither Western nor Chinese historians of medicine in China have considered the hospital in China per se worthy of close scrutiny. There is no history of 'The hospital' in China which approaches the scope of Guenter Risse's grand survey of Western hospitals from pre-Christian houses of mercy and refuge to the late twentieth-century temples of medical technology. Lindsay Granshaw and Roy Porter's collection of studies, *The Hospital in History*, which ranges from medieval England through Renaissance Italy to twentieth-century America, also has no parallel dealing with hospitals in China.[11] Nor is there anything comparable to Charles Rosenberg's or Rosemary Stevens' studies of the history of America's hospital system.[12] Maybe this is not surprising, since Balme's opinion—that the hospital, as a new concept and concrete reality, was introduced into China—was shared by his contemporaries and by scholars who have written of the medical missionary enterprise in China. In their pioneering work on the history of medicine in China, K. C. Wong and Wu Lien-teh, whilst acknowledging that "the germ of the hospital idea may have existed in China from the earliest times," went on to assert that the "development of such establishments had never been marked and could not be compared with those of Europe or America which were organized on an elaborate and extended scale."[13] Crozier comments, in his 1968 study of traditional medicine in modern China, that the "most conspicuous institution brought by the medical missionaries was, of course, the hospital."[14] Karen Minden echoed his view, almost thirty years later, in her study of the development of western medical training at Chengdu 成都, in Sichuan.[15]

What follows from such a premise is, firstly, there will be no 'history' of the hospital in China to investigate up to the time of the missionaries arriving and, second, no need to investigate its subsequent history in China. The Western hospital has a long and continuous history within Western scholarship: every instance of institutional—that is away from the family home—care is routinely cited as an element in a slow evolution into the highly specialized health care facility we now call a hospital. By contrast, an institution deemed to have been introduced has, by definition, no local antecedents. It follows, then, that its history will be the same as that from which it was copied. It is more difficult, though, to account for the almost total neglect of the history of the hospital once it was 'introduced' into China. Harold Balme did include an interesting chapter on missionary hospitals in his 1921 study of medical missionary development and, in the 1930s, Wong and Wu documented the establishment of these hospitals.[16] A number of Chinese medical historians, relying on missionary sources, have done the same but these works are little more than simple chronologies and contribute hardly at all to an understanding of the nature of these hospitals.[17] The various early histories of the missionary enterprise in China usually included some details of medical work but the authors paid scant attention to the hospitals in which that medicine was practiced.[18] Early biographies of several of the more prominent medical missionaries tend to fall into the category of hagiography but are useful for their descriptions of conditions in the hospitals. It is the hospitals of nineteenth-century Shanghai with which we are most familiar and for this, we are indebted to Kerrie MacPherson who devoted a chapter of her book dealing with the history of public health in Shanghai to the facilities and operation of the London Mission Hospital, better known as the Chinese Hospital.[19] This hospital, established under the auspices of the London Missionary Society (LMS) in 1844, provided medical services to the Chinese population of the Settlement. MacPherson also deals with the controversies surrounding the establishment of two other hospitals whose purpose was to treat foreign, rather than Chinese, patients. The Shanghai General Hospital served the visiting naval and military personnel and foreign residents of Shanghai and the relatively short-lived and troubled Shanghai Lock Hospital was established to treat foreign sufferers of venereal disease and monitor and treat the prostitutes who worked in brothels frequented by foreigners.[20] A few Protestant missionary hospitals have been the subject of individual histories and others have made incidental appearances in recent scholarship dealing with various facets of Western medicine in China.[21] For example, the Canadian Methodist hospital is part of the setting for Karen Minden's study of Western medical education in West China and Paul Howard's analysis of medical missionary responses to opium addiction includes mention of the hospitals that offered treatment. Missionary hospitals make fleeting appearances in Caroline Reeves' history of the Red Cross in China as they do in Carol Benedict's work on the plague and State Medicine.[22] Ho Tak Ming weaves the role of medical missionaries into his study of the encounter of Western medicine with Chinese Traditional Medicine but the hospitals the missionaries established are not dealt with in any detail.[23] Hospitals, under both missionary and Chinese auspices, occupy a substantial place in Ruth Rogaski's examination of public health in Tianjin. She discusses both the Hospital at Tientsin for the Treatment of Sick Chinese (set up by the British Army in 1861, "the first hospital of Western medicine, and arguably the first 'hospital' in Tianjin's history") and the Mackenzie Hospital established in 1880 under the auspices of the LMS.[24] It was her interpretation of an incident at the Tientsin Hospital which alerted me to a possible explanation for scholars' apparent disinterest in mission hospitals as distinct from those found in the West. Rogaski writes, "the Tianjin hospital allowed British military doctors to apply a detached clinical gaze upon the suffering of the Chinese body." According to her account, the "hospital . . . introduced a new and radically different site for cure. The sufferer who stayed in hospital became an individual, removed from the context of the family and the mediating role the family played between the patient and the practitioner. The sufferer became the patient, defined solely through his relationship vis-à-vis the doctor. Within the institutional setting of the hospital, the doctor had constant access to the patient as an object of study."[25] As we shall see, just because the hospital in nineteenth-century China was Western it did not mean that it was directly comparable to the eighteenth-century French clinic as characterized by Michel Foucault in his *Birth of the Clinic*.[26]

The fact that those who have gone to China with the intention of changing her were themselves changed in the process has been well documented. Jonathan Spence, in his book about Western "advisers" to China over three centuries, ably illustrates the phenomenon.[27] Anyone who left America to go as a missionary to China, as Paul Cohen has observed, was transformed from a "Westerner pure and simple [into] a Westerner-in-China." The missionary learnt the language, adopted some Chinese customs, interacted with his environment and "was metamorphosed in the process of encounter."[28] It seems entirely probable that the hospital he brought with him would also be changed. Any institution operating 'away from home' needs to adapt. It is always a balancing act where one has to make the best of what is available, satisfy the standards and expectations of one's sponsor, and accommodate the needs and culture of the client group. I wanted to find out how being in China serving Chinese patients had affected this particular institution, the hospital.

The notion of 'adaptation' permeates the record of the missionary enterprise in China and elsewhere but the terminology used by those who interpret that record can vary significantly. For instance, those who take 'colonialist' or 'orientalist' approaches tend to use pejorative terms for what others may describe as simple pragmatism. In his discussion of the role of Western medicine in colonial India, David Arnold, for instance, invariably attributes negative motives to British physicians. When they adopted Indian remedies or researched Indian medicine, it was plunder, and what's more, a "plundering of parts, not a wholesale incorporation [of Indian *materia medica*] ... appropriation, subordination and denigration were the processes by which Western medicine marked its conquest over indigenous medicine."[29] When doctors took account of Indian beliefs in their practice it was "this type of colonial accommodation of indigenous values (or what are taken to be indigenous values) [which] was thought to be an important part of the growing acceptability of these institutions. It was another example of the way in which Western medicine in India found it expedient to Orientalize itself in order to gain cultural and social respectability."[30] When Indians were employed in responsible positions in hospitals and dispensaries they became, in Arnold's words, "enthusiastic propagandists for Western medicine ... as actively involved as their European colleagues and ... arguably more influential" in the hegemonic enterprise.[31] One wonders what the physicians, or Indians they trained, could possibly have done to satisfy Arnold.

Arthur Schlesinger Jr. pointed out in the early 1970s that the missionaries in China were not agents of classically defined Western economic or political imperialism.[32] In his view, a more fruitful line of inquiry might be to engage and develop the notion of cultural imperialism, which he defined as "purposeful aggression by one culture against the ideas and wishes of another. The mere communication of ideas and values across national boundaries is not in itself imperialism ... it becomes aggression only when accompanied by political, economic or military pressure."[33] In more recent scholarship the term cultural imperialism has been used rather more benignly to mean "the encroachment of cultural practices and values that reflect ... political and economic power" rather than requiring Schlesinger's aggression.[34] It was this notion of the term that Gael Graham had in mind when she wrote that "the issue of American cultural imperialism" had been her initial focus when she started out on her examination of Protestant missionary educational work in China. She discovered, however, that it was overtaken by a story of "cultural exchange and interaction, of borrowing back and forth across a selectively permeable cultural border."[35] And, as Andrew Porter has demonstrated more recently, "highly effective as missions were in promoting cultural change, they were among the weakest agents of 'cultural imperialism.'"[36]

Lian Xi uses the term *conversion* to explain what happened to many early twentieth-century American Protestant missionaries and their work in China. Drawing on the stories of three missionaries including an American medical missionary (Edward Hume), he documents how "the courses of their missions changed as they were changed. They began to cast doubts on their Christian missions as they developed appreciative understanding of Chinese religion and of the culture they had set out to displace."[37]

In choosing a title for this book, I initially used the term *accommodation* to refer to the actual accommodation of patients in the hospital. As I explored further I came across so many examples of 'accommodating' behavior on the part of missionaries that it seemed even more appropriate. Later, I realized the word carries a lot of baggage. In mission studies it tends to be used to describe missionaries taking into account, or incorporating, the local culture, practices, and belief systems in their work. But it is not a neutral term. This mainly stems from the characterization of the modus operandi of the Jesuit missionaries who came to China at the end of the sixteenth century as *accommodationist*.[38] The policy of accommodation they adopted meant, for them, that they would do all they could to adapt to Chinese ways without compromising their Catholic beliefs. Unfortunately their views were not shared by all and led to the infamous "Rites Controversy," first between Jesuits, Dominicans, and Franciscans and eventually between the Kangxi Court and the Vatican.[39] The conflict centered around two main areas where Catholic belief clashed with Chinese practice: the veneration, or worship, of ancestors and the 'proper' name for God in Chinese. In the case of the first, the Jesuits determined that so long as the Chinese observances of Confucian rites could be defined as civil, and not religious, their continuation would not be a bar to conversion to the Catholic faith. As to the name for God, the Jesuits, mindful of the place held by the classics in the Chinese mind, had selected two words from them, Shangdi ("Lord on High") and Tian ("Heaven"). The Vatican, however, found them unacceptable. According to Joanna Waley-Cohen, some Chinese also thought it inappropriate: to them it was "insulting or deceptive to equate the Sovereign on High of the Chinese classics" with the West's God.[40] Incidentally the question about how to translate God into Chinese was still being hotly debated by the nineteenth-century Protestant missionaries we meet in this book.[41] The Jesuits' policy of accommodation did not cause conflict in all areas however. Because they were able to predict astronomical events more accurately than their Chinese counterparts, the Jesuits' skills were appreciated at Court. Adam Schall von Bell, for instance, produced the most powerful legitimizing symbol of state power for the Qing government, the first official imperial calendar of their rule.[42] Their use of secular scientific skills, despite the fact they were put to use in the service of Chinese astrology, was encouraged by the Vatican.

Since the 1970s, the term *inculturation* has been used to describe the situation where 'the other' in an interaction with missionaries takes an active, rather than passive, role. This can involve the recipients giving the introduced institution, say, a new form as though it had arisen out of their own culture. Writing from the viewpoint of the Chinese customer, James Watson puts this construction on the process when he describes the singular way the Chinese use that quintessentially American institution, McDonald's, as "leisure centers and after-school clubs." He speaks of the Chinese *appropriating* or *localizing* McDonald's.[43] I have found that none of these words encapsulates the whole of the process whereby foreign institutions are negotiated both by the importers and the intended recipients. I prefer, therefore, to view the process as one of indigenization, which implies neither specific actors nor agendas: it is more a matter of 'becoming.' I think we should focus on the form of the resulting institution while seeking out the reasons and motivations for actions taken—by whomever—which led to that form. This way we avoid fitting all of the various modifications into the straightjacket of a single overarching ideology. Rather, the process encompasses many motivations—accommodation, appropriation, appreciation, admiration, cynicism, disgust, disdain, fear, hatred—as well as the purely pragmatic responses to lack of funds, staff, and technical resources. Examining, in detail, how this process of indigenization specifically manifested itself in missionary efforts to introduce the hospital into China will, I hope, shed light on the process and contribute to the larger field of the cross-cultural transfer of institutions.

The most rapid expansion of the Protestant medical missionary activity in China took place between the years 1880 and 1910. It started slowly, the first medical missionary having arrived in China in the mid-1830s, but there were fewer than fifty arrivals up until 1870. In the next ten years, to 1880, an average of 3.8 arrived per annum and the rate increased to 13.2 per annum for the next twenty years. It accelerated again to 19.7 per annum for the five years to 1905.[44] Of the one hundred and twenty-six Protestant missionary hospitals established between 1880 and 1910 the ratio of American to British societies was almost two to one.[45] The timing of this arrival of medical missionaries from America in large numbers coincided with the period in which America experienced an extraordinary expansion of hospital provision (from a mere 178 in 1873 to some 4,359 in 1909[46]) and hospitals themselves were undergoing rapid change. Just as there was no "typical hospital" in Britain or America there was even less chance of there being one in China. Thus, I draw on information from a wide range of institutions in terms of their size, clientele, missionary society auspices, location in China, time of establishment, and stage of development and while I focus on American missions I have included some British societies where appropriate. The American mission societies, ranging as they do from Southern Baptist to New England Presbyterian, afford the opportunity to make generalizations about the 'American' hospital that would not be possible in a more restricted study.

Medical missionaries have left us a rich repository of primary sources since they wrote and published prolifically. They did not confine themselves to medical matters but discussed all aspects of their time in China. They exchanged ideas about learning the language, translating medical terms, the nature of Chinese medicine, administrative and clerical systems they had found useful, methods of financing hospitals, and designs for hospital buildings. I draw on the words of these medical missionaries published in the organ of their Association, the *China Medical Missionary Journal* (*CMMJ*) established in 1887, as well as their memoirs and biographies. They also communicated with each other and the wider public in China via missionary-run journals such as the *Chinese Repository* and the *Chinese Recorder and Missionary Journal* as well as the newspaper, the *North China Daily News*. The annual reports which most hospitals published for the benefit of their colleagues and, more significantly, for their supporters in America and Britain are another important source of information. I am aware that the hospital annual reports had to fulfill many purposes, not the least of which was to convince benefactors at home that medical missionary work enhanced the evangelical goals of the missions; as with all such propaganda tools, they must be treated with caution as primary sources. According to Sidney Forsythe the "missionaries in his sample were, on the whole, poor observers of the Chinese scene." He implies that physicians would be even less reliable when he describes them as being, along with married women, the most "mission-centric" of the missionaries. That is, they lived in "the highly organized structure of the mission compound, which resulted in their effective segregation—psychological as well as physical—from surrounding Chinese society."[47] But Forsythe's study was narrow: to assess missionaries' knowledge of and attitudes towards events in contemporary China, he relied mainly on correspondence between a relatively small group of missionaries (based in one province, Shanxi) who wrote to their mission Board. His most prolific commentators were thirteen "ordained male ministers" who provided two-thirds of the comments he analyses. Paul Howard, on the other hand, notes that the work of medical missionaries has been "less thoroughly studied" than that of those involved in other aspects of missionary work and argues that "the medical missionaries in particular were . . . comparatively more reliable observers of Chinese society. As 'men of science' as well as 'men of the cloth,' they were somewhat less likely than their non-medical counterparts to view the Chinese in purely moralistic terms."[48] After examining hundreds of reports written by medical missionaries, both male and female, I am inclined to agree with Howard and would argue that Forsythe's conclusion does not apply to most *medical* missionaries. A survey of the writings of physicians reveals men and women who did interact extensively with the Chinese and in various capacities: all physicians had to be able to speak Chinese; they visited people when they could be expected to be at their most vulnerable—sick or in labor—in their homes; they traveled the countryside dispensing medicines in villages and at fairs; and corresponded with each other through their medical journal. Many, as we shall see, built their own hospitals and personally let the contracts, sourced the materials, and supervised the building by Chinese labor. In addition, single women, who Forsythe classifies as being moderately "mission-centric," comprised a significant proportion of medical missionaries. They were not among the main correspondents with their mission Board but they were active members of the China Medical Missionary Society (CMMA) and frequent contributors to its Journal. This book is based, then, on evidence provided by the reports and photographs of what medical missionaries actually put into practice in hospitals in China. For comparative purposes, I draw on annual reports of a number of hospitals in America covering a range of sizes, auspices, locations, and times along with the wealth of secondary material available on hospitals in the West.

Hospitals, even the smallest, are complex institutions with a multiplicity of aspects each worthy of examination. I decided to concentrate my efforts on those aspects of the American hospital in China that have been almost totally neglected to date but which allow me go beyond superficial appearances. As mentioned earlier, scholars have investigated various aspects of the practice of Western medicine in China but have paid little attention to the sites and organization of this practice. For example, as far as I am aware there is no published analysis of the ways hospitals were financed. And, since Balme carried out a statistical survey in 1919, there has been no comprehensive architectural investigation of the buildings used for hospitals, comparable to the one by Jeffrey Cody of mission educational buildings.[49] I have not found a study that attempts to describe the policies and administration of Western hospitals in China that would have had an impact on the experience of a Chinese patient. Neither have I come across any which have examined the non-medical management of patients in relation to such things as their physical accommodation, diet, and so on.

The book is arranged both thematically and chronologically in five sections. In the first section (chapters 1 and 2) I attempt to place the hospital that the missionaries took with them to China in its historical context. I have surveyed the secondary literature dealing with the development of the hospital in Europe, the Roman East, and the Middle East, and set it alongside comparable, but much less prolific, scholarship chronicling institutions in

China. One result is the timeline (Figure 1) which demonstrates that institutions that would have been included in a history of the hospital had they occurred in the West have existed throughout Chinese history.

In the second section (chapters 3, 4 and 5) I trace the development, from the use of rented Chinese buildings to the advent of Western architects into the field of hospital design and construction, of the physical form of hospitals in China. The 'doctor-builders' who took on the task of designing and building their own hospitals dominated the period between these extremes. The China Medical Missionary Association played a crucial role as a forum for exchanging information and advice about all aspects of hospital construction relevant to China. It did this by collecting photographs and plans, which missionaries could consult when they wanted to build. Many of these were published in the *CMMJ* and have proved invaluable in this study, as evidence of what was actually built rather than what was merely talked about. I am interested principally in the ways in which medical missionaries sought to integrate what they knew about healthy buildings with a desire to make the hospitals approachable by the Chinese they wanted to attract.

In the third section (chapters 6 and 7) I explore the issues relating to guaranteeing ongoing financial support for hospital work without being forever dependent on the home churches. Missionaries were faced with the dilemma of, on the one hand, balancing the desire to use medicine as an example of Christian benevolence, charity, and science without deterring Chinese patients by charging fees, and, on the other, the belief that providing free treatment "pauperized" their clients. A model of financing hospitals emerged in China that varied substantially from the situation in contemporary America.

In the fourth section (chapters 8 and 9) I attempt to imagine the hospital from the point of view of a Chinese patient. Firstly, I follow a patient from their first contact with the hospital to their eventual release (or death) by exploring what is known of the hospital policies and procedures. By comparing the policies and procedures in hospitals in America and in China, I can draw conclusions about the extent to which hospitals in China were indigenized as a consequence of being in China, serving Chinese patients. Secondly, a general picture of missionary hospitals emerges from an examination of their size in terms of beds, the patient mix (men and women, surgical and medical), and the staff—with a special emphasis on the role of women as physicians. Lastly, I compare other aspects of life in hospital including, the rules and regulations, hospital food, the role of friends and relatives, how long one stayed, and one's fellow patients with the situation in America.

The book finishes with a discussion of a number of hospitals established by the Chinese at the end of the Qing, including the government hospital which first attracted my attention. Including these Chinese hospitals will, I hope, locate them firmly in the history of "The Hospital" while at the same time enhance our understanding of the mechanisms involved in transferring an institution from one culture into another.

Section I

The Historical Content

> The sweeping charge against the Chinese, as having no notion of, and never providing means for relieving the poor and destitute, is unjust—it is unfounded . . . it must be obvious, that the dictates of human instinct have been whispering in the hearts of the Chinese, long before China was open to foreigners, and have suggested schemes of philanthropy really judicious and appropriate.
>
> —William Milne 1857

The missionary who wrote this, William Milne (1815–1863), arrived in China in 1842. Like many of his colleagues, he was interested in Chinese culture and society and made Chinese benevolent institutions "one of his special topics of inquiry."[1] Whether they praised or condemned the Chinese welfare institutions, all the missionary observers provide us with an insight into the institutions themselves but also into the missionaries' biases and attitudes. We can thereby get some inkling into the effect the Chinese examples might have had on those about to set up their own dispensaries and hospitals. However, before considering the nineteenth-century Chinese institutions we need to explore the idea of what is meant by the term *hospital* and hence where these Chinese establishments fit into its history.

THE HOSPITAL—A PROBLEM OF DEFINITION

According to the prominent historian of the hospital, Guenter Risse, there is no such creature as *the* generic hospital. It is merely an abstraction drawn from the set of individual hospitals each with its own staff, location, clientele, buildings, and policies.[2] And, as we shall see, neither is the hospital a creation of any one country, society, or religion. Rather, it belongs to a long tradition of welfare institutions established in response to the needs, beliefs, economic conditions, technology, medical theories, and culture of the societies of which it is a part. It is not a static entity but is modified continuously in response to changing conditions, including ideas from elsewhere.

It is difficult, therefore, to arrive at an unambiguous definition of the hospital and somewhat easier to define it by what it is not rather than by what it is. It is not a dispensary or charity pharmacy where patients are seen and prescribed for; it is not a hostel which provides accommodation for people in need, where sickness is incidental rather than a defining feature; it is not a hospice which can provide most of what a hospital does but whose central aim is to ease suffering rather than cure ills; it is not a convalescent home that provides medical care to those who are recovering from illness but, for whatever reason, are unable to return home; it is not an asylum where people, who may have some form of illness, are provided with sanctuary; it is not a clinic where patients can consult and be treated by professional (or para-professional) medically trained personnel but who do not require a bed; it is not an infirmary that does what a hospital does, but for a specified group of people such as monks in a monastery, soldiers in the field, or employees of an organization; it is not a refuge, foundling home, orphanage, or aged care home all of which might provide medical care, and even treatment, in addition to their primary purpose of providing accommodation, food, and protection. A modern hospital is none of these but it has aspects of all of them and all of them have contributed to its evolution.

At its most basic, a hospital has to have food and bedding, nursing care day and night, and physicians to minister *to people who are sick or injured.* The 'modern' hospital was first distinguished from other institutions when it became the focus of medical research and training.

HISTORY OF WESTERN HOSPITALS—THE ANTECEDENTS

When I read histories of the hospital I am struck by the fact that those dealing with the West invariably start by discussing the very distant past and institutions that did not necessarily possess medical staff. The *Asclepieia,* or temples to the God of Medicine, *Asklepios,* originating in Greece in the fifth century B.C.E. and found throughout the Mediterranean world by Roman Imperial times, are usually the first to be cited as having a place in its history.[3] These temples, or shrines of healing, provided a place where the sick sought divine intervention rather than secular medical treatment. Visitors could stay overnight—a process referred to as *incubation*—either in the temple itself or in a special building provided for the purpose. The god might cure them miraculously or, via dreams, instruct them to perform particular rituals or recommend a medical treatment.[4]

The elaborate infirmaries, *Valetudinaria,* provided by Romans for their soldiers at the front or for their plantation slaves are another type of institution that has earned a place in the early history of the hospital.[5] The third category of institution of the ancient world to be dealt with by historians of the hospital comprises the *Iatreia,* or offices from which the physicians and surgeons of classical Greece and Rome operated. It is surmised that under some circumstances beds would have been provided for patients recovering from surgery. Although they are commonly mentioned, no one claims that any of these three types of institution were hospitals as such and not all agree that they are legitimate antecedents of the hospital.

Risse, using a broad definition of 'hospital,' recognizes the *Asclepieia* and *Valetudinaria* as *forerunners* of the hospital on the grounds that they meet his criteria as places where healing is expected, the buildings are imposing and special, and where rituals and companionship contribute to spiritual and physical recovery. They were also centers for medical advice, prognosis, and sometimes, treatment.[6] Timothy Miller, on the other hand, skirts the issue of whether or not these institutions should be included in the history of hospitals. For inclusion he requires a direct line of evolution from one form to the next. On this basis, he argues the case for the sixth- and seventh-century Byzantine hospitals as being the true precursors of the early twelfth-century Byzantine *Pantocrator*—his first "modern" hospital. He argues that *Asclepieia* and *Valetudinarii* were neither hospitals nor did they evolve into hospitals. He justifies ruling out the *Asclepieia* based on the source of healing: divine, rather than secular, intervention. While acknowledging the role of *Valetudinaria* in caring for and treating the sick, Miller excludes them on the grounds of their limited clientele: soldiers and slaves. He uses yet another criterion to dismiss the claim by some for the Greek *Iatreia* as a harbinger of the hospital; although surgery could be performed in them he claims there is no evidence that patients were provided with nursing care or a bed. He does acknowledge that *Iatreia* were subsequently transformed into institutions more recognizable as hospitals—providing food and board along with medical treatment—but only after the emergence of the Christian era.[7] Michael Dols, on the other hand, challenges Miller's "distinction between caring and curing" in relation to medieval hospitals on the grounds that, at the time, "care [was] as important as cure."[8] He defines a hospital as "a public charitable institution that affords care to the sick over an extended period of time" and dismisses the institutions of the classical period arguing that they were "neither charitable nor public." Depending on the aim, institutions can be ruled in or out of the history to suit the story. It will become clear that, although institutions analogous to these early Western examples existed in

China's past, historians have not considered them worthy of inclusion in the history of 'The Hospital.'

As can be seen from the foregoing, the hospital is not an easy concept to grasp. One knows when one is in one but it is hard to pinpoint the feature that sets it apart from an array of other institutions. It is this slippery and constantly changing concept whose evolution I needed to trace so that I could understand what it was the mid-nineteenth-century medical missionaries are said to have introduced to China. At the same time I wanted to seek out what is known about the history of *institutional* medical care in China. I was not looking for evidence that the hospital had either existed in China or that the modern hospital would have arisen spontaneously there without Western influence but, rather, sought to understand the effect that Chinese institutions may have had on the introduced hospital. I needed to locate the institutional hospital in time and space in China as well as in the West. Thus, the first chapter sets the Western hospital within its historical context alongside comparable, though not necessarily equivalent, institutions in other parts of the world, including China. In the second chapter of this section I introduce the reader to the range of Chinese welfare institutions that Protestant medical missionaries encountered when they arrived in China in the mid to late nineteenth century.

Chapter One
The Hospital—in Time and Space

When I started this project I found it difficult to visualize the history of medical institutions across time, let alone across space, so I constructed the comparative timeline (Figure 1 and Appendix A) based on a wide variety of secondary sources.[1] As no history has been written of the hospital per se in China, the question arose: which Chinese to include? I resolved this issue by incorporating any which, had they occurred in Europe, would have been included by a historian of the hospital in the West. In fact, I have been more rigorous in the case of China by counting only those institutions that had some association with the provision of medical care.

Regarding the Chinese institutions, there is a very limited scholarship in English or Chinese. I draw on three articles: one by Angela Leung, one of the most prolific chroniclers of Chinese welfare institutions, who has written about organized medicine in China in the Ming and Qing dynasties. Hugh Scogin has described the provision of, and analyzed the impetus for, poor relief in the Song.[2] Asaf Goldschmidt, who argues that Scogin's "charity system" is more properly a "public health system," has provided the most recent contribution to the literature in English on the medical institutions of the Song dynasty.[3] Chinese scholarship, particularly for the earliest period, is scant and of variable quality and as such needs to be treated with a degree of skepticism. Most general histories of Chinese medicine that mention hospitals are no more than simple chronologies. Similarly, I have found the few Chinese language articles purporting to deal with the history of Chinese medical institutions, with the exception of an article on the Song institutions by Song Jiong 宋炯, to be of limited value.[4] Zhen Zhiyi's treatment of the subject contains more detail than an earlier paper by the Chinese doctor and historian, Ren Yingqiu (1914–1984), and both are useful as summaries of the various medical initiatives and institutions but, unfortunately, they lack analysis.[5]

COMPARATIVE CHRONOLOGY: The Hospital in Time and Space

	500 B.C.E.	400 B.C.E.	300 B.C.E.	200 B.C.E.	100 B.C.E.	100 C.E.	200 C.E.	300 C.E.	400 C.E.	500 C.E.	600 C.E.	700 C.E.	800 C.E.

Western - incl Christian

1. 5th century BCE: Asclepieia : Healing Temples - Greece

2. From 3rd Century BCE: Iatreia - Physicians' Offices - Greece

5. 1st century CE: Valetudinaria - Rome

8. 370 CE Institutionalized Christian Refuges for sick, elderly, travelers   eg Basilias at Caesarea

16. 660 Hôtel Dieu - Hostel - Paris

China incl Buddhist

Zhou Dynasty: 1027 B.C.E - 221 B.C.E.   Qin   Han Dynasty 206 BCE - 220 C.E.   Three Kingdoms ... Norther Dynasty 220-581 C.E.   Sui   Tang Dynasty 618 - 906 C.E.

3. 5th - 2nd Century BCE Rudimentary State Medical Service

4. 4th - 1st Century BCE : Refuges for Deaf, Blind, Dumb, Lame - in Capital

6. 2 CE: "infected persons" taken to "empty outhouses" where treatment will be provided

7. 60 CE Proclamation: establish hospitals for the sick poor, orphans, widows. Doctors to treat sick

10. End 5th Century : " Liu bing guan " and " HuI' - charity hospitals established by individuals

11. 1 CE: "the first permanent hospice with a dispensary" - Buddhist

12. 510 CE: building "government hospital for poor or destitute suffering from disabling diseases".

13. "House for the Sick" set up by Xin Gong'i

17. Buddhist Temples - Hostels

18. 701-717 CE State-sponsored welfare

19. 717 CE Beituan yuan ass. with Buddhist monasteries - "medical care for indigent sick"

Eastern Christian

9. c.380: Xenon at Antioch - for the care of the sick

14. 5th century Nosokomeion developed, in late 6th century (or early 7th), into "elaborate hospitals"

Middle East - Muslim

15. 4th - 6th Centuries: Various Charitable Institutions: Orphanotropheia - for orphans (4th); Gerokomeia - aged homes (early 5th); Brephotropeia - foundling houses (6th)

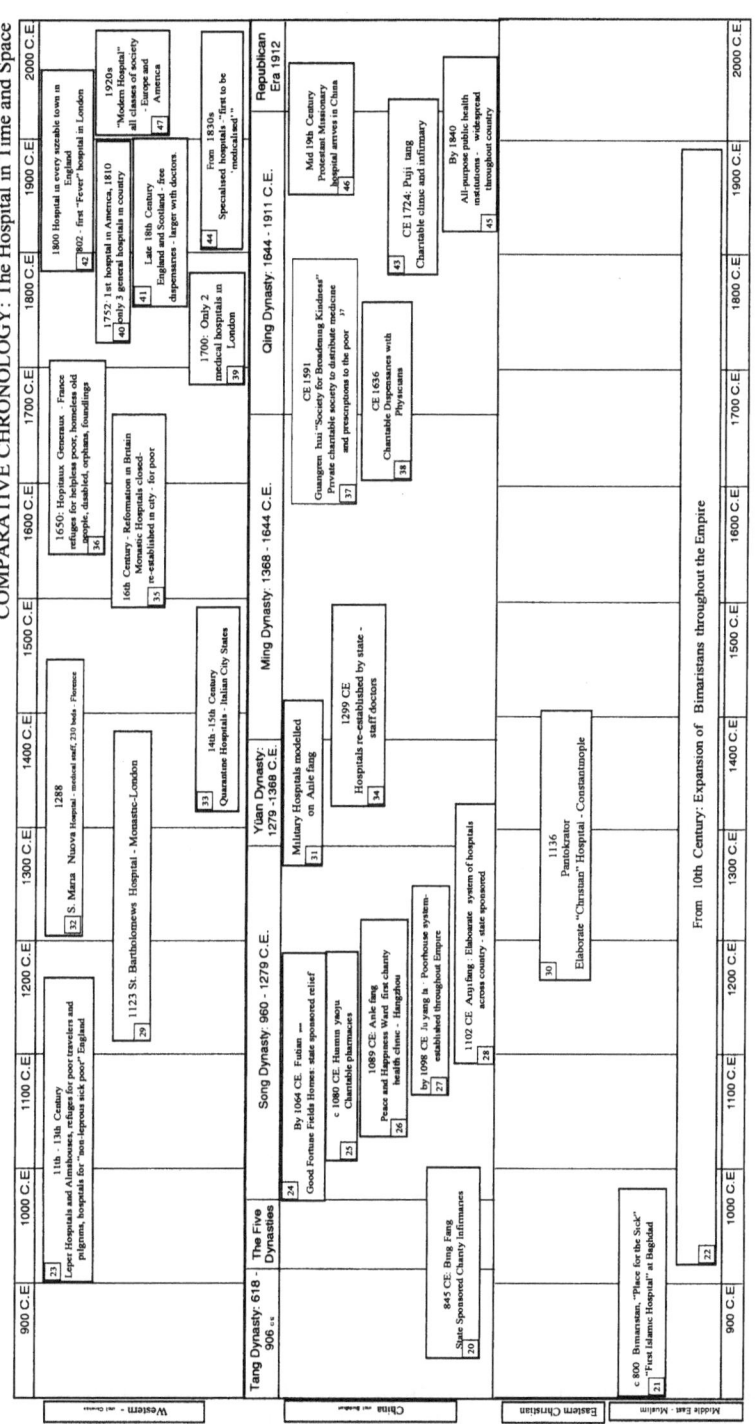

Figure 1. Comparative Chronology: The Hospital in Time and Space
For Sources, See Appendix A

The most striking thing that emerges from even a cursory examination of Figure 1 is that China is not absent. Chinese medical institutions, equivalent to those found elsewhere in the world, are found throughout the period from antiquity to the Present. This is not to say that that the hospital was indigenous to China, or that the 'modern' hospital would have arisen in China without foreign influence.

Four very broad categories of institution based on the degree of their medicalization emerge from the data: the hostel, poorhouse, 'early-medical' and modern hospital; the first three occur in each part of the world under consideration, including China. The 'hostel-type' provided accommodation or refuge to travelers, pilgrims, and the destitute. They were the most ubiquitous and lasted longest but were not always the earliest. In Europe hostels, associated with monasteries, emerged in the fourth century and were still there, little changed, into the thirteenth and fourteenth centuries.[6] In the early part of the Tang Dynasty (618–907 C.E.) in China, comparable institutions, also associated with monasteries, existed and provided refuge or accommodation to similar groups of people.[7] In the Byzantine Empire, and in the West, the monasteries were Christian; in China, they were Buddhist.[8] In these institutions medical care, if provided at all, was tangential to their main purpose.

The second type of institution, poor houses, existed by the sixth or seventh century in the Byzantine Empire; at the turn of the ninth in the Middle East; in the late part of the Tang and early Song (960–1297 C.E.) in China; and the thirteenth century in Western Europe. Although sickness was not a precondition for admission, medical care was among the services offered to the poor, homeless, or destitute. An example of such an institution in the West was St Maria Nuova, established in 1288 in Florence, to give "hospitality and sustenance to the poor and needy." It did not specialize in the care of the sick until the Black Death hastened its medicalization. By the late 1320s it had six visiting physicians, a surgeon, and 230 beds for patients with acute illnesses who only stayed for short periods of eleven to fifteen days.[9] By the fifteenth century, Florence had thirty-three welfare-type institutions that provided some form of medical care for the poor, widows, orphans, or pilgrims.[10] Only seven were hospitals devoted to the sick.[11] In England at the end of the fourteenth century (1390s), although there were some 470 institutions (the majority administered variously by guilds, fraternities, or parishes) most were small and barely medical.[12] Chinese institutions that fall into this second category range from a number of isolated instances of individuals responding to a local natural calamity (such as famine or epidemic) through state-sponsored welfare initiatives[13] to institutions, known as *fields of compassion* (*beitien* 背田), associated with Buddhist monasteries in the Tang dynasty.[14]

Thirdly, there was what I call the *early-medical* hospital where relatively sophisticated care, given the constraints of medicine at the time, was provided, increasingly, to people who were sick rather than merely poor. In Constantinople the Christian twelfth-century hospital attached to the monastery of the *Pantocrator* represented the height of Byzantine medical care. It catered for lay patients, both men and women, as well as sick clergy. Physicians were employed and, according to Miller, it was the world's first "modern" hospital.[15] Meanwhile, in the Islamic world, by the tenth century a hospital in Baghdad had twenty-five physicians on the staff who, in addition to treating patients, taught medical students.[16] According to Toby Huff, it was "with regard to hospitals that Islamic medical practice advanced beyond other cultures."[17] The tenth-century hospital at Baghdad was the descendant of the first *bimaristan* (in Persian literally "a place for the sick"[18]), the foundation of which Dols attributes to a member of the Barmakid family, at the beginning of the ninth century.[19] The model was not immediately emulated and hospitals emerged widely throughout the empire only in the tenth century but were well established in all major cities by the twelfth.[20] Huff cites two further "notable hospitals" in addition to the 'Abudi' hospital, founded in Baghdad in 987. The Nuri in Damascus (1154) and the Mansuri in Cairo (1284) were examples of the sophistication of Islamic hospitals; they separated patients depending on their ailment and had rooms equipped for specialists.[21] Dols distinguishes the Islamic hospitals from their Christian counterparts in some significant aspects. In particular, they were "exclusively medical" and secular, being administered by a "highly-placed government official" rather than by religious foundations. Although they were private, in the sense that they were supported by endowments, they enjoyed considerable imperial patronage, usually in the form of monumental buildings. Some served as sites for clinical teaching (apprenticeship) but were not integrated into the Islamic higher education system so that "doctors were relatively free to develop a professional institution far beyond the constraints of the seminary infirmary."[22]

Although similar developments occurred in Western Europe, it was not until the sixteenth or seventeenth centuries that the very few hospitals in London had medical staff. St Bartholomew's had three surgeons in 1549 and a physician in 1568. As late as 1700, London had only two medical hospitals and there were none anywhere else in England.[23]

In China, the Tang relief homes were further developed in the Song and culminated, at the beginning of the twelfth century, in a system of hospitals throughout the country.[24] Scogin provides textual evidence that physicians attended, patients were separated according to their illnesses, and food and drugs were provided.[25] There is no evidence that these hospitals matched the sophistication of those in Constantinople or Baghdad but they mirrored the pattern of increasing medicalization found elsewhere in the world and would appear to have had a greater medical focus than their contemporaries in western Europe.

Lastly, from early in the eighteenth century, but accelerating dramatically from the middle of the nineteenth, the number of hospitals in Europe and America not only increased greatly but hospital-based medicine began to occupy a central, rather than peripheral, place in society. Hospitals, especially those in major cities with large contingents of patients suffering a wide range of ills, started to become indispensable as sites of the new, scientific, medical research and training.[26] They continued to cater for, in the main, the poor who happened to be sick rather than the sick who happened to be poor.[27] Hospitals were potentially dangerous places to be avoided if possible, and besides, the medicine practiced in them could be equally well provided in the homes of those able to pay.[28]

Thus, just when Protestant medical missionaries arrived in China, in the middle of the nineteenth century, hospitals in their home countries were on the verge of a dramatic increase in number, size, scope, and reach. They were about to come into their own as the principal site for medical practice, research, training, and professional advancement.

THE EARLIEST CHINESE INSTANCES

Li Liangson locates the beginnings of the idea of a Chinese hospital in "bronze inscriptions dated 3,350 years ago"; extrapolating from a single character, he claims that patients with infectious diseases were accommodated in isolation wards.[29] Most Chinese histories of medicine, however, start with reference to the utopian text, the *Zhouli* 周澧,[30] which details what purports to be the government and administrative structure of the royal state of Zhou— China's *golden age*.[31] Tradition has it that the text is the work of the Duke of Zhou, brother of the first emperor of the Western Zhou (1066–771 B.C.E.), and as such represents the orthodox tradition to which later dynasties have turned for inspiration and guidance. K. C. Wong, in "Chinese Hospitals in Ancient Times" published in the *China Medical Journal* in 1923, translated the relevant section: "Physicians attend to the sickness of the people. There are particular diseases in the four seasons of the year. Headaches and neuralgic affections are prevalent in spring, skin diseases in summer, fevers and agues in autumn, and bronchial and pulmonary complaints in winter. The patients are sent to the different departments to be treated."[32] He goes on to claim that this means "government free clinics were known as early as the tenth century B.C." Wong, here, is drawing a long bow. Firstly, concerning the antiquity of the idea, William Boltz's analysis of the origin and authenticity of the text convinces *him* that, although the *Zhou li* is "a genuine pre-Han text" and was definitely in existence in its known form and scope by the middle of the second century, it most likely dates from the Warring States Period (480–222 B.C.E.) rather than Wong's "tenth century B.C."[33] Secondly, concerning Wong's interpretation, Lu and Needham conclude from their reading of the same text that a medical service was envisaged for the general community as well as the imperial family but neither they, nor Ilsa Veith, go so far as to describe the service as *free clinics*.[34] These uncertainties not withstanding, what is significant about this quotation is that it provides evidence that the *ideal*, if not the manifestation, of the Chinese state being responsible for the medical welfare of its people existed by the second century B.C.E.[35] In common with other early scholars, Wong also cites a reference in the *Guanzi* (管子) to illustrate the antiquity of the notion of a *hospital* in China which he translated as: "In the Capital there are institutions where the deaf, the blind, the dumb, the lame, the paralytic, and the insane are received [and] when ill they are cared for until they have recovered."[36]

In a survey of the history of Chinese medicine published in the *Lancet* in 1929, Wong, again citing the *Guanzi,* makes the bold claim that hospitals "were established more than 600 years before the celebrated Basilian monasteries."[37] Wong's interpretation implies the actual existence of facilities in the capital whereas Rickett, who has translated the complete text, stresses "that such a program of social service . . . ever existed in practice is, of course, highly doubtful."[38] The relevant section, which Rickett thinks could date from the beginning of the fourth century B.C.E., forms part of a chapter of the *Guanzi* that deals with "a virtuous ruler's compassion" towards the old, the young, the orphaned, the alone, the sick, the destitute, and the distressed.[39] "Providing for the disabled" is one of the "nine compassions" which the new emperor, on entering the capital, should address. The text elaborates on what is meant, in practical terms, by the instruction issued by an emperor. For example, "'Providing for the disabled' means that in the capital and in all administrative centers, there shall be officials charged with looking after the disabled. The sovereign shall gather together and provide for those who are deaf, blind, dumb, lame, partially paralyzed, or have deformed hands and are unable to live on their own. The disabled shall be placed in hostels so that they may be clothed and fed for as long as they live."[40]

T. J. Preston, in 1907, also cited the *Guanzi* when he addressed his fellow missionaries on the topic of Chinese benevolence. He considered it "manifestly unfair in looking for benevolence among the Chinese to expect to find such well-regulated and well-equipped charitable institutions, either in the past or at present, as are to be found in the cities of Western lands." He interpreted the *Guanzi* as demonstrating that "early in their history the Chinese were seeking through public bureaus and institutions to alleviate suffering and distress among their people."[41] In contrast to the *Zhou li* reference, the *Guanzi* more clearly refers to a specific place where people were not only treated but also taken in and cared for.[42]

In the absence of either supporting textual or archaeological evidence, there is no way of knowing whether or not these institutions actually did exist, much less having any idea of their operation. What *is* clear is that in China the notion of a place where the sick could be cared for away from their own home and family—a hospital—was current around the time of the institutions of classical Greece and Rome, which are considered by many to form part of the history of the hospital.

That this idea was current in the early part of the Common Era is reinforced by a number of references in dynastic histories. For example, in the summer of 2 C.E., in response to a drought and locust plague with its associated famine and disease, commoners stricken by epidemics were accommodated in empty guesthouses and mansions, medicines being provided for them.[43]

K.C. Wong cites another proclamation, issued in 60 C.E., which, according to his translation, ordered the master of the Grand Banner to establish a hospital: "there are orphans, widows and sick poor in the country and we do not take care of them. Is this our true intention in thus being the father and mother of the people? Therefore be it ordered that the Master of the Grand Banner shall establish a hospital in some suitable place and send all the suffering people there. Be it further ordered, that the Medical bureau shall assign doctors to treat them. Examinations will be held on the work of these physicians and promotion made according to the results shown."[44] The mere issuing of proclamations in no way proves that the orders were carried out widely, if at all, but does reinforce the belief that the concept, at least, existed in the first century.

THE HOSTEL ERA—THE WEST

The characteristic that institutions of classical Greece and Rome (*Asclepieia* and *Valetudinaria*)[45] had in common was the existence in them of people who were sick. This is not the case for the Christian institutions. Although there is virtually universal agreement among historians that Christianity was pivotal to the development of hospitals, the earliest Christian institutions to be included in standard histories of the hospital lacked both sick people and medical care. Granshaw, for example, after acknowledging the existence of healing shrines, infirmaries, and doctor's surgeries, states that "there is no evidence of buildings devoted to the reception, care, and treatment of the sick among the population at large until well into the Christian era, around 350 A.D."[46] He is, here, referring to Christian institutions that first appeared in the western part of the Roman Empire where monasteries took in pilgrims, travelers, and the poor. Medical care though was not their principal purpose. Monasteries had had infirmaries whose primary function was to care for sick monks. They developed these into medical facilities offering minimal care, and some treatment, to outsiders who happened to be there under other circumstances. The earliest of these monastic infirmaries is said to be the Basilias at Caesarea founded in the 370s C.E.[47] By the sixth century, Christian hostels able to accommodate large numbers could be found in all the major pilgrim towns such as Rome, Antioch, Alexandria, and Jerusalem.[48] Any medical care continued to be incidental, rather than central, to the services they provided. According to Henderson, in his survey of the hospitals of late-medieval and Renaissance Florence, the "term 'hospital' covered a wide variety of institutions, and only some of these were intended to cater exclusively for the sick."[49]

In the Byzantine Empire, where Christian charitable endeavor received the patronage of the first Christian Emperor, Constantine, a quasi-welfare-state developed, with a variety of specialist welfare institutions, between the fourth and sixth centuries C.E. The majority of these institutions provided refuge or accommodation to a particular class of client. The first, *xenodocheia* or *xenones*, offered shelter to the homeless poor, clergy, widows, or travelers; *orphanotrophos* looked after orphans (from the fourth century); the *gerokomeion*, dedicated to aged care, arose in the early fifth century, and *brephotropeia*, or foundling homes, dated from at least the sixth century. The only ones devoted specifically to the care of the sick or injured were the *nosokomeia* (from *nosos*—disease and *komeo*—to care for).[50] In the latter, physicians conducted daily rounds of examination and recommended medicines, diets, and regimens for individual patients, and nursing care was provided.[51] By the tenth century, the term came to mean a place for people suffering "acute diseases as opposed to a refuge for those with some chronic problem."[52]

In Constantinople, the first of what Miller calls "elaborate hospitals" emerged during the late sixth, or early seventh, century.[53] In these, men and women were segregated; separate wards were provided for patients depending on their disease (for instance those suffering from eye disease or requiring surgery); attendants kept watch at night; and medical assistants worked alongside doctors, who were graded hierarchically. These hospitals, though, were an aberration; the phenomenon was confined to Constantinople and not imitated elsewhere.

In the West, the most common institution continued to be the hostel and of these the most significant were the *Hôtels Dieu*, the most famous being the one established in Paris in 660 C.E.[54] It was not until much later that the distinguishing features of the institutions that preceded the modern hospital included the presence of sick people—much less—physicians.

THE HOSTEL ERA—CHINA

There are any number of reasons why a society will offer medical care to its people but it is common to explain it in terms of charity or compassion, qualities which are often attributed almost exclusively to the Judeo-Christian tradition. Christians, though, have no monopoly on charity or compassion. Risse points out that the Egyptians' emphasis on charity for widows, orphans, the elderly, the homeless, and wandering strangers was a consequence of Egypt's hierarchical society where there was a clear distinction between the rich—pharaohs who owned land—and the rest of the population. The rich had an obligation to provide for the poor and temples offered hospitality, food, and asylum.[55] In Greece, on the other hand, citizens were considered equal and it was not seen as necessary, or a virtue, to assist the poor: there, the key to assistance was reciprocity. Thus *xenones,* or guesthouses in private homes, were common.[56]

Charity was not absent in Confucian China. Chinese history records a number of instances of individual charity related to medical care. According to Needham, "the first permanent hospice with a dispensary" was founded by a Buddhist king in 491 C.E.[57] This was quickly followed by a government hospital, in 510 C.E., in response to an imperial order to "select suitable buildings and attach a staff of physicians for all kinds of sick people who might be brought there." Needham describes this institution, simply called *biefang* 别坊 (separate buildings), as having "a distinctly charitable purpose, being intended primarily for poor, or destitute, people suffering from disabling diseases."[58]

A celebrated case of an individual responding to the Emperor's call, is provided by Xin Gongyi 辛公义, a prefect in Min Zhou 岷州 during the Sui dynasty (581–618 C.E.).[59] The *Sui Shu* 隋书 records that he set up his own house as a refuge for the sick whose families had abandoned them during a summer epidemic. It is said that at times several hundred people, whom he attended personally, were crowded into his courtyard, that he hired physicians, and spent his own income to buy medicines.[60]

At times in China's past it was often Buddhists, who flourished and enjoyed their greatest influence under imperial patronage during the Tang dynasty (618–907 C.E.), who provided welfare.[61] Annexed to Buddhist monasteries, there were institutions that took care of the "old and decrepit, the poor, the famished, and the sick."[62] These benevolent institutions were called variously *beitian yuan* 背田院 or *beitian fang* 背田坊, that is, "compassionate fields home."[63] Ch'en explains that in Mahayana (later) Buddhism, "instead of the laity offering gifts to the monastery and monks, it is the monks and monastery who are offering gifts, and the people are the recipients; the people are now the field of merit or compassion."[64]

Dispensing medicine for the sick among the people was one of seven avenues by which a Buddhist earned merit. According to Ch'en, the abstract Indian concept of the people as a "field of compassion" was made concrete in China where actual fields, donated by benefactors and connected with a monastery, provided the funds for their altruistic work. Like the Christian hostels discussed above, *beitian yuan* provided food and lodging for pilgrims and travelers as well as medical care to the indigent sick; they also distributed rations to the poor. Ch'en relies on a memorial, from Song Jing 宋景 to the Empress Wu, to date the entry of Buddhists into medical care for the poor to 717 C.E. The memorial advised that the relief homes, having been governed by officials since the *Chang-an* 长安 period (701–704), should be turned over to Buddhist monasteries to manage.[65] Even after the transfer to the monasteries, the state continued to play its part. In addition to the profits wrought from monastic fields, monasteries were subsidized by the early Tang government and, in 734, the state required them to take in beggars from the streets to be cared for at public expense.[66] According to a census ordered by the throne there were 4,600 Buddhist monasteries, more than 40,000 shrines, and several hundred thousand monks and nuns (some of whom ministered to the sick) when Buddhism, feared as providing an alternative source of authority, was proscribed by the state in 845 C.E.[67] Monasteries and their lands were confiscated but, having been persuaded of their necessity and that charity was a traditional Confucian virtue, and on the advice of an official, Li Deyu 李德裕, the government took over the operation of the homes and continued the relief work.[68] These state-run charity infirmaries or sick wards, called *Bing fang* 病坊, or Patients' buildings,[69] continued to use profits derived from the monastic fields but their administration was

entrusted to "a respected elder."[70] Scogin issues the usual caveat not to assume that just because an edict was issued it was implemented on a wide
scale.[71] There is no mention of the role of physicians in these institutions and
it is probable that the services were confined to providing food and shelter
to the indigent sick. If this were the case, they could be said to be analogous
to the hostels in the West and, accordingly, have a legitimate place in the
history of the hospital.

It is hardly surprising that medical care was not central to any of the
hostel-type institutions discussed above, whether in China or the West.
When family members and physicians can administer the current medical
therapeutics in the home, society has no need for an institution whose raison d'être is medical treatment.[72] The type of welfare institutions needed
were those that catered for people who had no family: the homeless, widows, orphans, foundlings, and the aged, or those without access to their
families, such as soldiers, pilgrims, and travelers. Thus, inns, refuges, hostels,
foundling homes, orphanages, widows' homes, and homes for the aged were
found whether the society was predominantly Confucian, Judeo-Christian,
or Buddhist. Just as the family provided medical and nursing care to its
sick members, so these institutions—surrogate families—provided some degree of medical care. This might involve simple nursing care, the ministra-
tions of a physician who visited regularly, the supply of medicines, or other
treatments.

Much has been made of the role of charity in the history of the hospital, particularly the Christian variety "expressed in commandments enjoin-
ing compassion, the foremost duties of compassion being to visit the sick,
to help the poor, to feed the hungry, and to clothe the naked."[73] Sometimes
the reasons for organizations or states to provide welfare are more prosaic.
Although compassion shown to the poor was seen in Jewish and Christian
communities as being particularly worthy, by the later Middle Ages the poor
began to be seen as more dangerous than holy: more of a threat to society
than "Christ's poor" or *pauperes Christi*.[74] Consequently, the focus of institutional care for the poor changed from care to control. For example, the
nationwide network of *Hôpitaux Généraux* was established in France to
"confine a wide variety of paupers and social deviants" in late seventeenth-
century France.[75]

As in the West, where urbanization, social dislocation, over-crowding,
and epidemics could all stimulate social action, Scogin suggests that political, social, economic and intellectual factors coalesced during the Northern
Song in China to create the climate in which poor relief institutions could
blossom; poverty amidst splendor, urbanization, natural disasters, and fear

of violence all played a role. The traditional Confucian bias was to seek to eliminate poverty through sound government rather than ameliorate its effects, but it also included the notion that the state had a duty to look after its people, including their health. In the state ideology of the Song, Neo-Confucianism, the Confucian conception of state duty was wedded to a Buddhist belief in a man's moral duty to all people (not just family) arising out of compassion, that is, charity. So, while Confucianism contributed the notion of the bureaucratic state medical service, Buddhism supplied the institutional precedent—the state-sponsored charity infirmaries.

THE GROWTH OF 'MEDICAL' INSTITUTIONS IN CHINA

Scogin and Goldschmidt, and to a lesser extent Leung, provide us with a comprehensive survey of the Song poor relief system, including its medical aspects. The Tang practices continued under the Song but with a new, still Buddhist, name, *Futian yuan* 幅田院 or Good Fortune Fields Home, of which there were originally two in the capital.[76] They were initially small institutions (accommodating only twenty-four people) that catered for the aged, the sick, beggars, and orphans. Rapid expansion in number and size between 1064 and 1068[77] saw accommodation in the capital rise to twelve hundred across four establishments.[78] In addition, an empire-wide system of poor relief, *juyang fa* 居养法, with the "primary duty of providing food and shelter," but including the distribution of medicine, was in place by 1098.[79] The components of the system were set up and administered by local officials with the forms of aid varying according to local and seasonal needs. Poor relief in the capital thus followed a different path from that in the provinces until 1105, when the Northern Song dynasty emperor, Huizong 徽宗 (r. C.E. 1101–1129), decreed that the provincial poorhouse system should be emulated in the capital.[80]

The earliest example of a specialized *medical* facility was the *anle fang* 安乐坊, or Peace and Happiness Ward,[81] set up by "the famous scholar-official," Su Shi 苏轼 (1036–1101), who arrived in Hangzhou in 1089 as governor of West Zhejiang province and commander of the military district.[82] Su Shi's *anle fang*, which Angela Leung refers to as the "first infirmary of the Song" and Scogin describes as "what may have been China's first specialist charity health clinic," treated over a thousand poor patients without charge over a three year period.[83] Scogin claims that Su Shi relied on Buddhist monks to staff the clinic (but it is not clear in what capacity) whereas Wong and Wu say that he appointed "doctors and servants to dispense food and medicine to the people."[84]

Alongside the poorhouse system and based on the example set by Su Shi, the Song State sponsored the establishment of other, more specialized, poor relief institutions. The formerly ad hoc health care measures which had been undertaken in the relief homes were concentrated in a new institution called the *anji fang* 安济坊, which Goldschmidt translates as *Peace and Relief Hospital*.[85] The first of these dates from 1102[86] and, in Scogin's words, "the system actually involved the construction of elaborate hospitals across the country." He describes one, recorded as having many of the attributes we would associate with a relatively modern hospital: it had "ten in-patient wards. Patients were separated on the basis of their illnesses, expressly for the purpose of preventing contagion. The clinics also included kitchens to prepare food for the patients and pharmacies to prepare drugs. Each physician was required to keep accurate records of the number of patients who were cured and the number who died."[87] Relying on the same source, the *Song huiyao* 宋会要,[88] Leung describes the *anji fang,* "in principle, infirmaries to segregate the seriously ill and minimize the spread of disease," as being set up in major towns.[89] As Leung notes, these may have been set up more to protect the healthy than to assist the sick, but that has been the purpose of isolation and quarantine everywhere.

To these two types of organization—poorhouses and public hospitals—Goldschmidt adds a third, a system of "paupers' cemeteries" (established by Huizong in 1104) to form what he describes as a "unique and innovative attempt by an emperor to employ his authority in order to install a government-sponsored and operated public health system."[90] Paupers' cemeteries not only provided burial for the poor and friendless but were also instrumental in removing corpses, which posed a hazard to public health, from the streets.

Another important aspect of the Song system was the network of charity pharmacies, *huimin yaoju* 惠民药局, and the free distribution of medicines promoted by the state.[91] These were extensions of the Tang practices of publishing prescriptions, fixing and publicizing prices for medicines, and giving money to the poor to buy them.[92] It is worth noting that the combination of *huimin yaoju* and *anji fang* bears an uncanny resemblance to the later missionary practice of a large dispensary, or outpatient department, associated with inpatient wards in a hospital. This was not a deliberate ploy on the part of medical missionaries—the practice was common in hospitals in Britain and America—but it would have meant that the model was not so alien to the Chinese as might be imagined.

Despite the scarcity of diverse sources for these early 'hospitals,' it would appear that they satisfy even Miller's restrictive definition of a place which was available to the general population, providing accommodation, food, and medical care. In a history of "The Hospital" they would seem to have qualified for a place at least as important as the Byzantine institutions of the sixth and seventh centuries and the monastic hospitals of the West.

During the Yüan Dynasty (1279–1368), according to Leung, the state-sponsored medical system reached its height with medical bureaus, hospitals, and benevolent dispensaries being established throughout the country.[93] However the Ming (1368–1644) State, rather than extending its role of caring for its peoples' health in institutions, neglected it and allowed the system to deteriorate. Other than the initiatives of a few energetic officials, the State's role was limited to distributing medicines, or the money to buy them, in times of epidemic.[94] The early Qing Dynasty (1644–1911) response to the welfare (including medical) needs of society was an acceleration of the trend, started in the late Ming, to turn increasingly to private philanthropic charitable organizations run by various guilds.[95]

By the time the missionaries arrived in the mid-nineteenth century with a notion of the hospital as principally an institution for the sick poor and only minimally medical, such institutionally based medical care as existed in China was provided by charitable dispensaries and clinics with limited accommodation for patients.[96] Foundlings, orphans, widows, lepers, and the blind were cared for in a variety of homes where some medical care was provided, much as it had been in earlier times.[97]

Chapter Two
Chinese Institutions
the Protestant Missionaries Met

Early missionaries would have been aware of the existence and nature of Chinese charitable institutions through the writings of a number of their brethren who took a particular interest in the subject. As early as 1833, a missionary journal, the *Chinese Repository,* published cursory accounts of a number of establishments in Canton. In the 1840s, these were followed by translations of almost complete institutional annual reports, which provided the missionaries with an insight into the Chinese rationale for the range of services they provided and details of the financing, administration, physical plant, and staffing. A foundling hospital in Canton dating from 1698 said to have accommodation for two hundred and three children, would seem to belie the description of charitable institutions as being "small in extent, and of recent origin."[1]

Also documented were the *Yangzi yuan* 养子院, a "retreat for poor, aged and infirm, or blind people, who have no friends to support them"; the *Mafeng yuan* 麻风院, a hospital for lepers; and a public dispensary that was rumored to have existed "centuries ago."[2] These institutions, the Chinese Repository noted, were financed not by "native contributions [but] every 'barbarian ship' which enters the port pays about nine hundred dollars towards their support, without even the pleasure of ever having been informed."[3]

William Milne, who wrote of his experiences during the 1840s, said that he had "not seen any medical charity in Ningpo" except for a dispensary associated with the Practical Benevolent Society but had been "assured they can be found in Hangzhou and other cities of first magnitude."[4] The benevolent society, for which he had found an 1836 report, had been set up in 1834 by "two influential gentlemen" to take in "outcast infants," provide "raiment for the poor" during the cold winters, furnish the poor with coffins, bury those found dead, and collect and rebury scattered bones. In addition they were to dispense medicine to the sick, distribute tea in summer and the firewood to prepare it.[5]

SHANGHAI

Detailed descriptions of Chinese benevolent institutions that did have a medical component were available via translations of annual reports of both the Foundling Hospital and Public Dispensary at Shanghai for 1842 and 1845 respectively. Members of the gentry had established the Foundling Hospital in 1710.[6] Apparently, officials had failed to act following an imperial edict directing them to "superintend the public contributions, and to await the voluntary subscriptions."[7] Angela Leung has observed that the "provision of medical aid to children had become one of the most widespread features of welfare in China from the nineteenth century on."[8] She identifies "special health care for the child [as] a conspicuous *new* element [my emphasis] of the nineteenth-century institutions"[9] but it would seem that it had been the case in this Shanghai institution from its inception. Wang Tsinchin, who had been the superintendent of the hospital since 1836, spelt out the duties of the hospital's overseer who, along with keeping and examining the books, "superintend[ed] the physicians and apothecaries."[10] The hospital had had a checkered history and the quality of care had deteriorated after the immediate successors to the founders died. New directors, with a brief to revive the institution, had been appointed in 1726. They had conducted a review of the regulations, which had "long been neglected," particularly in relation to the physician and apothecary. They were to "see that the infants had aid in time of sickness."[11] Children, after being received, examined, and having their details recorded, were to be allocated by lot (to avoid collusion and partiality) to a wet nurse. If a child was sick when received it was to be kept within the institution until "perfectly cured and afterwards sent out." Any who sickened with "small-pox or other diseases" were to have their details entered into a "sick register" and be issued with one ticket to request a visit from a physician who "upon seeing it will instantly come" and a second ticket for the apothecary who "will dispense the medicines required." Listed among the officers of the institution in 1842 there were three apothecaries and five physicians. The accounts include an amount of 16,605 cash for "physicians' fees" and additional sums (relating to treatment or prevention of disease) were spent on "apothecaries' bills—draughts, pills, powders and other medical ingredients"; 13,363 cash for "fire balls and medicine firing";

23,880 cash for mosquito curtains; and 8,905 cash for "children's rice cakes, shaving, smallpox [vaccination], lamp oil and medicines."

The Public Dispensary at Shanghai was of more recent origin, having been incorporated in 1844 as an aspect of the work of the *Tongren tang* 同仁堂, or Hall of United Benevolence, which had been in existence since 1804.[12] Medical care had not been included in the services provided by the original organization but, as the committee explained: "That part of the country called San-woo-te (anciently denominated the Kingdom of Woo, and now corresponding to the southern part of the province of Keang-nan) is very damp, and that portion of it which lies near the sea is salt and still more damp than the interior, and in the summer and autumn, is much exposed to strong winds. In the Hwang-poo and Woosung rivers there are day and night tides, but in the brooks, streams and canals which join them, there being no flow and ebb of the tide, the water is still or stagnant, and acquires a greenish color and brackish taste; the water of the wells is also affected in a similar manner, and as regards the people who live in these places, the dampness moistens them, the wind shrivels them, the stagnant water soaks them, and they are thus rendered liable to disease."[13]

The founders were concerned that, unlike those who had means, the "poor and destitute" among the people who worked long hours in cotton fields could not afford to consult a physician, and "their disease [would] speedily become severe." They decided to open a public dispensary, to be known as the *Shiyi gongju* 施医公局 or Establishment for Gratuitous Medical Relief, for three months during summer and autumn from the "18th day of the 5th month to the 18th day of the 8th month."[14] The dispensary was to open every five days and physicians (who were forbidden to charge a fee) would see patients between 8 A.M. and noon in the order in which they arrived. "Surgical" patients, who "must attend in person," were given "powders and plasters" but to the rest were given prescriptions for sufficient medicine for five days. Prescriptions were to be filled at a private pharmacy at the patient's expense unless a subscriber could be found to donate money to purchase their medicine. Over the nineteen opening days in 1845, 13,519 men and women had been seen and 6,199 prescriptions written. The dispensary had paid 265,710 cash to eight apothecaries' shops, and a further 169,335 cash on "pills, powders, boluses, and plasters."[15] Medical practitioners were requested to attend at the institution on the set prescribing days and "not absent themselves on account of wind or rain." In 1844 they reported that twenty-nine practitioners had responded to the call: fifteen for internal diseases, four for infantile, four for surgical, two for ophthalmic, and four to perform acupuncture. If patients were too ill to go five days between visits the treating physician was required to see them, for no fee, at his own house.[16] William Lockhart, who was in charge of the Medical Missionary Society's hospital at Shanghai at the time, did not consider this dispensary a threat to his own establishment since the "class of cases is different in great degree, and the patients in [his] hospital come chiefly from a distance." He saw the *Shiyi gongju* as having been inspired by the example of missionary work and hoped that it would be extended to operate for the entire year. In his words, it was "a most praiseworthy undertaking, and while in operation, was conducted with much spirit and energy, and were the medical men better informed in the principles of the healing art, a very large amount of benefit would be conferred on the patients."[17]

GUANGZHOU

In Canton, it was John G. Kerr who carried out the most extensive contemporary survey of benevolent institutions. He divided them into three classes: guilds, temporary or permanent companies, and "public institutions supported by the government."[18] He identified homes for old men, *Laoren yuan* 老人院, old women, *Puji yuan* 普济院, the blind, lepers, and foundlings. He thought that "these or similar establishments [had] existed in Canton and other Cities of the Empire for many centuries" but the first reference he could find to them in Canton was in the Records of the Province (*Guangdong zhi* 广东志) for the third year of Qianlong 乾隆, or 1739, which dated their establishment to the second year of Yongzheng 雍正, or 1724.[19] Kerr, who seems to have had a somewhat rosy recollection of asylums at home, was scathing about the physical condition of the Homes. He contrasted the "well-furnished and neatly kept rooms in Asylums at home [with the] hovels filled with rickety stools and tables, bedding, broken earthen vessels, furnaces for cooking, and rubbish, the accumulation of months or years [in Canton]."

In addition, Kerr accused those who ran the institutions of corruption arising from the fact that government officials sold the right to manage the institution. It was said that the manager in 1873 had paid $440 for the right to run the *Laoren yuan* for five years and that this gave him the opportunity to make money by charging men aged over sixty with no near relatives and no means of support for the right to live there. He then proceeded to provide the inmates with inferior rice and in place of the 55 *cash* per day promised for the purchase of meat and vegetables he distributed only 32 *cash* every five days. Instead of the regulation "wadded jacket" worth $1.07, which should have been issued every three years inmates were given 500 *cash* (45 cents), and the cheapest of coffins were supplied when they died. Selling the rights to practice to the physician ($100 for life) and the same sum for right to supply water provided additional avenues for graft with the result that "in one way or another, either directly or indirectly, all concerned get a percentage of what has, by imperial decree, been devoted to charity . . . and the inmates are under the necessity of begging in the streets or working at something by which they can earn the pittance needed to satisfy the wants of nature."

It is the medical aspect of these institutions that is of relevance here and the financial accounts reveal that there was provision to pay a physician and his servant at the foundling hospital. A physician was also employed at both the home for old men and that for old women but apparently medicines were not supplied. Beyond this, Kerr gives no indication of the extent of medical care for inmates. He had suggested to his readers at the beginning of his article that "we may find something worthy of imitation in their *modus operandi*" but by the end he was convinced that there was an "urgent need for reform in the management of these institutions." Failing the best solution of being "put in the hands of suitable foreigners" along the lines of the Customs Services, the Missionary Society should set up comparable institutions to act as models and to "shame the officials into some reformation of the abuses now practiced under the cover of charity."

It would seem that Kerr had mellowed by the following year when he described the operation of the *Aiyushan tang* 爱育善堂, or Hall of Sustaining Love, which comprised three service departments: the first operated free schools, provided coffins, and prescribed and dispensed medicines; a second department was responsible for observing religious rites, and a third for general and financial administration. The dispensary department, which had been started in the *Yanghang huiguan* 洋行会馆 or old "Consoo House" using $49,000 raised during 1871, was inspired, according to Kerr, by the example of the "native merchants and compradors" of Hong Kong who had initiated what he considered the "first establishment, by natives, of a permanent institution for the treatment of the sick."[20] Two years later, in 1873, the Canton dispensary was transferred to the "princely residence of Pun-tin-qua (the last of the old hong merchants) which had been confiscated by the Government."[21] Among the detailed regulations of the organization, seven rules were "devoted to the management of the dispensary"; a further seven "pertain to the distribution of medicines" and five "point out the duties of the physician." Patients were neither fed nor lodged but the dispensary was open daily between 10 A.M. and 4 P.M. and patients were examined by one of the three or four physicians on duty and given a prescription that they could have filled gratuitously at the in-house drug store or by paying for it at a shop. He still thought the Chinese lacked the necessary "disinterested benevolence, and self-sacrificing devotion to the interests of suffering humanity" and that they would not succeed until "the Christian Religion and Christian education have done for this empire what they have done for western nations." He was, though, impressed by the business acumen of the committee of management, particularly in their efforts to ensure an ongoing source of funds from commercial and residential property they developed.[22] S. Wells Williams, writing twenty years later, was not so sure about the quality of management but thought that "even badly managed establishments . . . are praiseworthy, and promise something better when higher teachings have been engrafted into the public mind."[23]

Few commentators on Chinese benevolent medical institutions were so encouraging. Kerr's own description of what he saw during the bubonic plague at Hong Kong is more representative of the reaction of most physicians who visited the establishments: "the Chinese rebelled against the measures of the government, and demanded that the sick be placed in Chinese hospitals and be under Chinese treatment. This was granted in measure, and the results showed the utter incapacity of the natives to deal with so terrible a visitation. . . . a hundred patients lying on the floor, almost without attention, in the midst of the filth of their own discharges was a condition of things which did not commend native methods, even to their own people."[24]

Five years later he took an even more jaundiced view when he posed the rhetorical question: was another Canton charity, the *Fangbian suo* 方便 所, established in 1873 to "provide a place in which to receive the homeless and friendless persons who are hopelessly ill," an advance? He likens the people of Canton who are setting up dispensaries "to render the dependence on foreign doctors unnecessary," schools for girls "with the view of taking away the scholars and saving them from contamination by false doctrines," and preaching halls "to counteract the influence of Gospel halls" to the "Officials of the Chinese Empire [who are modernizing by] building arsenals, making cannon, and equipping a Navy." However, he was not impressed by the the *Fangbian suo* whose regulations "provide as far as possible against being imposed on" nor with the generosity of the subscribers who "give five taels per month and under."[25]

A number of observers pointed out that, contrary to the view that they were the exclusive preserve of Christianity, the Chinese too were capable of charity, altruism, and compassion. S. Wells Williams found the basis of altruism and compassion in Chinese culture: "Good acts are required as proofs of sincerity; the classics teach benevolence, and the religious books of the Buddhists inculcate compassion to the poor and relief of the sick" but, in his view, "charity is a virtue which thrives poorly in the selfish soil of heathenism."[26] Arthur Smith, in his classic 1890 work "Chinese Characteristics," was more skeptical about Chinese altruism. He cites as an example of its absence, some literati, blocking the acquisition of land for a dispensary and hospital to be run by Chinese "on the basis it was suggested by foreigners— apparently." He appears not to have considered the possibility that their opposition could have stemmed from a range of reasons quite unconnected with any attitude to altruism. He did allow that he had seen evidence of altruism among the Chinese, such as a woman suckling "a motherless child," and he acknowledged the existence of foundling hospitals, and refuges for lepers and the aged. But to him, Chinese charitable activities, like the setting up (by individuals or government) of soup kitchens and distributing clothing to the destitute in response to calamities, were "few in number and narrow in range . . . and intermittent." He had found hospitals, in particular, to be relatively rare and found only in "many of the large sea-ports, and perhaps in the great cities of interior along the routes of trade."[27] Almost twenty years later, T. J. Preston cited the range of benevolent institutions and activities in one such city, Changde 常德 in Hunan in 1907 as examples of Chinese charity: a Foundling Hospital, work houses for the poor, and a Beggars' Refuge. Also, the United Benevolence Hall provided oil lamps for street lighting, a free ferry boat, the distribution of "healing ointment" plasters for the "sick or suffering," padded clothing, and coffins for the poor.[28]

It is clear that, even while they acknowledged the charitable impulse and the medical aspects of these Chinese institutions, these missionary observers did not consider them comparable to their own dispensaries and hospitals. While historians such as Risse, Rosenberg, and Granshaw distinguish early institutions in the West from 'proper' hospitals, all are treated and viewed as antecedents of the modern hospital. The modern hospital is seen as having evolved from them. For example, Colin Jones describes institutions that "offered hospitality . . . to a wide variety of social types: short-stay entrants such as pilgrims, traveling clerics, itinerant workers, travelers and migrants, and longer-term cases such as resident paupers—the chronically infirm, the aged, abandoned or orphaned children"[29] in medieval France as 'hospitals' and treats them as having a legitimate place in the history of the hospital in Europe. But, while some of the chroniclers of Chinese welfare accept that there has been a history of charitable and state sponsored institutional medical care in China, none of them sees these indigenous institutions as forming any part of a general history of hospitals.

It does not follow that the mere presence of 'welfare-type' institutions in a society constitutes sufficient cause for the emergence of the modern, medically-based hospital. Just *because* analogous institutions can be found to have existed in China, one cannot say that the 'hospital' either existed, or that it would have arisen there in its modern form without outside influence. What one can say is that the various welfare and medical institutions that have existed in China, at least from the Song dynasty onwards, are equally deserving of a place in the history of the hospital as many in the West. So we should not be surprised, then, if their existence and long history had some influence on the nature of the foreign hospital that the missionaries established.

Section II
The Physical Hospital

Hospitals are much more than the buildings which house them but an examination of the buildings—their location and siting, orientation, architectural style, internal layout, range of facilities, building methods, materials and finishes, and so on—provides a wealth of information for the social or medical historian. The health beliefs and practices of an era, or a society, are made concrete in hospital buildings: prevailing notions of health, sickness, death and dying find their expression there. When first built, they will reflect contemporary medical theories but may change as ruling medical paradigms change. Medical considerations though are not the sole, or even the principal, determinant of the physical shape of a hospital.

Even a rented building, designed for another purpose, can be interpreted and understood in a number of ways. The choice to rent could have been a simple matter of economics: just how much of scarce financial resources should be allocated to buildings? The decision, though, may have had nothing to do with a shortage of funds but could have been dictated by politics. At times medical missionaries rented because they were not permitted to buy land; at other times, while allowed to buy land, they could not find anyone willing to sell it to them. The decision to rent in those instances where they *could* have purchased can reveal much about the medical missionaries' approach and values; for example, some preferred to start work straightaway and build a relationship with the potential patients and converts before establishing themselves permanently. The politics of the mission could also play a role when, for instance, the physician did not have sufficient influence to affect funding priorities. Still others thought that using an existing building, familiar to their patients, would mean that the Chinese might not be so reluctant to approach them for treatment.

The location of hospitals, whether rented, purchased, or newly built, could have a variety of meanings. Mid-nineteenth-century Western medical orthodoxy afforded a salubrious location high priority and this might have governed the selection of the site. Ideally, it was believed, hospitals should be located on high ground near a river to gain the advantages of good drainage and clean, fresh air. This was consistent with the long-held belief that disease was caused and spread by miasmatic effusions thought to emanate from the ground, decaying matter, and the bodies of the sick.[1] Disease, thus spread, could take different forms depending on the constitution, physiology, gender, age, or morality of the person afflicted. Many missionaries did not have the luxury of choosing the best site from this point of view: a balance had to be struck between their needs for a healthy location and the necessity to be accessible to the Chinese they were there to serve. Sometimes, they had to decide whether to locate within the relative security of the foreign enclave, or compound, or cast their lot with their patients and establish themselves within the Chinese community.

The orientation of the building on the site can say something about the designer's values and attitudes towards China and the Chinese, as well as his beliefs about healthy buildings. Did it conform to the Chinese tradition of the longest side facing south, even when this meant that its back would be turned to the river or sea? When there was conflict, which took precedence—ideas about what constituted a healthy orientation to sunlight and fresh air, or Chinese geomantic beliefs?

In the case of new buildings, choosing to adopt a particular architectural style was a deliberate act. In nineteenth-century America, where, for instance, a new hospital building could symbolize the charitable impulse of citizens and serve as a focus of civic pride, external appearance was particularly important. The trustees of the Lancaster General Hospital, in Pennsylvania, chose the neo-colonial form of Georgian-Revival—popular at the time for public institutions—when they decided to build a new hospital in 1902. The elegant, perfectly symmetrical stone building with a hipped roof, eaves detailed as classic cornices, a central cupola, rectangular windows, and the main entrance taking the form of portico with freestanding columns and topped with a pediment ably represented the solid philanthropic citizens of the town.*[2] In China, too, builders' choices could send messages about how they viewed themselves and how they perceived the place of the hospital as part of the missionary enterprise. Did they see themselves as modest foreigners, colonialists intending to be in China for the long term, helpful friends inviting the Chinese to approach, or admirers of Chinese material culture? Missionaries also wanted their hospitals to be seen

*www.michellerenshaw.com

as a manifestation of Christian charity but also of Western, or what they termed, scientific medicine. It wasn't until the early twentieth century that 'the hospital building' in America came to incorporate notions of modernity, science, progress, and health into its complex symbology. This development coincided with the most active years of medical missionary work in China, and a similar evolution in hospital building was to be found there.

Contemporary beliefs about sickness and health are most clearly observed in the *layout* of the hospital building or buildings. In the early stages of the medical missionary work in China, hospitals in America (other than the large public hospitals in the cities) were no different from normal residences. In fact, many of these hospitals were established by physicians who set aside some rooms in their own house for patient accommodation. Arthur Hertzler, a nationally-known turn-of-the century Kansas physician who established his own private hospital in 1902, described the situation in Kansas in the 1880s: usually "half a dozen or fewer hospital beds found available space in these houses. The operating room was usually the bedroom of the former cook, selected for the purpose because it was not a desirable room for a hospital bed. The kitchen stove usually provided the heat for sterilization of the instruments and dressings. . . . Operating in such hospitals was but slightly removed from the kitchen surgery of any private residence"[3] As Rosenberg points out, if "a building could house a healthy family it could house sick men and women. Running one was like running a boarding house."[4] Americans who could afford it avoided hospitals and preferred to be nursed at home by their family under the guidance of a visiting physician. The small residential hospital offered them nothing in terms of greater safety or technology and, indeed, were seen by some as "a 'distinct evil,' since they offered the doctor the temptation of prolonging a patient's stay for purely economic reasons."[5]

Designers of new, large hospitals, having absorbed the lessons learnt from the experience of both the Confederate and Union armies during the Civil War, moved beyond the residential and utilized the pavilion style.[6] Civil War hospitals had catered for, and operated on, thousands of wounded and sick soldiers relatively safely in hospitals comprised of large numbers of wards based on the pavilion design. The long narrow pavilion, with doors at both ends and an abundance of windows, had the advantages of ventilation, segregation, and separation. Wards could be closed and opened in response to changing demand, and for disinfection. Florence Nightingale had also become persuaded, after her experience of thousands of soldiers dying—5,000 of the 12,000 men sent from the front during the first winter—that sanitation and construction had played a greater role in the high death rate in her hospital than had the poor health of soldiers when they arrived. The majority of her patients had been sick, rather than wounded, and they were crowded into unventilated, filthy building with defective sewers.[7]

As Rosenberg has pointed out, her ideas were "hardly original" and it was their familiarity that caused builders, physicians, and architects to take up the ideas in her famous treatise, *Notes on Hospitals,* so enthusiastically.[8] Not everyone, though, was convinced that architecture was the solution to the problem of *hospitalism,* a phenomenon comprising four specific infections—hospital gangrene, erysipilis, pyemia, and scepticemia.[9] Although the role of germs (bacteria) in disease causation was not yet understood, surgeons used a variety of empirically discovered ways to counteract infection, these methods included washing wounds, draining pus, and using antiseptics, yet they did not necessarily keep their hands or clothes clean. At Glasgow Hospital in the early 1860s, Joseph Lister had more success than most by operating in a mist of carbolic acid. He saw no merit in the architectural solution.[10] In 1869, he wrote that despite the fact that his hospital wards had been the worst ventilated and that he had crowded patients in—children sometimes two or three to a bed and others on mattresses on the floor—he had not had a single case of erysipilis, gangrene, or pyemia.[11] With Pasteur's discovery of the link between living organisms (microbes) and disease, the rationale for antiseptic use was established but some continued to maintain that the architectural approach was sufficient, and campaigned vigorously against the germ theory in general and Lister's methods in particular.[12] But as Milburn, writing in the *Journal of the Royal Institute of British Architects* so cogently pointed out, "bacteriology has not discounted the value of fresh air and sunlight; it has explained and emphasised it."[13]

The changing architectural response to the problem of infection in hospitals can be traced in late Qing China as in America. These included using small cottage-style hospitals, or existing buildings adapted to frustrate the flow of possibly contaminated air, as recommended by James Simpson; locating ancillary functions in separate buildings under the plan put forward by John E. Erichson; and building hospitals with pavilion-style wards.[14]

Lastly, studying the methods and materials used in hospital construction not only informs us about contemporary Chinese building methods, but also serves to chart the introduction of new materials into China, such as Portland cement and galvanized iron. The values, attitudes, and motivations of those physicians and architects who consciously chose to use Chinese methods and materials—over foreign alternatives—are brought into sharp contrast with others who just as consciously selected foreign methods, materials, and finishes.

Chapter Three
Early Days—Adapted Buildings

Sailing into any one of China's Treaty Ports at the turn of the twentieth century and judging by the skyline, one could be forgiven for assuming China, like India, was a European colony. Building and town planning are often the most obvious symbols of colonialism and in China, as in India, the foreigners had indelibly stamped their presence on the country by this time. China, though, at the turn of the twentieth century was not a colony of any European power.[1] That is, it was not a colony in the strict political sense: there had been no "establishment and maintenance, for an extended time, of rule over an alien people that is separate and subordinate to the ruling power."[2] The European powers had entered China and although they had fought and won military encounters and had exacted concessions under various treaties, the Chinese government remained in power. Similarly, the relationship between the European powers and China could not be branded simplistically as imperialism. Foreigners were certainly living in China, by far the majority of them in foreign enclaves they had established in the so-called Treaty Ports protected by (mainly British) gunboats, and in a limited number of major cities. Doubtless the foreign powers, particularly Britain, had imperialist designs on China and may have hoped, and indeed anticipated, that the situation would develop along similar lines to that which they had experienced in India. It did not. According to Murphey, in his book comparing the British experience in India and China, this was due in large part to the fact that China had a more highly developed economy, system of management, cultural pride, and sense of self-sufficiency than India. As well, the Chinese had "proved themselves adept at both diplomatic negotiation and at resisting the implementation of concessions once granted because of their conviction that foreign incursion was something to be resisted."[3]

As Osterhammel points out, although in late nineteenth-century China a large number of political, economic, and physical phenomena that a wide variety of theorists would include under the heading of *imperialism* were evident, the term does not adequately describe China's relationship with the West. He rejects the label *semi-colonial* and opts for a model he calls *informal imperialism* that, he says, reached its high point in the twenty years between 1911 and 1931.[4] Nevertheless, the built environment of treaty ports superficially resembled their Indian equivalents. Physically, the cities "looked like the alien transplants they were, a circumstance underlined by their orientation to the sea and, wherever possible to surrounding waterways."[5] Chinese cities rarely, if ever, faced the sea but were built looking inward, surrounded by defensive and protective walls.

The dominant foreign community in the various ports built in their national style. This tended to lend a particular character to each of the ports: Canton—British; Qingdao 青岛—German; Port-Arthur and Dalian 大连—Russian; Tianjin 天津—a blend of Russian, British and Japanese. Shanghai, although heavily influenced by the French and British, was "renowned for its international flavor."[6] Anthony King, in his treatise on colonial urban development, concentrated his attention on India where he described the foreign enclaves as being "occupied, modified and principally inhabited by representatives of the colonising society."[7] In contrast, in China, while they may have looked the same they were occupied by 'would-be colonialists'—mainly merchants. In China the foreigners' formal control was restricted both in space (to the area conceded) and in scope (of their own nationals).[8] As in India, foreigners in China, in the main, kept themselves separate from their 'hosts,' both visually and physically. They expressed pride in the straight, wide streets in the foreign concessions of Shanghai and compared them to the traditional narrow streets of the Chinese quarter. Comprising the tools of imported Western capitalism such as joint stock companies, trading houses, banks, and insurance facilities the settlements were, in Murphey's words, "'working models' of western nationalism, the Protestant ethic, the sanctity and freedom of private property, and the virtues of individual enterprise."[9]

Protestant missionaries, though, comprised a distinct class among the 'metropolitan' population and did not necessarily live within the foreign enclaves. Few of them mixed socially with their compatriot traders or their government representatives at the Legation. Firstly, the missionaries were not necessarily admired nor their work approved of by other foreigners. E. H. Parker, the American consul in Peking, for instance, considered the missionaries did do some good, like teaching "poor children to be clean, [to] speak the truth and behave themselves chastely." And, unlike many diplomatic employees and merchants who did not speak Chinese, missionaries could be useful as interpreters for "those legations who have no proper staff of their own." He thought that they discouraged vice but criticized their "vain endeavours to disrupt and discredit one of the world's richest and most ancient cultures." In his opinion, missionaries should "minister to drunken sailors . . . in the treaty ports who obviously require corrective discipline" and better still, they could "go back home and work among the thousands of lost ungodly souls that inhabit the slums of such cities as Manchester and Chicago."[10] Secondly, and more significantly, the missionaries—whose purpose was, after all, evangelism—needed to interact with the Chinese they hoped to influence. Medical missionaries, in particular, needed to attract Chinese patients into their buildings and many established themselves outside the foreign enclaves.

Medical missionaries were not alone in thinking it advantageous to be near potential church members, and apart from their countrymen. For instance, Charles Ewing, of the American Board of Commissioners for Foreign Missions (ABCFM)[11] at Tianjin in Shandong in North China, wrote in July 1906 about his decision to move the mission to a better location; the new property, besides being larger, had the added attraction of being away from other missionaries. He argued that: "in the beginning it was wise to be near the foreign concession for health reasons. Now we are too far from the Chinese residence sections and are four missions together."[12] The new location was accessible to the Chinese—being near two large villages and having a "public highway on one border and [being] just off the great road to Peking." Not only would he be nearer to the Chinese but, living away from foreigners, he looked forward to being relieved of the "many demands on our time."[13]

TREATY PORT HOSPITALS

After considering the desired location, the next task for a medical missionary was to find suitable premises. The earliest mission-based hospitals established in treaty ports used existing (Chinese) buildings, often outside any mission compound. For example, Peter Parker, the first *medical* missionary to China, in 1835 chose a warehouse in Canton for his first hospital in a street "not frequented by foreigners."[14] When John Kerr re-opened Parker's hospital in 1858 (closed in 1856 because of war and subsequently destroyed by fire) it was in a rented Chinese building in the southern suburbs. He stayed there for eight years.[15] Similarly, Dr Dauphin Osgood and his wife, representing the ABCFM, "rented a small native building and received inpatients" when they arrived in the port of Fuzhou 福州 in Fujian Province on the southeastern coast of China in 1870. Later that year they established a second dispensary in "that part of Foochow called Ponasang 保福山" and another "native building . . . was rented for hospital use."[16]

The accommodation situation facing newly arrived missionaries in treaty ports changed as time went on. Although the earliest hospitals were housed in Chinese buildings, the hospitals they later built in the port cities tended to be in either a 'colonial,' or modest foreign style. One particular colonial architectural style was popular with the British and, later, the Americans. It had emerged in colonial India and the British brought it with them to China and was common to all the nineteenth-century treaty ports in Central and South China. Built in Chinese brick, with white plaster, open verandahs and wide arches running around the outside, and over-hanging roofs, it was designed to counter heat and humidity.[17] The style was referred to as *Compradoric*: like the comprador, a person engaged by a foreign firm as a go-between between them and the Chinese hong merchants, it was a blend of the Chinese with the foreign.[18]

The Gregg Hospital for Women and Children, built by the American Presbyterians in 1903 at Canton, was an example of this style.[19] A more modest, but still foreign, building housed the Hua Mei 华美 (literally the China-America) Hospital, operated by the American Baptist Foreign Missionary Society (ABFMS), at Ningbo宁波.[20] It replaced the rented Chinese house that served as both residence and hospital accommodation for Dr D. J. McGowan, the first foreign medical missionary there in 1843.*

The hospital established by the Board of Missions of the Methodist Episcopal Mission (MEM) at Suzhou 苏州 in 1883 was an interesting exception.[21] The most striking thing about the design (see Plates 4 and 5) is the human scale and the extent of coherence and integration of the buildings on the site. It is unmistakably Chinese while at the same time clearly influenced by Western ideas. The hospital consisted of a series of buildings of similar proportions: long, low, and rectangular. All had simple tiled flush-gable roofs, identical square windows on the long sides, and taller rectangular windows, with shutters, on the ends. They were set on a grid and all the wards shared the same orientation, at right angles to the main entrance and outpatient department. The whole was contained in a walled compound with a main gate into the dispensary and a small gate into the residential area. The buildings were connected by covered walkways, forming a series of square courtyards, and took up most, but not all, of the area within the enclosure wall. There is quite a large open space with trees in the northeast corner that was used as a kitchen garden. The hospital was described in the

*www.michellerenshaw.com

booklet published in 1933 to mark fifty years of medical work in Suzhou as the "most carefully planned and worked out along the most up-to-date ideas of the time . . . Dr. Lambuth aimed at giving the very best in scientific medicine."[22]

Why was this set of buildings so different from others built at this relatively early stage in the development of purpose-built hospitals? The answer may lie in the experience and history of the young man who built it. Dr Lambuth was different from most American medical missionaries in that he had been born in Shanghai, in 1854, and spent his early life in China. He was educated in medicine in America and returned to China as a medical missionary in 1877.[23] Before he arrived in Suzhou in 1882 and built this hospital, he had undertaken further study in America. At the time of his second sojourn in America a vigorous debate about how to make hospitals safer had reached some measure of consensus. Rather than a single, block-type building, a healthy hospital should be formed from a set of individual pavilions connected by the "equivalent of a long gallery."[24] An early example in America of such a hospital was the one designed for the Protestant Episcopal Church in Philadelphia in 1860 by an architect, Samuel Sloane. It was "widely praised for implementing in full—for the first time in America—the (1788) recommendations of the French Academy [that is] the pavilion-plus-link system."[25] The layout of Lambuth's buildings would have allowed air to flow freely around them and to expose them to sunshine. The

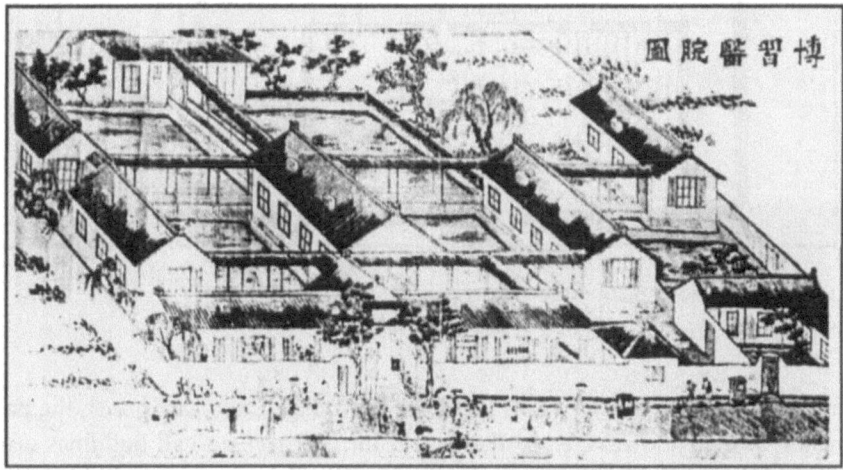

Plate 4. **Methodist Episcopal Church (South) Soochow Hospital as built in 1883**

Source: *Soochow Hospital, 1883–1933: Fiftieth Anniversary: Methodist Episcopal Church, South*, 1933: n.p.

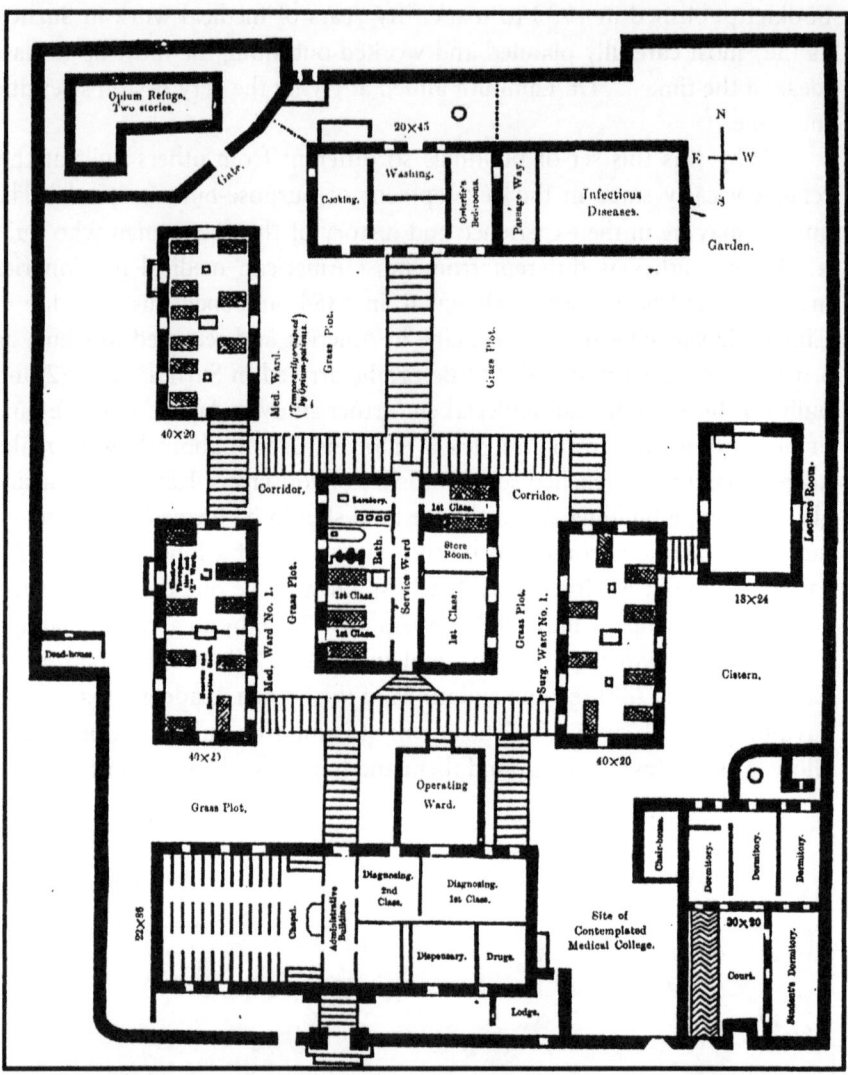

Plate 5. **Ground plan, Soochow Hospital, 1883**
Source: *CMMJ*, Vol. 18, no. 2 (1904): foll.56.

rectangular plan of the wards leant the advantages associated with the pavilion design, and covered walkways meant that access to all buildings was
easy and safe from the weather. The ward buildings were raised above the
ground and, with the chimney-like vents set into the roofs, ventilation would
have been assured. I think that the combination of growing up in China and
receiving a medical education in America could explain this pleasant and

practical complex. Not only would he have been acutely aware of the latest thinking on hospital construction but also would have been familiar with traditional Chinese building style and layout. The use of these Chinese design principles made his hospital fit comfortably into the Chinese landscape and presented a familiar face to potential patients.

MOVING INTO THE INTERIOR

The situation developed somewhat differently when the missionaries started to move into the interior of the country. They, like their predecessors in the treaty ports, rented and adapted existing Chinese buildings as 'first' hospitals. When they did build, rather than using the architectural style of buildings to symbolize Western superiority, science, or modernity, many builders of mission hospitals thought that the hospital should blend in with its surroundings.

Once China had signed the Treaties of Tianjin in 1860 foreigners were allowed, for the first time, to travel throughout the country and "reside and preach in the Chinese interior under treaty protection."[26] As in America when a young doctor decided to set up a practice in a small town, the medical missionary arriving in a Chinese town or village made do with whatever he could find in the way of accommodation. In China this accommodation was invariably more humble and basic than he would have had in America: an early dispensary at Ping-yin in Shandong is a case in point. (see Plate 6)

The anti-foreign sentiment and, in particular, anti-Christian activity, which was at its height in the period 1860 to 1900, also constrained the choice of building and location. Many missionaries describe the long and convoluted negotiations (including subterfuge) they conducted to be allowed to rent buildings. J. Howie's account of the first six or seven years of the English Presbyterian Mission at Zhangpu 漳浦 in Fujian reflects the experience of many others: "the first attempt to purchase land was met with wild opposition from the literary men and the Yamên people. The man who sold us the ground was seized and beaten, and for several months kept in prison; false witnesses were whipped up, who swore that the ground belonged to another man." The case went before a magistrate and the mission ended up with a small piece of land, one quarter the size of the original. When, in 1889, they built a small house so quickly that "the wise old men of the place were only rubbing their eyes and looking around the wee cottage when we began to inhabit it," they were surprised to encounter no outcry.[27] Another medical missionary, R. J. Davidson, wrote to the Chinese Recorder

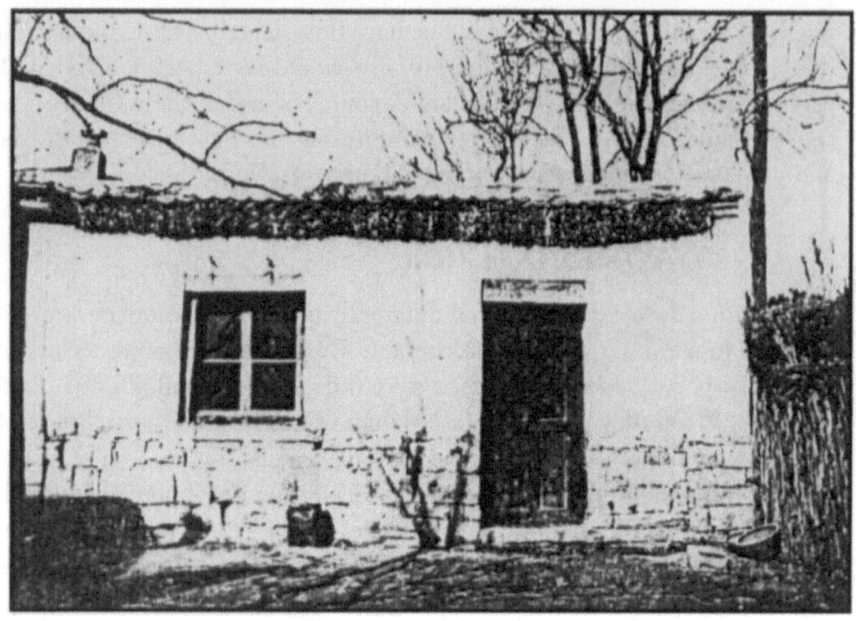

Plate 6. "Our First Mission Dispensary" at Ping-Yin, Shantung, c.1909

Source: Mary. A Moline, *Threatened Hospital in China*: London: Society for the Propagation of the Gospel in Foreign Parts, 1933: foll. 6.

in 1889 recounting his experience and seeking advice. He had first tried to rent a building to use as a dispensary in T'ung Ch'wan Fu 潼川府 in Sichuan. The first prospective Chinese landlord had opted out of an agreement to rent him a house without "a proclamation from the mandarin, saying that he would be free of molestation" so he had rented one from a "Mahommedan." A little time later officials had visited him to question him about the rental agreement and he received a letter from a Chinese official, Chief Officer Li, of San T'ai Hsien, in T'ung Ch'wan. Li claimed that under the Tianjin Treaty foreigners wanting to rent outside of the "open ports" had to notify him, and that he would investigate whether the local people agreed before granting permission. Any Chinese renting to a foreigner without notifying the local official was "to be punished." He further informed Davidson that he had been instructed by the Governor General of Sz Ch'wan to charge the person, a Mr. Gin, who had rented the property "without notifying his superiors" and to inform the missionary "to withdraw the rental and leave the place without the slightest delay, lest you further violate the Treaty."[28] Most missionaries, though, did manage to acquire premises, and existing

Chinese buildings, including inns, houses, factories, and temples all figured as sites of 'first' hospitals.

'FIRST HOSPITALS'—MAKING DO

When Henry T. Whitney of the ABCFM started visiting Shaowu 邵武 (250 miles from Fuzhou) he worked out of a "Chinese inn." Three years later he built a "small half foreign house" from which he started dispensing.[29] Even as late as 1906 when Edward Hume settled in Changsha 长沙, in Hunan, on behalf of the Yale Foreign Missionary Society (YFMS) to establish the Yale Medical Mission, an inn was his first hospital. He describes it in his biography as having "outhouses at the back where pigs were fallowed for market" and wells in the front and rear courtyards, which provided "plenty of water." He used insect powder, whitewashed the walls, replaced paper with glass panes in windows, added new gutters and was ready for business.[30] This picture is somewhat at odds with the one he furnished to the *CMJ* in 1908 when he reported on the official opening. Then it was "but a rented Chinese house, remodelled" which provided accommodation for fourteen patients (eighteen at "a stretch")—two wards with three patients, and four two-bed wards. There were also quarters for a missionary-trained Chinese doctor, a "good doctor's laboratory, a clean operating room, and good accommodation for the dispensary work."[31] It may be that time had somewhat colored his memory of that first building but there is no doubt that it was far from purpose-built. Judging from photographs, the hospital was entered directly from the street through gates in a six or seven foot high cast-iron fence. The exterior was plain, with wooden shutters and a sign in Chinese above the main entrance, typical of others in the crowded street.[32]

Elliott Osgood followed his father, who had died in 1880, as a medical missionary. He wrote about beginning medical work in 1899 in Chuzhou 滁州, in Anhui, a relatively small town of 20,000 people. His first hospital building was "a little thatched-roofed chapel." Despite the lack of sophisticated accommodation he was not dissuaded from amputating a boy's lower arm in the early days.[33] After returning to Chuzhou in 1901, having been driven away during the year when the Boxers were active, he built a small dispensary and another building to house sixteen inpatients. Unfortunately, we do not have a description of the style, plan, or materials of these buildings beyond the fact that the dispensary measured thirty-five by twenty-two feet and had a verandah running the entire length. He gives more details of his next venture, a mortgage on a set of sixteen buildings that had served as a grain *hang* 行 in which he could accommodate forty inpatients.[34] Only four of the buildings had (presumably timber) floors and brick walls and others were no more than open sheds. Roofs were thatched or tiled and floors were dirt or brick. In his estimation, these buildings provided him with a "very poor place to do operations, but a very fair place for housing in-patients." The first building that he considered a 'real' hospital was the two-story building with a "roomy attic and verandah the entire length" which he put up next.[35] Another who set up in makeshift accommodation was the founder of the Hope Hospital in Huaiyuan 怀远, Samuel Cochran of the APM (N), who carried out his first operations in "straw-roofed native houses."[36]

When Claude Lee of the American Church Mission (ACM) established a dispensary in Wuxi 无锡 in Jiangsu in 1908, he described it as the "first Western style building ever erected in Wusih ... a model strictly of utility and not at all of beauty."[37] The small grey brick building described as being "well built and well planned, extremely neat, and in the very best of taste" certainly lacked any pretension but is not particularly 'foreign-looking' as is clear from the photograph which accompanied the story of its opening.[38]* Almost immediately, he was faced with the problem of what to do with patients who required more care than he could provide in a dispensary visit. His novel solution was, for those who could afford it, to hire one of the numerous houseboats available and moor it on the canal in front of the hospital. For those so poor they could not afford the houseboat option, he built the "Chinese equivalent of a tent" made from matting spread over bamboo frames in the space between his house and the dispensary.[39] His next move was to purchase a "tiny Chinese house" that he renovated to accommodate a few patients: three men and two women—in one room divided by a wooden partition. Unfortunately he makes no mention in his diary of any effect this change of accommodation—from the open air to a crowded room—had on the health of his patients. Two years later, in 1910, he was given the money to build a house and added his own dwelling to the hospital stock.[40] By 1913 he was able to build "a real hospital" with four wards (each of fourteen beds), an operating room, and office: he was determined to "run this building along modern and scientific lines as far as I possibly can." He, like many others, had joined the ranks of 'doctor-builder.' He had to become knowledgeable about theories of healthy buildings, plans, building methods and materials, and to develop skills in contracting and supervising Chinese labor.

*www.michellerenshaw.com

Chapter Four

Putting Down Roots—
The Doctor-Builder

> We are here to conciliate, to win confidence and to present western improvements in as attractive garb as we can; let us see to it that this garb does not startle them by its strangeness.
> —Kenneth Mackenzie 1889

Whether propelled by a peculiarly Western belief in progress and expansionism or by nothing more than the desire to provide a safer and more stable medical environment, most missions progressed from renting and adapting to building anew. Not only did they have to acquire the land, they had to resolve a number of practical and theoretical questions. What was the optimum size, given their location, medical resources, and clientele? Should the hospital be a general one catering for both men and women and providing a range of clinic, medical, and surgical services? Once they had decided to build, the factors to be considered included selection of a suitable site and orientation; the design and layout; the materials, building methods, and style of the buildings. Affecting these decisions were considerations of cost; the local environment in terms of climate and topography; and the availability of water, materials, and craftsmen. The political environment and current attitudes to foreigners could also influence these decisions, as could local reaction to the design and siting of buildings because of their effect on *feng shui* 风水.

As well, through their own and imported medical journals, they were aware of the on-going debate in the West linking hospital design and health. They sought out salubrious sites. H.N. Kinnear's description of the factors affecting his choice of a new site when he returned to Baofushan 保福山 in Fujian in 1902 was typical of many others. He had rejected the old missionary site for being *low* and had judged that the "proximity of a number of idol paper tin foil shops, from which the black, resinous smoke poured at intervals" also detracted from the site. He chose, instead, a site on a hill which "for healthfulness . . . is one of the best locations in the suburb. It is elevated and faces in a way to receive the prevailing summer breeze."[1]

Their counterparts in America, who moved beyond the adapted residence to a custom-built hospital, faced similar questions but were rarely required, single-handedly and physically, to build their own hospital. In America, a new hospital building could symbolize many things—progress, philanthropy, civic pride, or charity; its style—often neo-classical—symbolized order, certainty, stability, and science. In China, too, missionaries had to consider how potential patients, whom they did not necessarily understand, would perceive the building: they had to take account of the nature of coded messages the building was sending.

The missionaries' need for information, advice, and guidance about the design and construction of hospitals was catered for by their journal, the *CMMJ,* and it became a significant topic for discussion at conferences. At a meeting on July 24, 1903, the members of the CMMA unanimously agreed to ask the editors to collect together copies of plans, specifications, and costs of every hospital in China so that they could be made available to newcomers. It was further suggested that they "publish in each issue one or more ground plans of hospitals already in existence."[2] A call for papers for the 1907 conference drew attention to "that big subject which we failed to touch upon in our last meeting—hospital construction—with the discussion of plans, materials, ways and means. Of what vital interest it is to many who are looking forward to its future usefulness."[3]

Despite their distance from home, medical missionaries in China actively participated in the ongoing international debate on hospital design.[4] In 1887 Dr Kenneth Mackenzie, at Tianjin with the London Missionary Society (LMS),[5] compared the peculiar problems faced by medical men in China when establishing a hospital with a rather romantic view of what their counterparts experienced at home. In the West, he said, "a committee of influential men is formed, plans are invited from several architects, sanitary engineers are consulted, and everything is done regardless of expense to ensure a handsome and perfect building." In China, on the other hand, the medical missionary "generally has to be his own architect, and as to the sanitary engineer—well, his time has hardly come yet."[6]

This aspect of the situation continued well into the twentieth century; the doctor, and in one case the nurse, acted as architect and builder. Charles Lewis of the APM, who arrived in China in late 1896, was one such doctor. In 1902 he built the Taylor Memorial Hospital at Baodingfu 保定府 in Hebei to replace one destroyed by Boxers in 1900. Despite having "no knowledge of architecture or of drawing"—he did both. He was more fortunate than many others to have some "assistance from one of the railroad engineers, who was also an architect and who drew the elevations."[7] Charles Lewis demonstrated his commitment to building again in 1914 when he "took a course in truss building, and one in engineering and surveying" and added an annex to the hospital.[8] Not all the builders were men or doctors. A rare instance of a woman builder is found in Miss J. E. M. Lebens, "a graduate pharmacist and nurse of experience [who] was the architect and also superintended the building" of the Margaret Eliza Nast Memorial Hospital in 1905 for the MEM at Xianyou 仙游 in Fujian.[9]*

It was to men and women such as these that James Butchart, of the Foreign Christian Missionary Society (FCMS) at Luzhoufu 盧州府 in Anhui, directed his paper, "Hospital Construction," read to the Shanghai Medical Missionary Association conference in January 1901.[10] In it he addressed the decisions facing missionary builders when contemplating a new hospital. He covered the full range from the choice of style, materials, building methods, plans, and furnishing and he did so within a clearly defined philosophical framework. He cautioned his audience to consider the feelings of their Chinese patients so as not to alienate them but to use the building to make them receptive to Western medicine and, ultimately, the Christian message: "We must not forget that in the interior at least that we are building for the Chinese—whose feelings are often the opposite to our own. If in the construction of a hospital we can plan it to be convenient and clean and yet provide those things that they consider as comfort, we conduce to the number of cures and success with a good impression made on the minds of those that we meet."[11]

Translating this sentiment into bricks and mortar was left to individual builders. They took a range of approaches: paying attention to Chinese sensibilities when siting the hospital and ancillary facilities; incorporating Chinese design principles into the building; using local and familiar materials; and including facilities designed to appeal to Chinese patients or make them feel comfortable. Parallel with these considerations, hospital builders also aimed to make their hospitals conform as far as possible to the good health and sanitary requirements being introduced into hospitals in the West.

CONSIDERATIONS OF STYLE

Despite the fact that medical missions had been operating in China since the mid-nineteenth century, no comprehensive survey of hospital buildings was

*www.michellerenshaw.com

carried out until Harold Balme and Milton Stauffer conducted one during 1919.[12] The researchers did not visit the hospitals but relied upon answers to a detailed questionnaire sent to some 289 hospitals for which they had addresses. The final report was based on the 200 returns received from the 250 missionary hospitals found to have been operating in China during 1919.[13] This survey is the only source of comprehensive, comparative, information about the architecture of foreign hospitals in China.[14] The history of foreign architecture in general in China is also very sparse. Chinese architects, Liang Ssu-ch'eng and Su Gin-Djih, who write about the history of Chinese architecture, deal with the phenomenon in a broad sense but their emphasis is on traditional Chinese architecture.[15] A search of the literature reveals that the only current scholarship specifically dealing with missionary architecture is that by Jeffrey Cody, who confines his study to churches and educational institutions built during the Republican period—1911 to 1949.[16] He concludes that many missionary architects and clients were "consciously trying to make their buildings superficially appear more 'indigenous' and less western. As they sought to educate, proselytize and convert Chinese, they tried to strike a culturally harmonious chord with their buildings."[17] Cody dates this trend as starting, slowly, in 1911 and accelerating after the May Fourth Movement in 1919.[18] It was led mainly by American architects who had set up practice in China after the fall of the Qing.[19]

In the case of hospitals at least, this trend started much earlier and it sprang from more than a simple desire to create a *superficial* resemblance to Chinese building styles. As early as 1887, A. P. Peck of the ABCFM at Pangjiazhuang 庞家庄 in Shandong; writing (in the first issue of the *CMMJ*) about the style of his hospital, explained "our aim is to keep the style of building and all arrangements as near to that of the vicinage, to which the people are all accustomed, as is consistent with needful sanitary precautions."[20]

He was not relying on the mere *appearance* of the building, but attempting to make the arrangements, or *procedures,* as familiar as possible. In the same year that Peck described his situation others were encouraging readers of the *CMMJ* to consider the effect of the design of their hospitals on potential Chinese patients. Kenneth Mackenzie, in the second issue of the *CMMJ,* recommended a number of principles that should govern hospital building. As well as advocating the pavilion style, which as we have seen was considered the most efficacious design in America at the time, he paid particular attention to the appearance and the likely effect on the Chinese. Even when the hospital was to be built in a port city, where a foreign building style was normally preferred, he advised against pretension and thought that the medical missionary "should bring his western ideas as much in line with Chinese feeling as possible without sacrificing efficiency."[21]

His description of his own hospital as "being erected in the best Chinese architecture [with] an extremely picturesque and attractive appearance" is borne out by the lithograph reproduced in his biography. (see Plate 7) The design of this hospital was more than merely imitation or façade. The front building, which was entered through a covered gateway, was enclosed within its own courtyard and had a verandah with "massive wooden pillars running along its whole length." The interior was distinctly Chinese: as well as a waiting room with benches there was the "usual Chinese reception-room ever to be found in a native building [and] the rooms were very lofty, without ceilings, leaving exposed the huge painted beams, many times larger than foreigners deem necessary, but the pride of the Chinese builder."[22]

He gives the impression of admiring the Chinese architectural style and seems to have believed that trying to impress the Chinese with his Western superiority would have been counter-productive. He also recognized the importance of taking account of Chinese feelings and advised any missionaries attempting to move into the interior where "the prejudices of the people have to be consulted before everything [that] he may be compelled by the very exigencies of his position to utilize an ordinary Chinese dwelling as his hospital."[23] Dugald Christie was another who was very clear about his reason for choosing to build in the Chinese style in Moukden in

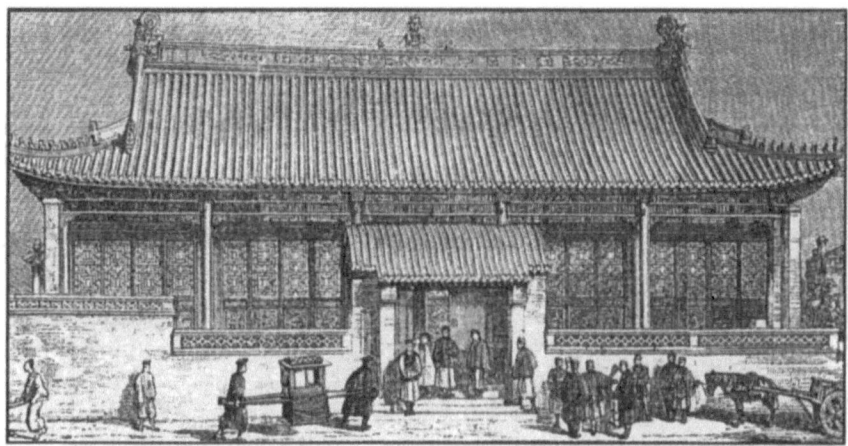

Plate 7. **Mackenzie's LMS Hospital at Tianjin, Shandong, 1879**

Source: Mary Isabella Bryson, *John Kenneth Mackenzie: Medical Missionary to China* (London: Hodder and Stoughton, 1891): facing 379

1887. (see Plate 8) As he explained it, "to build a foreign house in those days would have been to court trouble; a two-story house would have meant a riot. So the *compounds* were Chinese to outward seeming, with massive gateways. . . ."[24]

Robert Speer quotes Charles Lewis describing the McIlvain Hospital he built at Jinan 济南 in Shandong as being "in Chinese style with good bricks." On reflection, Lewis had concluded that the decision to use a Chinese-style building had been instrumental in making the hospital approachable by the Chinese: "such buildings, though perhaps less efficient from our point of view, in connection with medical work, in those days were doubtless more effective in introducing modern medicine into China, because the patients felt more at home than they would have felt in a typical western hospital building."[25] A similar interpretation had been put on the role of the small proprietary hospital in America. According to Hertzler, one of the "chief services of the hospital was that it broke the patients of hospital shyness. They learned to go to the hospital for relief of minor ailments and for the beginning of the more serious ones. Patients were much more willing to go to a hospital at home near their friends, under the care of a doctor known to them, than to go long distances to a city to be placed under the charge of a strange doctor and in strange surroundings."[26] Harold Balme shared Lewis' view when he explained, a "hospital which looked exactly like their

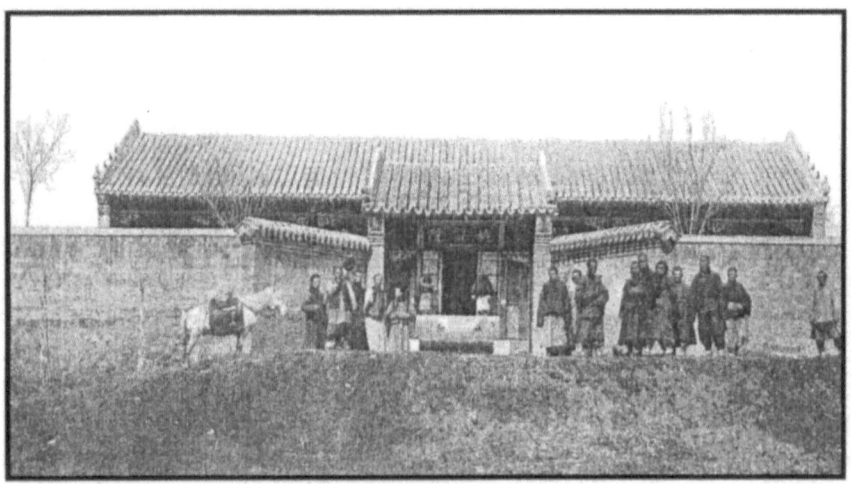

Plate 8. "Moukden Hospital before the Boxers." Opened 1887
Source: Duguld Christie, *Thirty Years in the Manchu Capital.* New York: McBride and Nast, 1914, facing 136.

own Chinese house and in which they could live and eat and sleep very much as they did at home could not after all be such an uncomfortable or foreign place. Thus their apprehensions were allayed. . . ."[27]

H. D. Porter, writing about the medical aspect of missionary work in 1895, provided a colorful description of a Chinese building taken and adapted for use as a hospital in North China. The building had been a tea warehouse and the missionaries were not simply relying on the familiarity of the building-style to convey a message of welcome but had appropriated traditional Chinese scrolls to present their Christian message. He described a "courtyard with wooden pillars covered with crimson scrolls. On one the Ten Commandments are written, on another is the Lord's Prayer."[28]

In the cases cited above it would seem that rather than, as Cody suggests, adopting a Chinese architectural style simply to harmonize with their surroundings, these medical men aimed to beguile the Chinese. After all, their principal aim was evangelistic, albeit through the medium of medicine, and unless they could persuade the Chinese to put themselves and their families into foreign hands, they would have no opportunity to demonstrate Christian charity and Western (in their belief, Christian) scientific superiority.[29]

Not every medical missionary shared the view, however, that a Chinese-style building would more readily and positively influence the Chinese. W. Hamilton Jefferys and Edmund Woodward, for example, both considered native buildings inappropriate for adaptation. Jefferys thought that the Chinese recognized the hospital as a "foreign institution and there is no harm in living up to that reputation." Nevertheless he did allow that a "concession could be made to Chinese ideas" by way of rooflines, decoration on walls of compounds and the external surfaces of the building." He was also sensitive to Chinese geomantic ideas and had observed that tall buildings tended "to raise up the native prejudice" and recommended confining buildings to one or two stories.[30] The designer of the two-story CMS hospital at Hangzhou 杭州 in Zhejiang was one who relied on the roofline to lend a Chinese appearance to his building. He appears to have used the "tail feather corner" style roof end that, according to Knapp, was peculiar to east central Fujian.[31] Placed as it was above an apparently flat roof, the overall effect is suggestive of the *matouqiang* 马头墙 (horses' heads wall), which *was* common in Zhejiang. (see Plate 9)

On the other hand, Woodward, who built two hospitals at Anqing 安庆 in Anhui for the ACM, could see no reason to accommodate the Chinese as regards style of building or materials. He had had experience of both Chinese and Western buildings. The layout of his first buildings (1901) had been "all Western" but the architecture was "strictly oriental," with an

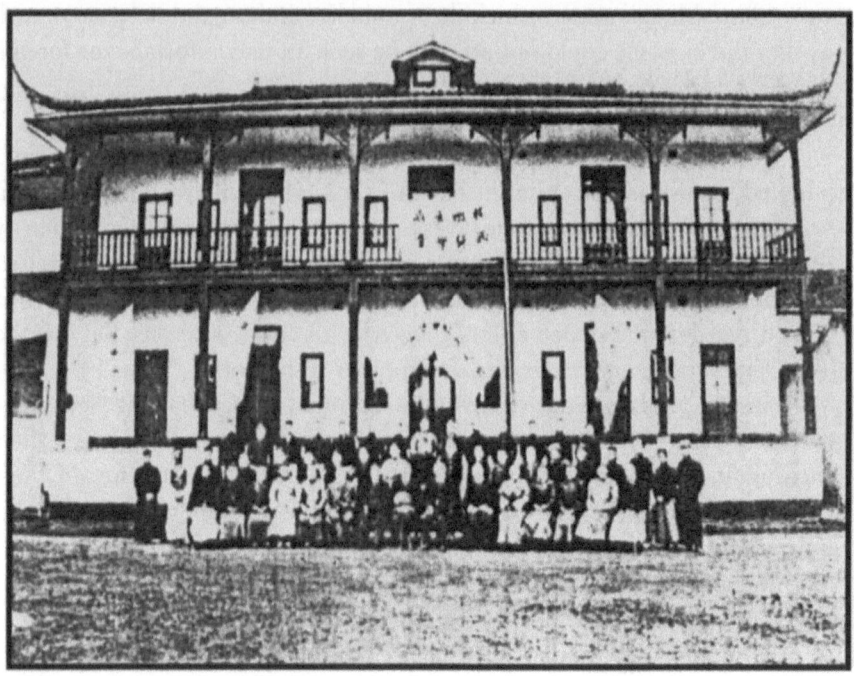

Plate 9. Church Missionary Society Hospital, Hangzhou, Zhejiang, 1910
Source: *Story of the Hangchow Medical Mission: in connection with the Church Missionary Society*: n.p., 1910: 16.
Courtesy of the Burke Library, Union Theological College, New York

"imposing gateway [which] forms one of the features of the city."[32] He had not been impressed with Chinese materials, tradesmen, or building methods. He thought that "except for brick and mortar, local building materials are inferior and very dear ... constant supervision prevails but little with the local workmen to improve upon the *'c'ha puh to'* (which is elegant Chinese for 'jack-leg') building methods of their immemorial forefathers."[33] When he was provided with adequate funds to replace this hospital he determined to use the Gothic style that, he thought, "embodies, as nothing else does in architecture, the noblest historical ideals of the Protestant Christianity which we endeavor to exemplify in China." He disagreed with Jefferys and characterized the practice of "foreign buildings in China retaining the distinctive Chinese roof" as a departure from good taste. Also, in his view, "the former prejudice against buildings of foreign architecture is rapidly passing away, as is shown by the frequency with which the better class Chinese residences are being built two storey with various imitations of Western architecture."[34]

In a report on the opening of a new hospital, St Agatha's (for women and children) at *Pingyin* 平阴 in Shandong in 1909 by the Society for the Propagation of the Gospel (SPG), the granite building was proudly described as being "constructed upon foreign lines, having a plentiful supply of foreign doors and windows, board floors, plastered white-washed walls, and plaster ceilings, which are all new to the Chinese around here."[35] Despite this description, the photographs which accompanied the announcement tell a rather different story. (see Plate 10) The finishes may have been foreign but the walled compound, simple lines of the hospital, roof profiles, the entrance gate—"designed entirely by a Chinese workman"—and south facing orientation all conformed to Chinese design principles.[36] (see Plate 11)

Similarly, when Stephen C. Lewis, the builder and physician in charge, announced the opening of a new hospital at Changzhou 长州 in Hunan for the APM, he described it as the "first hospital of foreign construction in the southern half of Hunan."[37] The accompanying photograph shows a two-storey brick building with (possibly concrete) pillars supporting a Chinese-style tiled overhanging roof covering a verandah. The materials may have been foreign but the style was not and is reminiscent of Chinese two-storey buildings, common in southern China.[38] (see Plate 12)

Before 1910, Woodward, with his uncompromising views on Chinese building style, appears to be an exception among American medical missionaries. Both Cody and Gael Graham paint a different picture as regards attitudes to church and school buildings. For example, Cody summarizes his understanding of the situation: "Up until the end of the 19th century, Europeans sought to erect buildings that unequivocally felt and looked European." Both he and Graham quote the Rev. P. W. Pitcher, who "lambasted the 'rottenness of the whole scheme of Chinese architecture' [and urged his compatriots] to erect unabashedly Western edifices of several stories and with towering spires in order to destroy [this] nonsense about fengshuy [or fengshui], the Chinese art of geomancy."[39]

The available primary sources would seem to suggest that most *medical* missionaries followed Butchart's advice, and Mackenzies'. In contrast to the situation today, America did not see itself as either an unassailable world leader or an imperialist power in China. America, founded on a belief in religious freedoms and lacking a state religion, may have been expected to produce missionaries who were more tolerant and understanding of Chinese beliefs and sensibilities. For instance, Butchart advised modesty and the "avoidance of any display in excess of the actual working needs conducive to a good effect on the minds of the people that we seek to influence . . . [because] it is the Christian influence for which the hospital work is carried

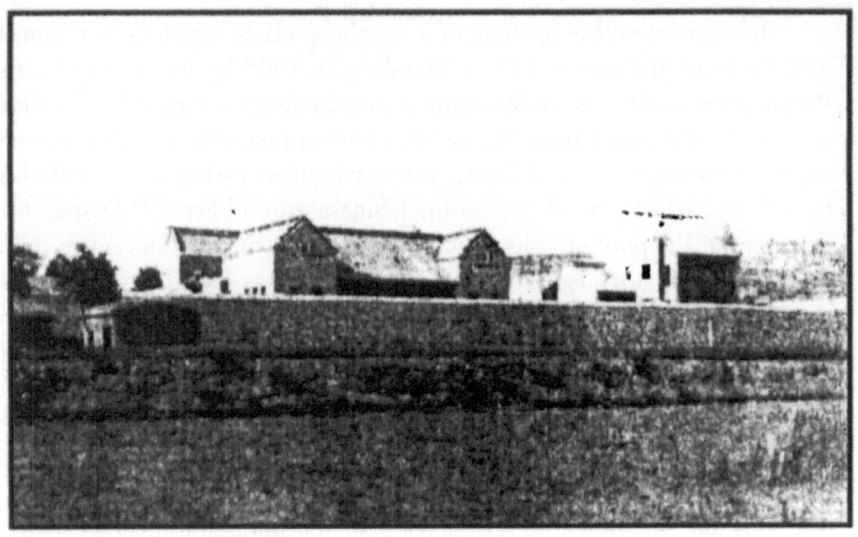

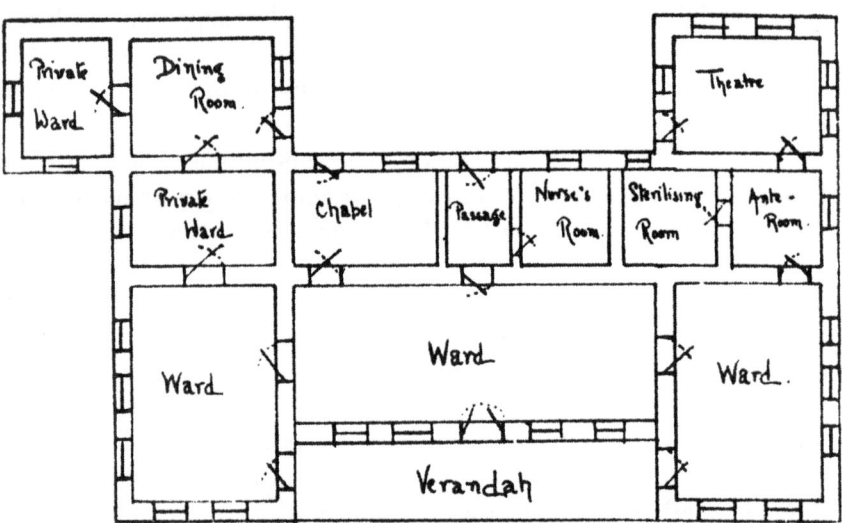

Plate 10. **St. Agatha's Hospital Pingyin, Shandong, 1909**
Source: *CMMJ,* Vol. 23, no. 6 (1909): facing p. 407.

on."[40] It was more than a desire to merely project an *image* of modesty and frugality. The availability of finance was obviously a significant factor. Charles Ewing wrote to Judson Smith in November 1904 warning against making the same mistakes with new building at Tianjin and Linqingzhou that had been made at Peking and Tongzhou 通州.[41] He was referring to mission buildings in general, rather than hospitals, and addressed "the whole

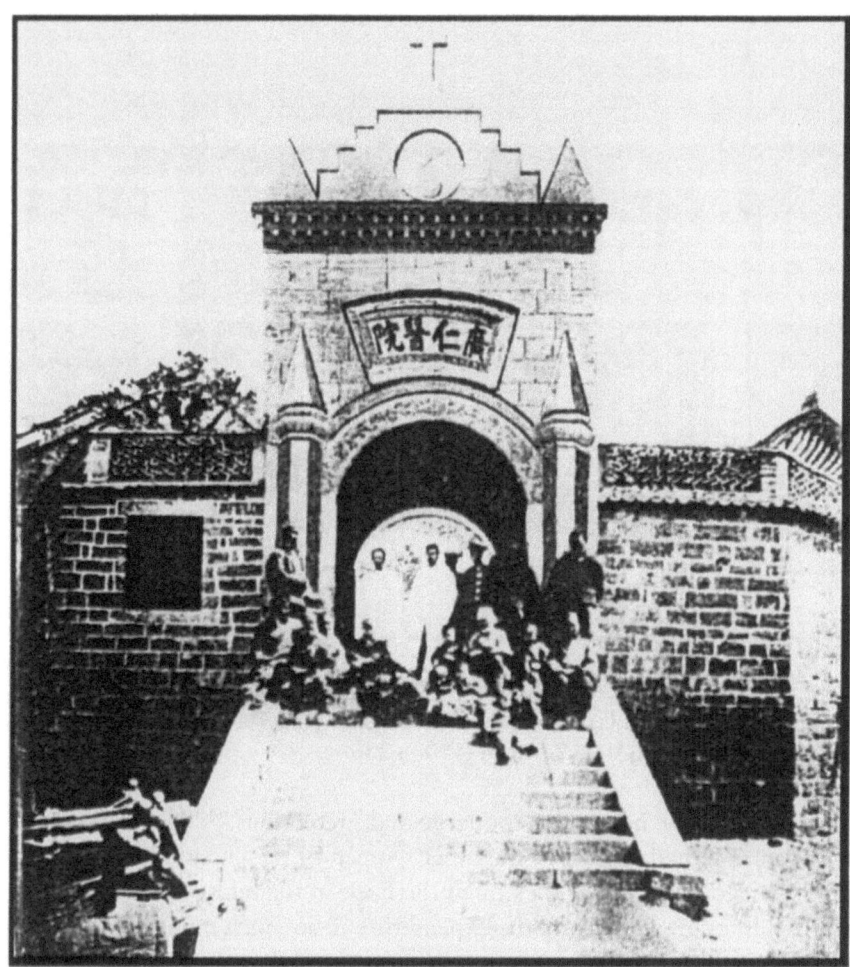

Plate 11. **Main Entrance Gate, St. Agatha's Hospital**
Source: Mary. A Moline, *Threatened Hospital in China: Being the Story of St. Agatha's Hospital, P'ing Yin, London: Society for the Propagation of the Gospel in Foreign Parts,* 1933: front cover.

question of the style in which the mission property should be rebuilt."[42] Although he thought it "an excellent thing to have in a capital city a church building that is imposing," he did not doubt "there may be others who think the church building too fine." He considered the mission houses as "modest as they should be." However, at Tongzhou, fifteen miles from Peking, he thought that "the whole property is many times as large as it ought to be, and it would very likely be wise, even at this late date, to dispose of some

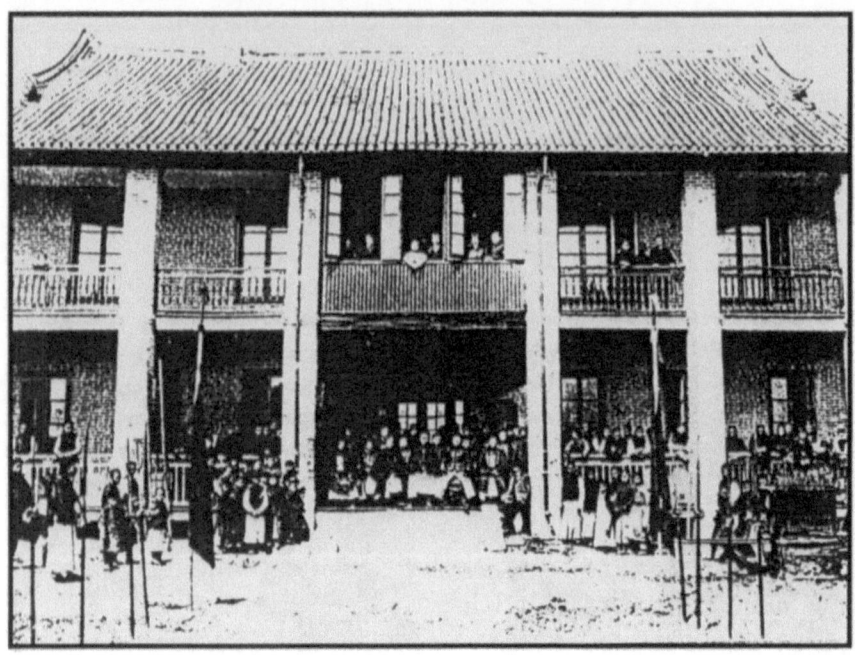

Plate 12. **APM Hospital at Changzhou, Hunan, 1908**

Source: Stephen C Lewis,. "Opening of the American Presbyterian Hospital at Chenchow, Hunan." *CMMJ* 22, no. 4 (1908): 256.

of it, and that the houses are too large and pretentious."[43] His wife agreed with him. She had spoken to the other women of the mission and reported that "the ladies wish that they might be back in the midst of more modest surroundings . . . they regret the expenditure of so much money."[44]

There were exceptions of course. Some sought to impress, and the Alden Speare Memorial Hospital, built by the MEM at Yanping 延平 in Fujian in 1906, was one such. A photograph, reproduced in the *CMMJ*, was of a hospital "located on an eminence in the very heart of the city of Yen-ping, and its gray brick walls and white verandahs give it an imposing and airy aspect."*[45]

How then is one to characterize the medical missionaries' attitudes? Firstly, it is important to take into account that these missionaries were the products of their time and place. It is clear from their writings and actions that American medical missionaries, along with their countrymen at home and their British counterparts in China, were what Ling Oi Ki describes as "encumbered by the cultural biases of their age."[46] They took for granted that Western ideas, values, technology, and political and economic structures

*www.michellerenshaw.com

were superior to those of the rest of the world, and this belief affected their perceptions of what they encountered in China. Most damned traditional Chinese medicine as *unscientific,* folk medicine as superstition, and believed they were practicing a superior, rational, scientific medicine. They equated science with civilization and both with Christianity. Secondly, it is clear that those who advocated building in the Chinese style were motivated by a desire to attract, or at least not repel, potential Chinese patients. They had no power to coerce and in this their situation differed from that of a colonial power seeking to introduce Western medicine or to impose Western sanitary measures. There is nothing in what they wrote to indicate that their advocacy of Chinese stylistic features in hospital buildings was born out of a deep respect for the Chinese, although several did admire Chinese architecture, but then neither did it reflect disdain.

CHOICE OF BUILDING METHODS

When it came to the method of building, the builder had a choice between Chinese and Western. A traditional Chinese building method, common throughout China (but more so in the south), does not use the load-bearing walls used in Western buildings. Rather, timber columns and lintels form a frame that holds the roof up on a set of timber brackets.[47] In both the north and south of the country, regardless of the type of wall, the arrangement of internal spaces is similar: columns are set at standard centers producing a building that consists of modules, referred to as *bays,* the numbers and arrangement of which are varied depending on the purposes for which the building is intended.[48] Spaces are created using lightweight (often timber) movable screen-walls. This design principle is extremely flexible and is used for a wide range of purposes, from dwelling houses to temples. External spaces are designed with as much care as internal: the dimensions are varied according to the arrangement of building elements.

Butchart was even-handed in his approach vis-à-vis the foreign and Chinese methods. As he explained: "there are two styles of wall—the solid brick of the foreign way and the hollow or *teu-tsiang* of the Chinese made with foreign sized brick. The latter may be used where there is only one story or where cheapness is desirable. In this style the roof and floors are entirely supported by a timber framework and the walls filled in. The hollow between the bricks can be filled, Chinese fashion, with broken brick and mud plaster, which makes it a solid wall and prevents any danger of a brick being driven in by a blow as one sometimes sees done for mischief in compound walls where this precaution has been neglected."[49] It was not 'mischief,' when the missionary Claude Lee "pushed down one whole wall of the dispensary with his stick." He blamed a "dishonest contractor [who had used] plaster made of simple mud."[50]

Peck, whose hospital at Pangjiazhuang was also of this construction, saw distinct medical advantages to be had from Chinese building methods. It enabled him to effectively implement the strategy, which had been found so effective during the Civil War, of housing patients in temporary sheds or tents. His surgical experience with the Chinese has convinced him that: "notwithstanding their filthy habits, it is comparatively easy to secure good antisepsis. Our hospital buildings all have independent frames to support the roof, and the walls are filled in with adobe brick which can be torn out at any time if they become infected."[51] He improved ventilation by adapting and installing another Chinese device, "ventilating frames like Chinese windows in the north wall." He did not eschew all foreign design features however—the windows in ward buildings were of glass (rather than paper) with transoms over them.

WARDS

It was knowledge of the current thinking about healthy hospital building rather than consideration of Chinese sensibilities that dominated the recommendations regarding ward design. Mackenzie, in line with the most up-to-date thinking in America and Europe, promoted the pavilion design for his ideal ward.[52] He could see advantages—beyond those discussed earlier concerning the ease of treating surgical cases safely—in this style of building. He saw it as appealing to the Chinese because it "adapts itself readily to Chinese taste, especially as the roof may be modelled after the native pattern, while the grounds around and between the wards can be planted with shrubs and trees."[53] Chinese roofs, being supported on a series of brackets above the building frame, allowed additional ventilation by allowing air to pass out of the building through the space created.[54] The plan also offered the flexibility important in an uncertain political climate: it was difficult to know whether a mission was to be allowed to grow or be hindered. He asserted that his plan "combines simplicity with economy—economy in that, instead of erecting a large block of buildings which will not be required in their full capacity for many years to come, you are able to add ward to ward as the needs of the work develop."[55]

At Tianjin his large twenty-four-bed ward and four three-bed wards in buildings "entirely detached and separated by courtyards," set behind the main building, conformed to his ideal ward, which should be "single storied buildings, entirely detached; for example, wards of the following dimensions, 48x24x14 feet, with opposite windows in the sides, capped with transoms, and reaching nearly to the ceiling."[56] A couple of examples will serve to illustrate that Mackenzie's call did not go unheeded by those who were starting to build their own hospitals. One of the earliest examples of the pavilion design used in China for a new hospital building was the one James H. McCartney, of the American MEM, established at Chongqing 重庆 in Sichuan province. He had arrived as a "young physician" in Chongqing in 1891 and, in 1893, moved from temporary Chinese buildings into a hospital consisting of two brick pavilions, 65 by 26 Chinese feet.[57] Each contained a public ward, two private rooms, a medicine room, and a clothes press. He also used a two-storied "native building" to house twelve wards and a bathroom.[58] In 1889 Mildred Phillips reported on the building of a hospital for women at Suzhou 苏州, for the MEM (South), to complement the men's hospital which had been opened six years earlier.[59] Again the pavilion was the preferred ward design, being "calculated to allow satisfactory separation of the sick, and to secure good ventilation." As she described them: "the buildings are of brick, plastered inside and out, and connected by open corridors. They are finished neatly inside with high ceilings and special ventilating pipes. [Then there are the] medical and surgical wards in two separate pavilions, each containing a bathroom and a room for special cases. [These] are single-storied, raised three feet from the ground, with good ventilation underneath and the ground beaten down with a cement of sand and lime."[60] When Butchart delivered his address in January 1901 he still recommended pavilion-style wards where "with the use of simple antiseptic dressings in order to isolate the wound, with plenty of fresh air and cleanliness of the ward, you are largely independent of tidiness in the person of the patient, and may have a ward full of surgical operation cases while the air is perfectly fresh."[61]

Conscious that money for buildings was scarce, Butchart advised on how to save it. For example, building two stories rather than one could keep down the cost of roofs. Eliminating corridors, and locating the stairway at one end of the verandah could save space, and therefore money. Another advantage of this arrangement related to hygiene: hallways, where dirt tended to accumulate, were difficult to plan so "they shall not be dark." Butchart's advice would also have been compatible with the plan and style of Chinese buildings that commonly used verandahs, connected by covered walkways or galleries, and lacked corridors.

SANITATION

The main consideration, beyond availability, in the choice of building materials for internal finishes should be the ease of maintaining cleanliness, according to Butchart. He started with roofs. Chinese buildings had tiled roofs
without ceilings but, in his opinion, corrugated iron, sufficiently lapped, was
the "best roof by far." He counseled against tiles unless either "board sheath-
ing" or "flat tile with plaster" was used in any room that needed to be kept
clean because "in windy weather great quantities of dirt will blow through
the tile in those parts of the country that are dusty." The roof design should
follow the Chinese custom and have eaves that project eighteen inches to
protect the wall from the weather. However, Balme's survey of hospitals, undertaken during 1919, revealed that Chinese tiled roofs continued to be the
norm, being reported in seventy two percent of the hospitals.[62] A number of
possible reasons for this choice: Chinese tiles were plentiful, Chinese builders were familiar with laying them, imported corrugated iron was in short
supply or was too expensive, or the tiles used on familiar Chinese-style roofs
would be attractive to the Chinese.

For floors and walls, ease of cleaning was the key. Peck recounted
that he suggested that Mackenzie use Portland cement for floors, which
was less porous than the "native bricks," standard in Chinese buildings.[63]
Mackenzie duly recommended it in 1887, and, according to Butchart in
1901, the best floor was "oregon pine, or . . . Portland cement" because it
could be "swabbed over daily, and thus cleanliness will be ensured while ab-
sorption is prevented."[64] Cement, with the advantage of hardness compared
with porous bricks or simply tamped earth common in Chinese buildings,
proved popular. It was recommended by Woodward for those parts of the
dispensary "through which streams of patients must pass" to avoid damage
wrought by the "nail boots of patients in wet weather."[65] The ever-enterpris-
ing Charles Lewis, sacrilegiously perhaps, ground up a "great stone ancestral
tortoise" and mixed it with cement to "get a perfectly smooth finish on the
operating room floor."[66]

Many who described their new hospitals pointed with pride to the
foreign flooring.[67] Where timber floors were used they were often varnished
with Ningbo varnish, as described by Mildred Phillips at Suzhou: "the wood-
work is of the best Chinese red-wood and camphor-wood, and the floors of
foreign pine—varnished with the commonly used Chinese varnish."[68]

Butchart identified an interesting safety problem associated with laying timber floors in China. He exhorted builders to "insist on seeing that
none of the floor timbers are run into the chimney and beneath the fire place,

but at that point are separately supported." He explained that "even good contractors are careless here, and fires are a consequence." As a solution he recommended to "have the chimney built entirely outside the wall like the southern cabin, in which case it may be used to strengthen the wall and even be made ornamental."[69] It should not have surprised him that Chinese contractors had difficulty with this building technique: wooden floors were a novelty and chimneys were not a feature of Chinese buildings. Inexperience and unfamiliarity on the part of Chinese builders may have been a better explanation than carelessness.

Sewerage, of course, was a concern but many hospitals simply discharged waste into the river on whose banks they had conveniently located themselves. Jefferys noted that latrines were a serious problem in a "land where running water is unknown and difficult to provide and where there is no sewerage water-closets are impossible (in Shanghai even forbidden by law)."[70] Butchart considered it "next to the impossible" to achieve a clean latrine in a Chinese hospital. He suggested having a cement floor elevated three or four feet above ground level with a drain for a urinal at one side, and with oblong apertures opening into Chinese *gang,* or galvanized iron cans, below: "The Chinese can then adopt the natural squatting posture which they prefer and the floor having nothing on it, can be easily flushed with water and the *gangs* removed at the back and cleaned."[71] His suggested solution provides further evidence of his ability to come up with solutions that were sensitive to Chinese custom while not sacrificing the hygiene he knew to be necessary.

ARRANGEMENT OF BUILDINGS

The other feature commonly found in mission hospitals, whether or not they adopted the pavilion ward, was the location of ancillary hospital functions in separate buildings. Most often these included the kitchen or cooking area, dining rooms, bathrooms, laundry, sometimes the operating theatre and, always, the morgue. McCartney's first Chongqing hospital provides a good example. All non-ward facilities were located in a series of separate buildings. These included an operating room with instrument room attached and a two-storied building with a dining room, kitchen, bathroom, and room for the patients' cast-off clothing on the first floor and rooms for assistants and students on the second. St. Agatha's at Pingyin was another that comprised a number of separate buildings within walled compounds. The main hospital building contained only wards, a dining room, the chapel and an operating suite. A kitchen and bathroom were located—as far away from the main building as was possible—in the northwest corner of the compound and the latrines were in the southwest corner. In an adjoining compound there were buildings for the outpatients department and guesthouses for those men who had accompanied their womenfolk to hospital.*[72]

The separation of ancillary facilities could have been based on the belief that harmful vapors emanated from various activities and so was in tune with the recommendations of surgeon and clinical professor at University College London, John E. Erichsen (1818–1896). In his 1874 lectures on hospitalism, he noted that the majority of hospitals were just large houses of three or four stories with interconnected stairways and corridors. These did not lend themselves to simple modification as Simpson had suggested. Erichsen's solution was to move "ancillary facilities, such as kitchens, cellars, washing facilities and dead house, to separate buildings." He also advocated the establishment of independent isolation wards for patients with erysipelas or suppurating wounds and regular closure of wards for disinfection.[73] Certainly, the reason could also have been the practical one of adding a series of smaller buildings as time, money, expertise, and need manifested themselves. Equally, it could have been that in China it was traditional practice to build a series of buildings, each with a specific use, around a courtyard. For example, in a Chinese domestic situation cooking was most likely to be done out in the open, on a verandah, or in an outhouse. Privies, also, were located in separate sheds from which sewage was collected at night to be used as fertilizer.[74] Chinese houses rarely had rooms set aside for bathing: those well-to-do who did bathe had water basins and tubs brought to them by servants.[75] It may be no more than serendipitous that congruence existed between the Chinese traditional arrangement, of separate buildings for different functions, and the separation recommended by Erichsen. If McCartney located ancillary facilities in separate buildings to avoid having *contaminated* air circulate through the hospital wards, he did not articulate it. The practice would not have appeared at all strange to the Chinese and may, in fact, have served to make the hospitals more familiar.[76]

ACCOMMODATION—CLASSES OF PATIENT

Another related issue facing hospital designers was the proportion of total beds that should be set-aside in private rooms. Medical missionaries made the same assumptions in China as did their counterparts in America and Britain—the poor could be herded together and the rich had to be provided

*www.michellerenshaw.com

with privacy. As Butchart expressed it: "there are two classes of cases; one set that are poor and come perhaps with no friend. These like to be in the large ward, where they are not so much afraid of the magic of the foreigner. Others are used at home to retirement, and fret at being with the common herd. Private wards should be arranged for these, and are much appreciated and may be a good source of revenue to the hospital, as they are willingly paid for."[77]

Single rooms, though, were necessary when it came to dealing with patients with contagious diseases, particularly typhus. Butchart suggested using an isolation ward "large enough to hold one patient, on the plan used in the separate pavilions in the women's hospital in New York." He went on to describe its construction: "four corner posts with a floor, and the sides and roof are made of corrugated iron fastened to frames so as to be rigid and yet to be easily entirely re-moved, exposing everything to the sun and air ... ventilation will be free under the corrugations of the roof. The aim being to protect only from rain and storm." Given that he spoke of a one-person room he did not envisage significant numbers of people with contagious diseases being admitted. Unlike those in America, hospitals in China were not able to exclude people suffering from contagious diseases. Many mention that they could isolate patients: Osgood and Lewis utilized buildings separate from the hospital and McCartney used the second floor of the main building.[78]

When Balme conducted his 1919 survey, by far the majority of hospitals in China had been purpose-built as hospitals: a mere ten percent operated in buildings described as being adapted from Chinese houses. Given that, as we have seen, most missionaries started out in existing buildings, there must have been something of a boom in building in the first two decades of the twentieth century. In fact, Balme discovered that more than eighty percent (that is, 148 of the 177 for which details were provided) had been built since 1900: 72 in the first decade and a similar number, 76, in the second. Of the remaining 29, all but two had been built since 1880.[79]

American and British architects did not enter the field of hospital design in China until the mid-1910s and even then, only in rare cases of medium to large hospitals often associated with new medical schools. For example, when formal medical classes were started in Jinan by the BMS "a small hospital, administered on native lines, seemed amply sufficient." By 1914, when a Union Medical College was established to consolidate the medical educational work carried out jointly since 1904 by the American Presbyterian and the British Baptist Missions, it had become "quite apparent that nothing less than a large modern hospital, built and equipped on thoroughly up-to-date lines, could possibly suffice." A new hospital under the auspices of the Baptists and designed by Gilbert H. Perriman, one of the architects of the Shantung Christian University, was opened in September 1915.[80] Some smaller concerns, such as the Westminster Sunday School Hospital in Changde 常德 (Hunan), consulted an architect to solve particular esthetic dilemmas. According to O. T. Logan, who had initiated the medical work for the Cumberland Presbyterian Mission (CPM) in 1899 at Changde, "Mr. Stanley Wilson, Supervising Architect of the Yale Mission, who kindly furnished the drawings for the veranda, which in this case practically makes the front elevation [had succeeded in] diversifying the front of the building so as to give a pleasing appearance."[81] Given that sixty percent of all missionary hospitals operating in China in 1919 had been built prior to 1910, and architect-designed buildings are not mentioned before 1913, it is clear that the day of the doctor-builder in China lasted well into the twentieth century. It is likely that the understanding of Chinese preferences and customs these doctor-builders gained over the previous half-century would have influenced the architects' approach when they did arrive on the scene.

Chapter Five
The Arrival of Architects

The arrival of private architects in China ushered in a new era in mission building. According to Cody, by the end of the Qing there were at least a dozen foreign architectural firms operating from Shanghai.[1] These early architects were mostly British and none appear to have been involved in designing hospitals. One of the earliest examples of an architect-designed hospital was *Hsiangya,* the hospital component of the Yale-in-China (*Yali*) campus at Changsha 长沙 in Hunan, in 1913.[2] The medical school was established by the Yale Mission in partnership with the gentry of Hunan and administered by a committee with both American and Chinese members.[3]

HSIANGYA FOR YALE-IN-CHINA, 1913

The architects chosen to design most of the campus were Americans, Henry Killam Murphy and his partner, Richard H. Dana, Jr., who were experienced in designing for American educational institutions but, at that time, had no experience in China. Murphy, though, wanted his buildings to reflect the philosophy of Yale-in-China: to balance "deference to Chinese history and adherence to scientific progress."[4] He could use his buildings to demonstrate to the Chinese that adopting modern plans and methods of construction did not mean that they had to abandon their architectural heritage. Also, according to Cody, members of the Yale-in-China Committee were anxious to "downplay *Yali's* American roots by making some of the buildings appear as little 'foreign' as possible." Not only had there been "fierce [anti-missionary] riots in Changsha in 1910" but Edward Hume, who had been in charge of the medical work since 1907, would have been influential in adopting this policy. He had become what could be described as *accommodationist* in his approach to many aspect of his work, realizing, as Lian Xi puts it, that "it was a good idea to honor the Chinese dictum 'When entering a village, follow its customs.'"[5] Murphy took as his inspiration for his Chinese-style buildings in Hunan the Ming dynasty palaces constructed in Beijing during the fifteenth century.[6] He did not design the hospital component of the Yale complex, however.

When Edward Hume was on furlough in America he went to see his "good class-mate, the philanthropic Edward S. Harkness" to discuss his need for a new hospital.[7] Harkness offered to provide the funds to build and equip a hospital on condition that he not be approached for recurrent funding; that it be a teaching rather than purely medical facility; and that the people of Hunan would consider it their own and manage and support it. He directed Hume to his own architect, John Gamble Rogers, who, armed with the information and samples of building materials available in China that Hume had brought with him, prepared plans for a four hundred-bed hospital. In his autobiography Hume described the plans as being "like nothing thought of in Hunan before." It was to utilize reinforced concrete with "wards reaching out to the south toward the city, only a short distance away, like great arms beckoning the sick to come."[8] Hume makes no comment on the style of building but a photograph reproduced in his biography is of a monumental building very obviously built using foreign materials and building methods and relying almost exclusively on Rogers' interpretation of Chinese curved roofs to lend local character.[9] Architect and historian Su Gin-Djih describes such foreign attempts at incorporating Chinese style as having the appearance of "a western building wearing a Chinese roof as a hat."[10] In his opinion this arose because the American architects' "knowledge of the Chinese treatise and proportion of unit module to elements of construction, and the method of obtaining the proper curvature of the roof was pitifully lacking."[11] So, although the "Yale administrators were . . . committed to using Chinese-style buildings" and the rest of the medical school (Library, Chapel, School and dormitories) echoed Ming palaces, this modified Western-style hospital would have sent "mixed stylistic signals" to the people of Changsha.[12]

CHURCH GENERAL HOSPITAL AT WUCHANG AND THE PEKING CENTRAL HOSPITAL, 1916.

Another foreign architect, Harry Hussey, went further than the roof artifice and incorporated basic principles of Chinese design and orientation into his hospital for the ACM at Wuchang 武昌 in Hubei. His model for parts of the Wuchang hospital was not a palace or temple but the more modest mud-brick, or rammed earth, buildings of the Chinese countryside.

Hussey was a Canadian, a principal of the Chicago-based firm Shattuck and Hussey, who had been in China since 1911, when the YMCA moved into China and brought him in as their architect.[13] By 1915, when the ACM approached him to design a modern general hospital to replace their separate men's and women's hospitals (St. Peter's and Elizabeth Bunn Memorial[14]) at Wuchang, he was very familiar with building under Chinese conditions. His decision to establish an office in Shanghai in the autumn of 1915 had been welcomed by the China Continuation Committee (CCC) of the National Missionary Conference, which had been investigating ways to relieve missionaries of the burden of designing and overseeing the erection of mission buildings.[15] Of all the foreign architects it appears that he became the most prolific in hospital design. Between 1916 and 1920 he was responsible for the design of at least three significant hospitals: the Peking Central Hospital for a Committee of Chinese Trustees[16] (opened January 1918); the Church General Hospital at Wuchang (opened December 1918); and the Peking Union Medical College (PUMC) for the Rockefeller Foundation (opened September 1921).[17]

The published plans for the Wuchang hospital reveal some of the ways Hussey was experimenting with incorporating Chinese design principles into his architecture. First, the orientation and massing of buildings. Four main principles govern the manner in which traditional Chinese buildings are arranged on a site and grouped within a complex. They can be summarized thus: orientation to the cardinal directions; inward-looking and introverted rather than extraverted; axiality; and side-to-side symmetry. In addition, buildings are commonly surrounded by a wall, intersected only by an entrance gate, which emphasizes the sense of seclusion, and they are arranged so as to form internal courtyards.[18] Within the compound the most important buildings face south and are set hierarchically, one behind the other, along a north–south axis—the highest status building occupying the northern-most, most secluded, and most private position. In the traditional residential compound lesser status buildings are built facing east and west. South facing orientation, with a solid back wall to the north, not only protects the occupants from strong wind while opening the building to the winter sun but also has symbolic meaning. According to Peter Swann, the Chinese view the north as the "source of evil influences" and the emperor's palace "corresponds to the Pole star in the heavens" round which all stars appear to turn. The palace (like the emperor) turns its back to the north and faces south with all subordinate buildings—or the world the emperor rules—lying to the south of it.[19] The selection of sites and the arrangement of buildings are also influenced by geomantic considerations. Francesca

Bray discusses the role of geomancy on health at some length in her article on Chinese health beliefs. She describes the landscape, as well as the body, as possessing *qi* 气 that can be manipulated to improve the well being of its inhabitants. The Chinese science of siting is called, *dili* 地理 (the principles of the earth), "or in more vulgar terms" *feng shui* 风水 (wind and water). Firstly, a favorable location is determined by its orientation and the "configuration of streams, hills, boulders and trees" on and near the site. Then, the arrangement of buildings within the compound and the height of roofs and gates are "all designed to channel (not increase) cosmic *qi* for the benefit of the occupants and to exclude harmful influences."[20]

The orientation and plan of the Wuchang building conformed in large part to these principles. The first building patients encountered—housing the waiting rooms for men and women—was rectangular in plan and was oriented with its longest side facing south. The hospital-proper was symmetrical in design and was positioned, on a south–north axis, directly behind the dispensary. Both main buildings presented a long, low, rectangular elevation on the south that was perfectly symmetrical in every respect. When and if expansion became necessary, Hussey had anticipated that the multi-storey part of the building could be replicated immediately behind the first building—again in accord with the Chinese planning principle of "axiality." * The whole complex was set within a walled enclosure and as one moved along the south to north axis one entered increasingly private space. Other than pagodas, Chinese buildings in the Ming, and to an even greater extent in the Qing, were characterized by their 'horizontality,' and both the hospital and the waiting rooms conform to this tradition.[21] Still, there was no doubt that this complex was a Western creation: the most obvious deviation from traditional Chinese principles was the absence of enclosed courtyards. In this three-storey building, without direct access for patients and staff to the grounds, some of the functions of courtyards would have been performed by the solaria and roof gardens.

It is difficult to determine which hospital Hussey designed first, this one at Wuchang or the Peking Central. We know that he was engaged by a group of Chinese officials to prepare the Peking plans in the spring of 1915 and foundations were dug in June 1916.[22] The design for the hospital at Wuchang must have been developed at about the same time because his drawings (an isometric rendition and plans of the three floors) were reproduced in a fund-raising pamphlet published by the Rt Rev. Logan H. Roots sometime in 1916.[23] Although the hospitals were of comparable size—around 150

---

*www.michellerenshaw.com

beds—and shared a considerable number of design features, they also differed significantly. Drawings and a photograph survive for one (Wuchang) and a detailed description and photographs of the other (Peking).

The Wuchang hospital complex was set on land with a frontage of 400 feet and depth of 500 feet enclosed within the ubiquitous, in this case low, wall. (see Plate 13) The design called for two main buildings: a one-story building housing separate waiting rooms for men and women and, directly behind it, the two-story hospital proper with a roof garden. These buildings, both rectangular in plan, faced south with their long sides running east–west. A one-storey dispensary running south–north formed a link between the waiting rooms and hospital. The most striking thing about this design is the way Hussey clearly differentiated between the in- and outpatients' departments. The former was essentially Western in appearance, suggestive of the neo-classical style common in America at the time. It was constructed with "ferro-concrete and brick" exterior walls, a simple hipped roof with chimneys, and lacked the characteristic Chinese curves or overhanging eaves. The outpatients' department, comprising two main components (the waiting rooms and duplicate dispensaries) on the other hand, was housed in extremely simple, single-story buildings with Chinese tiled, flush-gable, roofs in a style more reminiscent of rural Chinese adobe buildings. The dispensaries consisted of examining rooms, bathrooms, surgeries, and offices for Chinese and missionary doctors—one set for men, on the west, and a matching set for women, on the east. These were, like the waiting rooms, single-storey with twin gable roofs—one over each section—continuing the low simple lines.

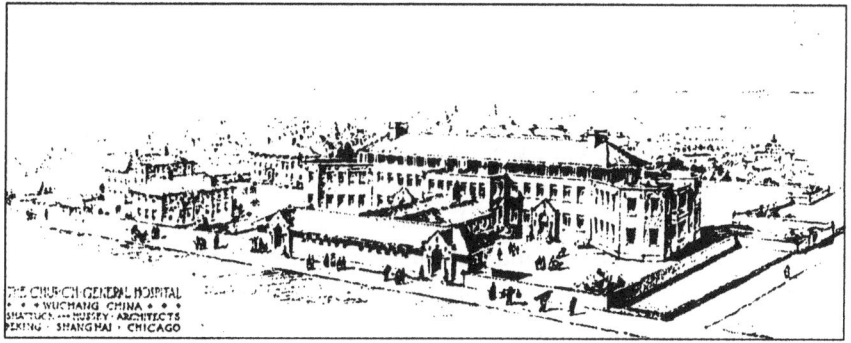

Plate 13. **The ACM Church General Hospital, Wuchang, 1916**

Source: Logan H. Roots, *Our Plan for the Church General Hospital, Wuchang*, New York: The Board of Missions, c. 1916: 2.

Courtesy of the Burke Library, Union Theological College, New York

The number of patients attending the dispensary was always far in excess of those admitted to hospital, and it was almost always the first point of contact between the Chinese patient and medical missionary. If Hussey, or the medical missionaries he was working with, adhered to the principle of 'not frightening the natives' discussed earlier, it would be appropriate that the dispensary be designed in keeping with local tradition. In Hussey's Wuchang hospital the entrances through matching gatehouses, waiting rooms, and dispensaries were all in line with this principle and would have been familiar and possibly even welcoming to potential patients. Presumably, by the time a patient was admitted to hospital he or she would be sufficiently familiar with the situation to be undeterred by the foreign appearance of the hospital-proper. Hussey does not tell us in his memoir, nor is it mentioned in anything published at the time the hospital opened, what drove his overall design nor what thinking shaped this component of the complex.[24] Was it purely an esthetic decision, governed by a wish that his building 'harmonize' with its surroundings; was he consciously trying to appeal to the Chinese; or was cost the deciding factor? It would seem that any or all of these might have been motivating factors. Unadorned Chinese-style buildings, constructed using traditional materials and methods, were less costly per square meter than using foreign materials. Adopting this style for the outpatients department would have freed scarce funds for the more expensive foreign-style hospital building. Hussey's ability to use local materials and provide the Chinese with buildings acceptable to them was demonstrated when he was commissioned by the Red Cross to solve the logistical problem of housing thousands of refugees from floods in North China at the end of 1917. With the help and advice of the man he had contracted to provide labor for building the hospital, Mr. Liu, he designed a hut made of locally available and cheap materials. He used reeds bent over a framework, plastered inside and out with mud, sealed with waterproof lime—"a material . . . known only in China"—and paper stretched over a light wooden frame formed the southern face. The huts not only let in light and heat from the sun but were also warmed in winter by a cooking stove, the smoke and fumes from which passed through flues under a brick *kang* 炕 and out through a chimney. His practical organizational skills and ability to work with Chinese tradesmen were also in evidence: he had taken the tradesmen who were to build the Peking hospital to Tianjin and there they built at least nine thousand "Hussey Huts" in the first seven weeks while teaching the local (refugee) farmers to build so that they could take over and complete the project.[25]

Now, to the hospital-proper. The plans Hussey drew make it clear that he was attempting to satisfy a number of conditions: efficiency of operation, segregation of the sexes, separation of medical, maternity and surgical patients, adequate ventilation and access to sunlight, a variety of classes of accommodation, and sensitivity to Chinese preferences. The desire for efficiency led to him place common services centrally. For instance, the drug rooms on the ground floor served both the outpatients' department and the hospital, and were accessible from either. Certain aspects of efficiency, though, were compromised by the need to separate men from women. As Lewis had explained, he had had to build his hospital at Baodingfu in 1903 exclusively for men because "in the early days separate hospitals were built for men and women to meet Chinese ideas of propriety."[26] Hussey's early twentieth-century general hospital was still effectively two hospitals. A central south–north axis split the hospital metaphorically and physically: a solid wall ran through the whole complex from the waiting rooms, through the dispensaries to the hospital-proper, on all floors, completely separating the men (west) from women and children (east). There was no way for staff to move from the men's hospital to the women's, except through the chapel which opened into both sections. Not only would this arrangement have been inefficient in terms of staff; it also meant that every facility and its equipment, including operating theatres, had to be duplicated.

Letters exchanged between Bishop Roots of Wuchang and Roger Greene of the Rockefeller Foundation in 1915 throw light on the reasons for this expensive design decision. Greene was concerned that establishing separate hospitals for men and women would hinder "Chinese [male] graduates in medicine [receiving] a general all-round training under proper supervision." He saw "great practical difficulty in using male internes . . . in a hospital devoted exclusively to women and probably managed by a woman doctor."[27] Partly, it was to satisfy one such "woman doctor" that the Wuchang General took its form. Doctor Mary Latimer James had arrived at Wuchang in 1914 to take control of the women's hospital and she was, in Bishop Roots' words, "an exceedingly capable and independent physician." Not long before she arrived, the Mission had decided that a Director should administer the institution formed by the union of St. Peter's Hospital for Men and the Elizabeth Bunn Memorial Hospital for Women. Dr. James had "some difficulty at once in observing [the] stringent provision that the Director supervise small details" and the Mission tried to ease the situation by creating two separate departments, still under a single Director, but giving her more autonomy. Problems persisted and eventually the Mission was faced with the choice of adhering to their plan and, "if she could not fall into it, let her go back to America" or acquiescing to her demands for "administrative independence and freedom." As Dr. James had the support of the majority of the hospital and Mission staff it had been decided that it was "better to change our plan of organization to suit the requirements of our staff rather than force the retirement of part of the staff."

A further consideration drove the separation of the sexes at Wuchang. It was not so much to cater to the sensibility of Chinese patients but, rather, to "control nurses who are being trained: young women in the Women's department and young men in the Men's Department [and] to relieve the general tensity among the hospital staff workers and especially the nurses." The Bishop felt that "in order to insure even a fair degree of safety, provision must be made to by which the necessity, and even the possibility, of any considerable contact between men and women nurses in training should be eliminated."[28] (see Plate 14)

The hospital was organized along departmental lines: there was separate accommodation for medical, surgical, and maternity patients as well as separate wards for children, eye patients and those with tuberculosis. There were also two small isolation wards. This arrangement was similar to that recommended for contemporary, medium size, hospitals in America.[29]

A particular feature of this hospital was the accommodation for patients suffering from tuberculosis, using roof gardens—both open and covered. At the time 'open-air' treatment involving exposure to fresh air and sunlight was a popular response to tuberculosis, and in 1913 architects were advised of the advantages: "External heating is reduced to a minimum . . . patients are indeed trained to live in as cold a temperature as the resisting powers of their bodies will permit with safety."[30] The flat roofs of the wards and their solaria, at the extremes of the east-west axis, were used as open roof gardens. Above the main east–west corridor there was a hipped roof supported by columns that formed a covered roof garden—open on three sides and with a solid wall on the northern side. Facilities, such as the pair of isolation wards, diet kitchens, storerooms, bathrooms, and an office for Chinese doctors, were located along this wall. There was accommodation for ten tuberculosis patients in separate cubicles: five men and five women. A further fourteen beds (for seven men and seven women) lined the southern side.

Hussey's architectural solution to ventilation and sunlight within the building was also innovative. His design diverged radically from the commonplace central core with pavilion wards forming the U, or the equally common, H plan. On each of the first two floors a corridor ran from west to east but at either end it was split into a "bipartite wing with an intervening verandah containing the main . . . wards and their solariums." Wu Lien-teh explained the thinking behind this aspect of the design of the Peking Central

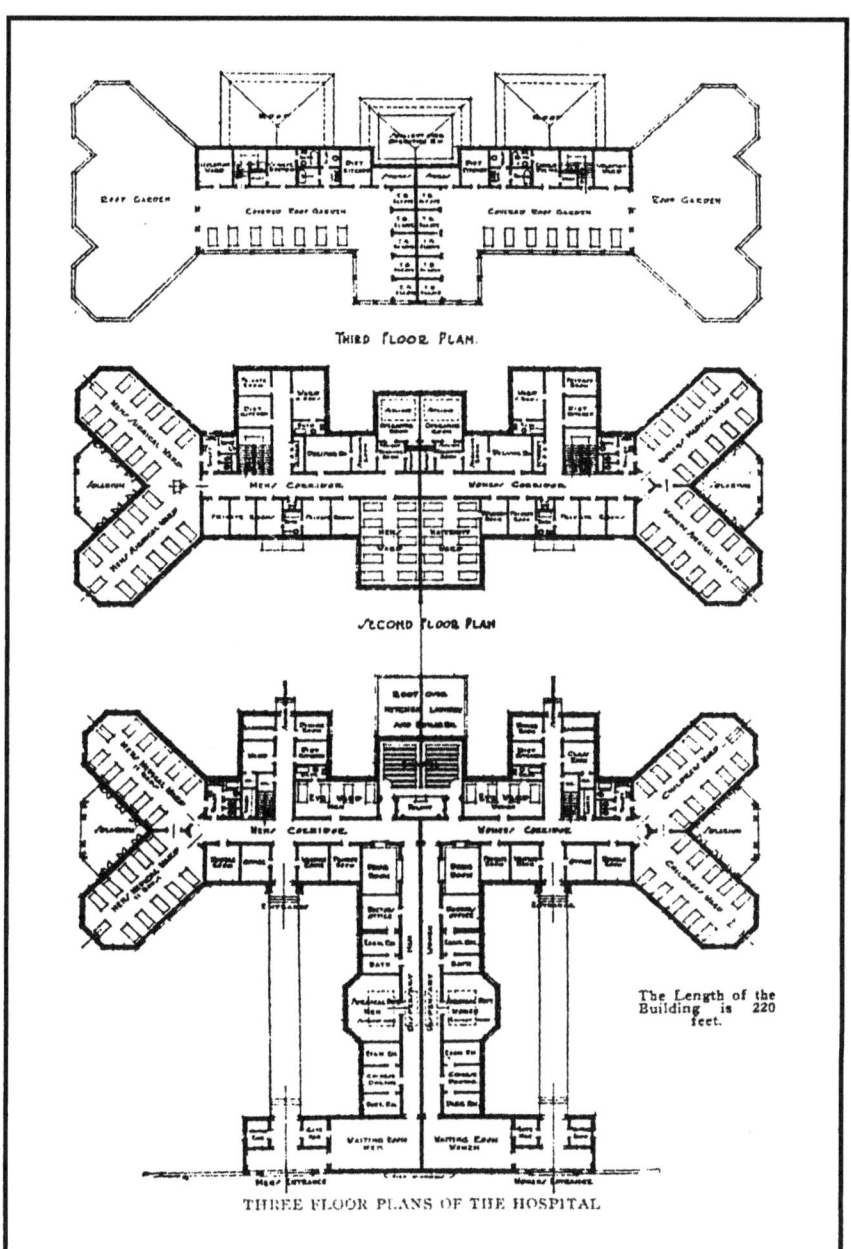

Plate 14. **Plans for the Church General Hospital, Wuchang, 1916**

Source: Logan H. Roots, *Our Plan for the Church General Hospital, Wuchang,* New York: The Board of Missions, c. 1916: 12.

Courtesy of the Burke Library, Union Theological College, New York

Hospital, which shared a similar ground plan, as having been "decided upon in order to gain maximum of light with a minimum of exposure to northern winds in winter, and also to meet the objections of Chinese patients to rooms facing directly east and west."[31] The plan reveals that Hussey's solution had a number of practical advantages over the standard pavilion as well as accommodating Chinese sensibilities. The resulting eleven-bed wards were octagonal in shape, with two long sides and six shorter ones. Breaking the wall into three was esthetically pleasing and allowed for three windows instead of one. Thus each ward had five walls that could accommodate a total of eight windows and three sets of French doors. This arrangement had the ventilation advantages of the pavilion cleverly incorporated into the building without sacrificing efficiency of staff movement or supervision. All patients "requiring the sun treatment" had direct access to a solarium through French doors.

The plan of this building is that of a modern hospital, comparable to what was being built in America at the time: it was "piped for steam heat, hot and cold water, sanitary drainage, and . . . lighted by electricity."[32] Surgery was undertaken in a pair of well-lit operating theatres (one for men and one for women) on the second floor on the northern side, above the chapel, and each had an atrium and skylight over half the room. The hospital fell short, though, in a number of respects. Firstly, the degree of separation was somewhat less than ideal: the bipartite wards were not isolated from one another, or from the corridor, since a door connected them and both opened directly onto the corridor. The toilet and bathroom also opened directly onto one of each pair of these wards. Secondly, compared to the facilities considered essential for the practice of 'scientific' medicine in a modern small-town hospital in America, the Wuchang hospital does not appear to have been well endowed.[33] Although there were plans for replacing the "crude and inconvenient" laboratory facilities (if $1,400 could be raised) there is no evidence of provision for a laboratory or X-Ray department within the new hospital.[34] There does not appear to be space set aside for administrative-type activities such as record keeping and charting. The kitchen and laundry were apparently housed in the basement but there appears to have been a distinct lack of storage and other utility spaces for the storage, for example, of clean and soiled bedding and clothing, cleaning equipment, or food supplies, or a work room for nurses. There is no indication, either, of the way death in the hospital would have been handled and there is no morgue shown on the plan. Although both clinical and classroom teaching was carried on at this hospital there was little provision made for teaching space—just one small classroom the size of a single private room.

The emphasis seems to have been on providing beds for as many patients as possible with the needs of staff or any students taking a lower priority. There is no way, given the available material, to know whether this emphasis was a function of wanting to treat, and influence, the maximum number of people for the amount of money available for building—after all ancillary services and amenities for staff would have been very costly—or whether there were other ideological reasons.

A mix of standards of accommodation was provided in wards, single private rooms, and small four-bed wards. This mix mirrored the growth in private accommodation in hospitals in America to provide for the middle and upper classes. In China, though, mission hospitals had, from the beginning, tried to attract patients from the official and gentry classes. The motivation was two-fold: a means of gaining official recognition and the opportunity to influence people in power as well as earning additional income. Consequently, in China, private rooms had been the norm rather than the exception.

While Hussey used the same basic plan and shape for the hospitals at Wuchang and Peking, any concession to Chinese design principles, other than symmetry (which was, after-all, a feature of the neo-classical architecture popular for public buildings in America at the time) was abandoned in the Peking version. (see Plate 15) The Peking Central Hospital, which Wu Lien-teh described as "thoroughly modern" and "distinctly American" in style, was far grander than the one at Wuchang.[35] Gone was the modest human scale outpatients' department providing an unthreatening introduction; the hospital-proper stood alone on high ground with a sweeping circular driveway in front of an elaborate entrance at the top of a flight of steps.[36] There was a small outpatients' department but it was incorporated into the basement of the eastern wing of the principal building.[37] There does not appear to have been a wall surrounding this hospital, and Wu does not mention one. It is also taller than the Wuchang building, mainly due to a basement floor with windows at least six feet above the ground. The façade of the Wuchang building was altogether plainer. Its simple rectangular windows lacked ornamentation compared to those at Peking and its roofline was simpler, not having the elaborate roofed entrance.[38]

The differences Hussey incorporated into the basic design can be explained in a number of ways. Firstly, the capital, Peking, was more cosmopolitan than Wuchang: Wuchang the "strategic center of China," located where the Yangzi River crosses the railway from Beijing in the north to Guangzhou in the south, had been more recently, and less extensively, exposed to foreigners and foreign buildings.[39] A grander, more substantial-looking, building

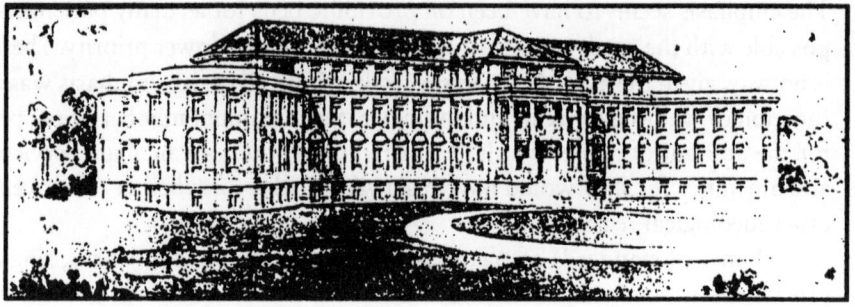

Plate 15. **Peking Central Hospital, 1916**
Source: *CMMJ*, Vol. 31, no. 4 (1917): 271.

suited the capital city site whereas a more modest, but equally modern, hospital was more appropriate in a provincial centre. Secondly, the aims of architectural clients are always an important influence and it would appear to be the case here: Wu Lien-teh, the honorary medical director of the Peking Central Hospital, wanted a "thoroughly modern hospital . . . as a reminder to America that her sister republic is forging ahead" and one which would act as "a model *civil* hospital of China . . . to promote the interests of scientific medicine."[40] The Wuchang ACM, on the other hand, expressed their rather less grand aims and focused more on the needs of the Chinese community; they wanted to relieve suffering and afford a model that the Chinese may "safely imitate."[41] Thirdly, Hussey's personal ambition probably played a part. At the time he was building the Peking Hospital he was courting the Rockefeller Foundation executives who were looking for an architect to design the Peking Union Medical College (PUMC); an imposing modern hospital worthy of the capital would have been impressive and would have demonstrated his credentials.

PEKING UNION MEDICAL COLLEGE HOSPITAL, 1920

Since arriving in China, Hussey had developed a passion for Chinese imperial architecture. When he settled in Peking in early 1917 he purchased a home that he described as having been being built for the "Keeper of the Imperial Archives under the Manchu." It was "within the red wall of the Imperial City, a stone's throw from the walls of the Forbidden City, and a five-minute walk to the British and American legations . . . a fine example of the Chinese architecture of the early Ming emperors, evidently designed by the architects who had built many of the palaces and public buildings in

Peking."[42] He improved his understanding of Chinese architecture during the years he spent restoring it, trying to "make it a good example of the best Chinese domestic architecture adapted to the requirements of modern life. It became the meeting place for the Oriental and the Occidental."

It was with the commission to build the PUMC that Hussey was able to indulge his enthusiasm for traditional *grand* Chinese architecture. The Rockefeller Foundation had purchased a twelve-acre property, close to the Forbidden City, surrounded by a twenty-foot-high wall.[43] Hussey described the buildings he was to demolish to make way for the main buildings of the medical school and hospital: "the palaces with their beautifully carved, white marble balustrades and steps; the beautiful gardens with small lakes crossed by white marble bridges, and the great number of old trees, all in a remarkably good state of preservation ... in destroying Yu Wang Fu we destroyed greater and more beautiful and more important buildings than we built. It was vandalism; we should have built elsewhere and kept the beautiful Yu Wang Fu, equal to any residence in the imperial city, as a national monument."[44] Despite this regret and self-recrimination he was to nominate the buildings for the PUMC as "the best I ever designed."[45]

The Foundation had approached Hussey early in 1916 while he was back in America: "they wanted to look me over a few more times" before commissioning him as "chief architect for all their buildings in China." He agreed to take on the dual roles of architect *and* builder of the PUMC. He moved to Baltimore, where he established an architectural office within Johns Hopkins Hospital, visited "all the new hospitals and medical schools in America" and, later, several in Europe." He was to draw up plans in consultation with Drs. Winford Smith and William H. Welch of Johns Hopkins and consulting architect, Mr. Charles A. Coolidge.[46] Never one to miss an opportunity or to fail to use his connections, and so that he could understand the requirements of the various departments, he was "given the privilege of attending all lectures, operations and autopsies held in the hospital. I took full advantage of this opportunity. The name of Rockefeller was a magic word at Johns Hopkins."[47] He also had access to all the hospital staff for advice. The hospital that Hussey designed would have the benefit of the latest findings on the best of contemporary hospital planning. For the exterior, though, he decided to use "the same style of Chinese architecture as was used in the beautiful buildings of the Forbidden City."[48] In this, according to his account, he was supported by the Rockefeller Foundation, Charles Coolidge, the American Ambassador to China (Dr. Paul Reinsch), and officials in the Chinese government. He reported that Coolidge had spoken to Chinese officials who told him "they hoped the Rockefeller Foundation would not build another foreign city, like the Legation Quarter." He also claimed that Coolidge recommended him to the Rockefeller Board not only because of his "connections with Chinese government officials" but also because of his knowledge of Chinese architecture.[49] The Minister for the Interior, an architect, Chu Chi Ch'ien, whom Hussey flattered as "the greatest living authority on Chinese architecture [and] one of the greatest living architects and author of one of the finest books ever written on Chinese architecture," apparently praised the Hussey design. "He told me how pleased he was with my designs; told me how relieved he was, as he had feared the buildings (so close to the beautiful Forbidden City) would be built in foreign style, the style of many ugly buildings the foreigners had already built in Peking."[50] George Kates described these *ugly buildings,* particularly in the Legation Quarter (built on land divided among foreign powers after 1901) as looking as though they had been lifted and set down in China—"a most oddly assorted juxtaposition of architectural *tranches de gateau.*"[51] By comparison, it is evident from the perspective he drew of the complex that the scale, massing and symmetry of Hussey's buildings all conform to Chinese design principles. (see Plate 16) Support for Hussey's design decision was not universal, however, and he cites missionaries as saying, on more than one occasion, that the "buildings should not be in Chinese architecture, they should have been designed like our American colleges to show the Chinese some good American architecture."[52]

Hussey did not concentrate, as others had, almost exclusively upon roof slopes, to lend a Chinese look to an otherwise Western building. Not only did he use traditional double-hipped, curved roofs but the Chinese appearance was further enhanced by his choice of materials, particularly bricks and roofs tiles. He found that the Chinese-manufactured bricks were not suitable. They were poorly made, too small, and too soft and he had "long before been converted to the idea of the Chinese architects that the bricks used in a building should be proportionate to the size of the building—small bricks for small buildings and large bricks for large buildings."[53] He found his answer in the two hundred-year-old bricks used in the wall of the compound. The wall was to be demolished and it had been built of the "same bricks that were used in the Great Wall of Peking." These were large, measuring sixteen inches by four and a half inches, and, although they were imperfect specimens, they were easily cut.[54] He had them split and used the good faces.[55] When it came to roof tiles he planned to emulate the roofs of the nearby Forbidden City buildings. He found that the glazed imperial tiles, made from a special, fine clay mined in "Men-t'ou-kai, a village in the Western Hills outside Peking," had not been made in China for fifty years.

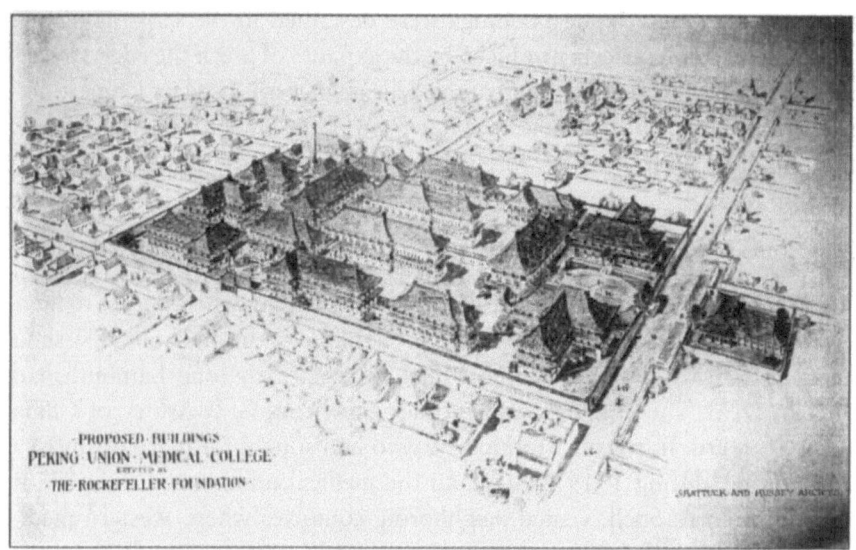

Plate 16. **Peking Union Medical College, Perspective by Hussey**
Source: *China Medical Board Third Annual Report, January1–December 31, 1919.*
Rockefeller Archive Center, CMB/PUMC, Folder 68–69
Courtesy of the Rockefeller Archive Center.

According to his account, he organized the re-opening of the mine and the rebuilding of kilns and then entered into a five-year contract for the supply of tiles.[56] His roof shapes and proportions also more closely resembled traditional Chinese roofs as he relied on Chu Chi Ch'ien to advise him on all aspects of roof design, including "the proper pitch of a Chinese roof, the amount of overhang for the cornice, the details of the huge ornaments on the ridge of the roofs, the proper design of the little figures (such as an emperor riding on a hen) on the eaves of the roof and the other mysteries of Chinese architecture."[57]

Hussey's motivation for using the Chinese architectural style was not necessarily the same as the medical missionaries' preoccupations discussed earlier. Nowhere does he, or anyone else, defend its use on the grounds that it would be more familiar, and therefore less threatening, to patients. Hussey's considerations were esthetic and borne of a fascination with Chinese architecture. He was trying to "combine the best of Chinese art and architecture with present-day requirements for a modern … hospital."[58] The PUMC buildings however, as is clear from photographs taken at the opening in 1920 and published in the *CMJ,* did closely resemble the imperial buildings to which the people of the capital were accustomed and thus blended with their surroundings.[59] The buildings were described in the *CMJ* as having "wonderful colour effects produced by the expanse of green tile edged by exquisite painting in many colours of the delicate patterns used by Chinese artists centuries ago."[60] His earlier Peking Central Hospital, on the other hand, fitted in more with the other foreign buildings of the Legation Quarter.*

SOOCHOW HOSPITAL, 1919–1922

Another example of a hospital designed by an architect who appears to have been consciously using Chinese design principles was the one built at Suzhou between 1919 and 1922 for the MEM to replace the one Lambuth had built in 1833. The architect was another American, G. F. Ashley of China Realty Co. Ltd. In contrast to Hussey, who had sought ideas from America and Europe, during 1919 Ashley and the medical missionary in charge at Suzhou, John A. Snell, visited neighboring countries where Western medicine had recently been introduced—Korea and Japan—to study "hospital problems and plans."[61]

Ashley's hospital complex, conforming to Chinese design principles, was built facing south with a larger, perfectly symmetrical, main hospital building set directly behind the dispensary on a south–north axis.[62] An aspect of his approach to the problem of building a modern hospital that would satisfy the needs of modern 'scientific' medicine and yet would harmonize with its environment was, like Hussey at Wuchang, to treat the two components—inpatients' and outpatients' departments—differently. Both of them adopted a Chinese style for the building where the majority of people would first encounter Western medicine. Hussey had used a simple Chinese building for his entrance—waiting rooms and clinics—whereas Ashley used a more formal, traditional Chinese style with a double-eaved, hip-and-gable curved roof for his outpatients' department. (see Plate 17) This two story building, housing the outpatients' department on the first floor with accommodation for interns above, was designed to give the appearance of being constructed using the Chinese column and lintel method and conformed to the traditional practice of being built on a raised platform.*

The main hospital building was a plain, rather severe, flat-roofed, three-story brick building with a large U-shaped plan. The clean, simple lines symbolized the supposed modern scientific efficiency of Western medicine. As at Wuchang, the dispensary was connected to the hospital-proper but, here, Ashley employed a gallery as traditionally used in Chinese architecture

*see www.michellerenshaw.com

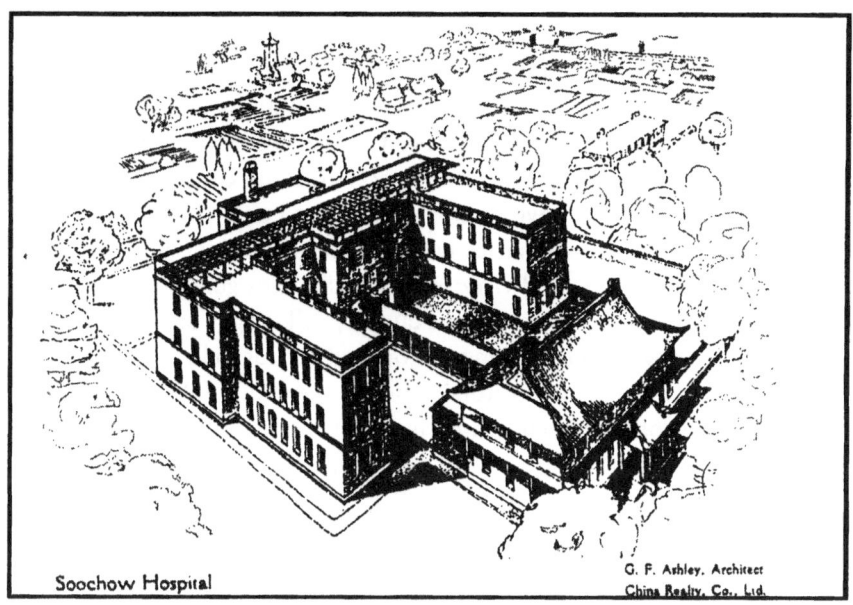

Plate 17. Architect's perspective, MEM(S) Soochow Hospital, 1919
Source: *CMMJ* 34, no. 5 (1920): 467.

to connect halls in both Buddhist and Taoist temples. This gallery, of brick columns supporting a Chinese-tiled roof, tied the two very different buildings together and, with the east and west wings of the hospital, served to form a pair of rectangular courtyards. Thus it extended the Chinese feeling of the complex beyond the dispensary.

Entering the outpatients' department building one would be struck by its similarity to a temple hall or the main hall of a large house. As Liang Ssu-ch'eng points out, the internal planning of a traditional Chinese building rarely needs to be spelt out because the form is eminently flexible and can be readily adapted to any purpose by erecting partitions or screens between any of the columns on the grid. This principle applies equally to secular and religious architecture.[63] Ashley's dispensary building, despite using non-traditional building methods, took this traditional form: essentially a traditional "three *jian*" building with (typically) the central *jian* wider than the flanking bays.[64] Internally, this was experienced as a large hall with internal columns, rectangular in plan (the ratio of the sides being approximately 5:2) with small rooms (formed by partitions) around three sides. The central area was given over to a single large waiting room. (see Plate 18) In marked contrast to the arrangement at Wuchang, men and women were not strictly segregated in the clinic at Suzhou. The series of rooms, all of which led directly off the waiting area, housed a variety of examination, minor operating, and dressing rooms as well as offices, a laboratory, and a drug room. While patients would not necessarily have been able to observe everything that was going on in these rooms they were accessible and consequently not as mysterious as they might have been if a plan based on a corridor had been used. Several medical missionaries have commented on the importance of allowing waiting patients and visitors to see what was going on as a means to allay fear and counter rumors. For example, O. T. Logan set out his "open door" policy of always encouraging visitors and friends to be present and his operating room included a "visitors' stand . . . generally filled with friends and well-wishers of the patient who is under the knife." He believed that the policy prevented a "great deal of bad talk" and accounted for "a good deal of the confidence the people show us."[65]

One section of the hospital-proper owed its character to Chinese style. This was the flat roof of the main building where patients with tuberculosis were accommodated. A low, lattice brick-wall ran around edge of the roof and a heavy wooden trellis held up on wooden columns topped by wooden brackets was constructed using Chinese techniques.* Like Hussey's at Wuchang, the rest of Ashley's building for the hospital-proper was obviously Western in style. Internally, it was laid out according to design principles that had been established in America by that time for a healthy, efficient institution.

The attitude toward indigenization, or sinicization, displayed by the architects and missionaries discussed above, whilst widespread, was not undisputed. The British Consul, J. T. Pratt, did not agree that China had anything to offer by way of architecture. At the opening of the Union Medical Hospital at Jinan, he was quoted as commending the foreign building: "Whilst China is the home of the fine arts, architecture, one of the noblest of them all, can hardly be said to exist in the country . . . the erection of such splendid buildings was in itself a fine piece of missionary work."*[66]

Balme's 1920 survey was silent on the prevailing attitudes amongst missionaries towards indigenization of hospital buildings. He found that only 8 of 177 hospitals were described as being of "pure Chinese style." There were 47 described as "modified Chinese" and the remaining 122 as "foreign." These self-descriptions can be misleading however. As we have seen in the examples cited earlier, many hospitals described as foreign by their builders reveal on closer examination many Chinese features or adaptations.

*see www.michellerenshaw.com

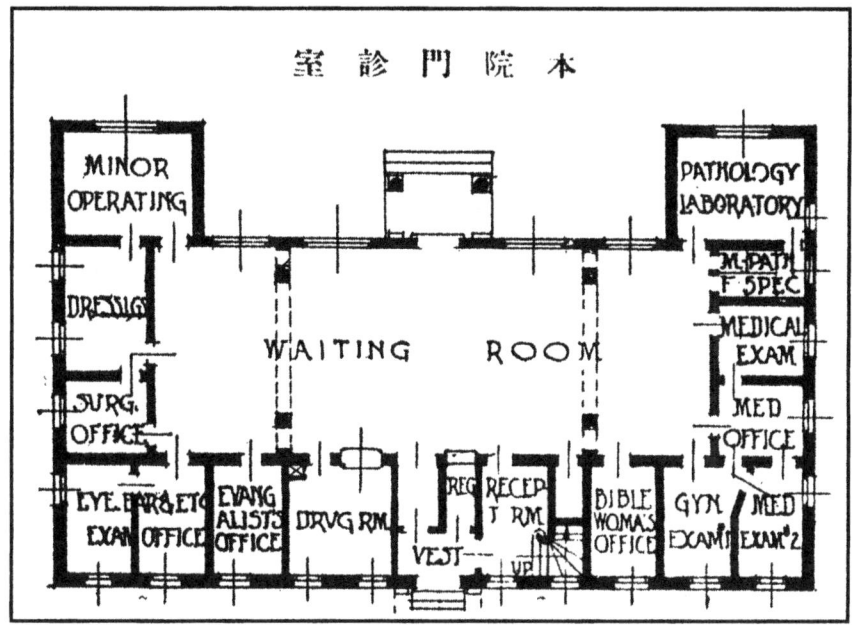

室 診 門 院 本

Plate 18. **Plan of the out-patient building, Soochow Hospital, 1919**
Source: *Soochow Hospital, 1883–1933: Fiftieth Anniversary.* Board of Missions of
Methodist Episcopal Church, South, 1933.

It is clear that whether the hospital was in a modified Chinese building; was built by a doctor; or was one of the few designed and built by
architects, the 'Western' hospital in China differed physically in significant
ways from its counterpart in America or Britain. Within the constraints of
available funds, materials, and skills builders did attempt to emulate the
amenities that were considered important from the point of view of health
and hygiene but this was not their only consideration. They were aware of
the effect a foreign-looking building might have on potential patients and
they also needed to accommodate Chinese customs, preferences, and sensibilities. The motives behind such desires were many and varied and are difficult to discern but the significant thing is that such accommodations were
made, and were manifested in the physical hospital. Medical missionaries in
China were doing more than adapting architecture in order to blend in: they
were trying to practice what they perceived as 'modern (Western) scientific'
medicine among a people who had their own medical tradition as well as
a traditional architecture which had preserved its essence—symbolic and
tangible—for more than two millennia.

Section III
Financing the Hospital Enterprise

> The *one* object and *the* great object in having Mission Dispensaries is, as we all know, to enlighten these people concerning the Doctrine of Christ and point them to the True God. By making them pay to listen to a doctrine they do not care for, it looks as though we are laying a trap for them. And some may maintain that we ought to give them the medicines for listening to our preaching.
>
> —Elizabeth Reifsnyder 1887

One of the last missionary hospitals to become financially self-supporting was the Peking Hospital run by the American Methodist Episcopal Mission. In 1910, after forty years of operation, it recorded that this had been the first year in which it had not had to call on the Missionary Society for a financial contribution other than for salaries of foreign doctors.

Even at this late stage the hospital did not establish a set schedule of fees and charges but had put up a notice alerting its Chinese patients that a contribution was expected from those who could afford it. Until this time patients had been charged only for medicines and doctors' home visits. The bulk of the hospital's funds came from foreign and Chinese annual subscriptions and the proceeds of an optical department that assembled and sold spectacles. This blend of sources of finance—patients, benefactors, and customers—mirrored the state of affairs in the majority of hospitals in China by the end of the first decade of the new century. What follows is the story of how they arrived at this situation, particularly in relation to patients' contributions.

FUNDING HOSPITALS IN AMERICA

Rosemary Stevens, in her authoritative book on the history of the twentieth-century American hospital, analyses hospitals in terms of their role as charitable institutions *and* business enterprises. This emphasis leads her to classify hospitals according to the nature of their ownership and control, viz. proprietary and non-proprietary. The first class comprised the purely private proprietary hospitals, often owned by physicians or surgeons. They charged patients for board and treatment and aimed to make a profit. It was estimated that these made up between forty and fifty percent of all hospitals in 1910.[1] The second class, non-proprietary, included hospitals run by the various levels of government or by voluntary organizations. Public, that is, local or state government, hospitals were fewest in number; 220 out of 1493 (or fifteen percent), according to a 1904 survey.[2] The non-government non-proprietary hospitals could be further divided into two types: secular, and those that were religiously based.*[3]

In America the most numerous and prominent of these types were secular charitable hospitals, twice as many as those run under religious auspices. However, patient numbers were equal in the two systems.[4] In other words, at the beginning of the twentieth century, when the largest contingent of American medical missionaries were establishing themselves in China, half of all the beds in non-proprietary, non-government American hospitals were being provided by bodies with religious affiliations. It would not be surprising if the medical missionaries had taken the prevailing philosophy of how these hospitals should be financed to China with them. But the lone medical missionary would have also felt himself akin to the sole practitioner who set up a private proprietary hospital in an existing, albeit modified, building. Stevens has put forward the suggestion, with reservations, that there could have been as many as 1,500–2,000 of the relatively new, private proprietary hospitals among the estimated 4,000 hospitals of all kinds in America around 1910–1911.[5] It would seem reasonable to suggest that these small proprietary hospitals provided an alternative organizational and, indeed, financing model for a *sole practitioner* medical missionary establishing himself in China.

The few large general hospitals in such cities as New York, Chicago and Philadelphia, financed through a mixture of substantial endowments and government grants and controlled by boards of management, catered principally for the poor well into the twentieth century. However, the hospital with which the great majority of Americans would have been familiar was the relatively small hospital run either by a local government, a secular or religious charity, or a private physician. Voluntary charitable hospitals relied on a variety of funding sources including modest endowments, donations in

*see www.michellerenshaw.com

cash or kind, annual subscriptions, contributions from various companies to provide care for their employees or from city and town governments on behalf of their citizens, fund-raising by hospital guilds, a variety of business enterprises and, lastly, fees from patients.[6] The published plans for the Lancaster General Hospital in Pennsylvania show the emphasis on maximizing accommodation for private patients. Private rooms accounted for fifty-seven percent of the total area allocated to patients and, indeed, patients' fees contributed a significant proportion, 35.7 percent, of the total income of $16,978 for the year 1905–1906.[7] These fees, together with a substantial grant from the government of Pennsylvania, constituted 84 percent of revenues. A great deal of work was required to raise the remaining 16 percent: benefactors had to be courted, rummage sales organized, and morning teas prepared. In addition to cash, the hospital received many donations in kind. For example, the 1906 list of gifts included "ice cream for the whole house" from Mrs. E.M. Cohn, seven dozen eggs from Mrs. John Eby, nine "garage cans" from the business of Shreiner & Stauffer and "83 jars of fruit, 8 cans of vegetables, groceries, 14 glasses of jelly, [and] 3 crocks of applebutter" from the energetic volunteer, Miss Alice Rengier.[8] The Lancaster General was part of what Rosenberg terms "the private patient revolution" that occurred in America between 1880 and the First World War. The phenomenon has been well documented.[9] All the studies canvass the strategies adopted by hospital boards to attract middle and upper income patients who could afford to pay for their care. Rosenberg, for example, argues that the increase in provision for private patients was as much driven by supply as it was a response to increased demand. The hospitals needed the money: endowments were no longer sufficient and costs were escalating. It was not simply that hospitals were becoming safer and thereby attracting other than the poor into hospitals. The well-off were courted because hospitals were becoming ever more costly to run: expensive medical technology, lighting and heating, and specialized nursing all cost money. They consumed more and more funds and paying patients were seen as a permanent well to be tapped.[10]

The 1904 survey, referred to above, revealed that it was church-run hospitals in America that recouped the highest percentage (71 percent) of their costs of operation from patients and, not surprisingly, government-run hospitals recouped the least (7 percent). Secular charities, on the other hand, relied on patient fees for 45 percent of their costs.[11]

Paying patients in a voluntary hospital were, in the main, *private* patients admitted and attended to by their personal physician. They were accommodated in small wards or single rooms and surrounded by the trappings of home. Often even the very poor who were admitted to charitable hospitals were not treated unless *some* payment was made: their city which, rather than fulfill their responsibility to the poor by setting up public medical services, entered into contracts with religious and charitable hospitals to provide the services—what would be termed *out-sourcing* today. The government purchase of care for the indigent effectively reduced the amount of charitable care actually provided in terms of free beds in charitable hospitals. As the proportion of paying patients grew, the principle of paying for care became accepted, so that, by 1900, a British hospital expert could describe America as the "home of the pay system."[12]

In 1910 a municipal hospital, the Auburn City Hospital in the State of New York, had a similar range of income sources as the Lancaster General but, in addition to the payment by the city authorities for city folk, a number of nearby towns and the county paid the hospital expenses for the townspeople of Seneca, Mentz, Ledyard, Brutus, and the County of Cayuga. They also had financial arrangements with five large employers to provide hospital care for their employees. In addition to charging private patients, this hospital board demonstrated its entrepreneurship by charging all patients additional fees for such extra services as the use of the X-Ray machine, the operating theatre, and the ambulance. The normal fees covered only *normal* nursing but special nursing could be had for a further charge. No amount was too small to be collected: $2.25 from the "sale of fats" and $3.15 from selling "old boiler pipes" in 1910.[13]

PHILANTHROPY AND ENTREPRENEURSHIP

One of the most popular avenues for generating a steady flow of funds was for hospital boards to encourage people to endow a bed, either by depositing an amount of money that would provide sufficient interest annually to cover the cost of a bed for the year, or by agreeing to make an annual contribution.[14] The Babies Ward Post-Graduate Hospital in New York City was skilled at this method of fund-raising. It charged no fees yet, in 1917, had thirty-five endowed beds, which at approximately $200 per bed per annum raised $7,900—or a little over half the hospital running costs for the year. The other half was made up from a much larger number of individual small donations and annual subscriptions and, in addition, there were many individual gifts in kind acknowledged in the annual report.[15]

In America, it was only from the relatively small number of patients who were actually admitted to a hospital that a fee was extracted. Others who required medical attention relied on outpatient departments and dispensaries, which, in the main provided gratuitous diagnosis, prescription, supply of medicines, and minor medical procedures. This latter group represented the majority of Americans. For example, of the total of 915,971 people who received free medical treatment in New York City in 1895 a mere 8.5 percent were treated in hospital as opposed to a dispensary. The situation had only changed marginally by 1913 when some 13 percent of those who were sick were treated in hospital.[16] It was this model of medical care which the medical missionaries took with them to China where the establishment of a dispensary almost always preceded the hospital and the dispensary continued to deal with the vast majority of patients once the hospital was established.[17] But the path taken by missionary societies to fund their medical work and hospitals diverged from the American model and the considerations which led to them adopting an alternative strategy is the subject of the next chapter.

Chapter Six
Who Should Pay?

> It needs no argument to show that practising for money, or fixing a price for services rendered, must of necessity present to the Chinese mercenary and selfish motives, thus taking away from the healing of the sick that which gives the missionary physician his power as a co-worker in Christian missions.
>
> —John G. Kerr 1895

Despite his best efforts, John Kerr failed to convince the majority of his missionary brethren of the dangers inherent in charging Chinese patients for medical services.

Not only did missionaries take the models of proprietary and voluntary hospitals to China, they also took a belief in philanthropy, entrepreneurship and *user pays* which characterized both the profit-making and charitable institutions in America. Avenues for fundraising or business in China, though, especially in the early days, were more limited. Unlike the seventeenth-century Jesuit missionaries to China, who favored a top-down approach and who had sought to influence imperial officials and the gentry, Protestant missionaries at the turn of the twentieth century concentrated their efforts on the lower, poorer classes.[1] Thus, in the beginning, as far as donations were concerned the hospitals had to rely on their friends and supporters at home. Support from Chinese city and provincial authorities was limited, as were fees from private patients.

In the initial phase of any medical mission, almost all patients were treated gratuitously regardless of their status or their ability to pay. Firstly, medical treatment was seen as the most potent tool in their Christianizing armament: in order to gain access to potential converts nothing should be allowed to stand in the way. The *New York Medical Journal* and the *Lancet* had criticized the fact that medical and hospital work in China were always accompanied by religious proselytizing, but, as the editor of the *CMMJ* explained to his readers, they did not understand the missions' purposes in being in China: "The prime object for which we are in China is to propagate the Christian religion and make it a power in the hearts and lives of these people ... much as we believe in the medical work for itself very few of us would be willing to endure the isolation and the expatriation for it alone."[2]

In addition, the missionaries wanted to impress upon the Chinese the unselfish and charitable nature of Christianity and believed that charging fees could damage their reputation in this regard. A pioneer medical missionary, John G. Kerr, expressed it thus in 1895: "In view of the fact that the work of the medical missionary is the evidence to the heathen of the exalted character of Christianity—the proof that it is a religion of love and mercy, and so differs from all other so-called religions—it is necessary that we should avoid everything which could in the least vitiate that evidence or weaken its force."[3]

Unlike the Auburn City hospital, discussed earlier, medical missionaries in China did not have access to funds from city authorities nor from large employers. They had to rely almost exclusively on funds sent from home, either through the various mission societies or from individuals and organizations, often from the hometown of the missionary. Raising these funds at a distance was a constant battle and required an enormous amount of effort on the part of the individual missionaries. For instance, whenever missionaries returned home on furlough they spent a significant proportion of their time visiting people, showing pictures, or speaking to groups to solicit funds. One of the most important functions of the annual reports issued by most hospitals was to keep in touch with benefactors so that they would continue to support the hospital with annual contributions, endowments, or non-monetary gifts. At home, often the most energetic fund-raisers were groups of women who organized themselves into guilds and committees that fulfilled a social role while providing a stream of hospital funds. Such (foreign) women were scarce in a Chinese town and those among them who could organize fundraising functions were already busy enough. It was only in the older established treaty ports that sufficient men of means could be found among the foreign merchant and banking contingent able to emulate the level of philanthropy commonly found in an American city. In these circumstances, and despite the misgivings of some, many missionaries concluded that the only solution was to collect money from patients. Where the practice differed from that in America was that the patients they targeted were not the private inpatients but *all* patients, including those who attended as outpatients at dispensaries.

The impetus for moving to a system of fee paying in China was not so much the increase in hospital costs (as it had been in America) as the paucity of alternative sources. If this phase in American hospital development can be characterized as the search for the paying patient, or at least someone to pay for the patient, then in China it was the era of finding out how to get most patients to pay. The most significant result of this difference in emphasis was that dispensary visits, made by the most *ordinary* of Chinese patients, were included in the range of services to which a fee might attach while in America dispensary services continued to be provided free of charge.

FEES—THE DEBATE

To introduce a system of fee-paying for a medical service, when the primary motives were to demonstrate "Christian charity" and to allay hostilities, was, however, controversial.[4] The debate, carried on within the letter and editorial pages of the *CMMJ*, at various regional conferences, and in the annual reports of individual hospitals, was multifaceted and nuanced. Any battle lines that were drawn were permeable and differences were mainly of emphasis and rationale.[5]

One of the earliest sallies into the debate was made by Elizabeth Reifsnyder, who ran Shanghai's Margaret Williamson Hospital for Chinese Women and Children for the Women's Union Missionary Society (WUMS)[6] In a paper read before the Medical Missionary Association of Shanghai, in April 1887, she canvassed the majority of issues that would emerge in the coming debate. She proposed charging fees for ordinary, as opposed to private, patients because, "in China it is not just the poor who come for treatment, as it is at home." She agreed that patients who were too poor should continue to receive free treatment and, at her hospital, she kept a "special stamp for charity patients." In her opinion, most "prefer to pay . . . no doubt the idea prevails that what is given for nothing is worth nothing." On the most practical level, she thought that charging ordinary patients for medicine containers encouraged them to actually take the medicine as directed and bring the containers back with them when they returned the next time. She advocated charging the rich the full cost of medicines. She mused that some dispensaries had "free days" for the poor but she thought it impractical, especially in the countryside where many had to travel long distances and would find it difficult to "keep track of the time." It could perhaps work in the cities but she worried that those who were not poor might take advantage of free days.[7] Reifsnyder's concerns would echo over the next twenty years as the debate about fees played itself out.[8] The notion that providing treatment without charge would lead to "pauperisation" or abuse of the system was as commonly held in China as it was in America.[9]

Although some participants in the debate opposed charging fees, few argued that they should not accept money or gifts from Chinese patients. One though, Horace A. Randle, did advise strongly against accepting gifts in kind, such as "chickens and ducks, eggs and confectionery," in place of money. He also recommended that doctors make it plain that they preferred cash to "scrolls and inscriptions [which] generally do satisfy the native givers more than the foreign recipients."[10] However, most seemed quite happy to accept gifts and boasted proudly to their home missions about the scrolls and letters of praise received from patients. Even one of the most vigorous opponents of patient fees, John G. Kerr, was sometimes ambiguous on this score and agreed that those who benefited should support the medical work financially, but any aid should be voluntary not enforced. In his opinion, based on experience, there was a "wide range for the exercise of judgment and tact in the methods which can be used to secure aid to medical work."[11]

Although no one argued for a shift to the American proprietary-style hospital catering largely for private patients, there was common agreement that private patients could be taken in, and provided for separate from the common herd, for a fee. Similarly, visits made to the homes of the rich should attract a fee. At the other end of the scale, all agreed that the extremely poor or destitute should be treated free of charge. The main issue of contention centered on the routine charging of the *ordinary* patient, either a dispensary outpatient or a hospital inpatient. In this respect the experience in China varied quite significantly from that in contemporary America. Although America could be referred to as the home of the paying patient, it was private patients who paid—not the common man, his wife or child. The debate in China was more wide-ranging: it concerned all patients, regardless of class, and the whole range of services, from dispensary visits, hospitals stays, particular medical procedures, and the provision of food and medicines.

CHINESE PERCEPTIONS

The main point of difference between those who supported and those who opposed charging ordinary, as against private, patients focused on the issue of the presumed perceptions of the Chinese. If the missionaries charged fees, would the Chinese see them as commercial, grasping, greedy, or worse, uncharitable, and, if so, would it detract from their evangelical purpose? One of the earliest to take up the cudgel against fees, A. W. Douthwaite of the China Inland Mission (CIM),[12] argued in 1894 that "any charge degrades the mission from charitable institution to being seen as the meanest trading with the aim of making money while professing to do good."[13] Sydney R. Hodge, who had entered the argument in 1891 as a representative of the British churches, agreed. He reasoned that the free treatment distributed to the poor and needy in the "large and wealthy cities of Europe and America" should be the least offered in "heathen lands where the hospital is professedly the practical expression of the Gospel."[14]

If, on the other hand, they did not charge fees would they be seen as fools, a 'soft touch' or to have an ulterior motive apart from the religious one? Omar Kilborn was one of those who contended that charging for their services would increase respect for missionaries and lead to a more "enlightened understanding of the position of the foreign doctor."[15] He was concerned that not to charge might create the impression that the foreigners had ample funds and, possibly "under foreign imperial pay for some mysterious and therefore sinister purpose." If such an impression was created, rather than generating gratitude for missionaries' efforts in the recipient it could give rise to the opposite response: the patients might then become less tractable and more demanding. Rather than *ask* for favors, they might be "apt rather to demand their rights in the shape of free board and lodging and free treatment. They may become very independent in their demeanour, and under the circumstances see no particular cause for gratitude."[16]

In 1897, the editor of the *CMMJ* invited discussion on the theory and practice of gratuitous treatment for patients in China. He outlined the main arguments put forward in "medical journals of America and Great Britain" relating to either the "the abuse of medical charity" by people who were able to pay or the "degradation" suffered by them if they were not allowed to. He reported the newly elected President of the Board of Charities of New York City, Dr Steven Smith, as saying "that hereafter not one person who is able to pay for medical aid will receive free treatment at any of the city institutions."[17] As these institutions were not permitted to charge any fees at all, this decision meant that any patient able to pay would not be eligible to receive treatment from the city and would have to seek out and pay a private physician. Horace Randle, who again stood out from the crowd, was the only one among the participants in the debate to argue against the very notion of using medicine in the cause of religious conversion. An enthusiastic champion of charging fees, he was asked to give a paper, "How to Encourage the Chinese to Subscribe Toward the Support of Medical Missionary Work Among Them," at a conference in Shandong in 1898. If he had had his way, he would have chosen a word other than encourage: to his mind, such subtleties would fail without external pressure. He advised that missionaries should simply charge everyone, except the "absolutely poor and helpless," for all medicines and all operations. He had stopped giving free medicine himself, seeing his "kindness [as having been] trodden on." He could have tolerated that—"had the salvation of souls followed—but that has failed." Rather than simply preaching, he thought that by giving the Chinese "secular and temporal advantages ... we have baited him instead, with almost every imaginable inducement to accept the Gospel" and the Chinese were like the fish that takes the bait but still gets away. He attempted to clinch his argument for fees with a novel rationalization. He contrasted the situation in China with that at home. There, he argued, medicine was "both rightly and advisedly" given free because of the benefit afforded the medical profession who owed much to charity patients by way of "abundant opportunities to study the course of disease, and the effects of medicine or other treatment." These advantages were not similarly available in China because the "Chinaman comes for his own benefit ... he can't be trusted to give the whole truth or his full history. He will eat what he likes, leave when he likes and not do as he is told."[18]

MORAL SUASION

By far the most popular argument made by the proponents of fees was couched in terms of the 'moral' effect on the Chinese. As in America, the proponents of fees argued that providing free treatment *pauperized,* or destroyed the self-respect, of patients. Some described it as positively evil in its effect. Roderick MacDonald, of the Wesleyan Missionary Hospital[19] at Foshan 佛山 (Fujian), expressed a commonly held belief: "Indiscriminate charity—as everybody knows—is injurious and unjustifiable; nor does the excellence of the motive which prompts it abate anything from the evil consequences."[20] George Stuart, of the Wuhu 芜湖 General Hospital (Anhui) which was operated under the auspices of the MEM, identified the pauperizing effect of free dispensing as causing the more well-to-do members of the community to avoid his mission. He also thought that it could lead to a lack of respect for the scientific medicine the missionaries were promoting in competition with Chinese medical beliefs. He had "noticed that there has been no increase in the patronage of the wealthy and official classes, nor indeed of the ordinary, well-to-do merchant class [and felt it was] in a large measure, due to the pauperizing method of free dispensing." In his opinion, "free dispensing is as unjustifiable in China as it is in America or England.

And further, it is suicidal to Western medicine, whether practised by foreigners or natives."[21]

The missionaries eventually convinced themselves that they were doing their Chinese patients a favor by charging them a fee. Paying a fee would improve the patients' self-respect: "he is not tempted to fawn upon us, or be hypercritical in his gratitude"[22] and, as Whitney added, it would teach the Chinese "the value of favors and their obligation in connection with the reception of them." They could not teach that lesson "by promiscuous charity to the heathen . . . their character is not bettered one iota thereby, nor have they learned from us a single higher motive to moral action."[23] Further, the Chinese were to be taught the real meaning and value of charity—"True charity lovingly supplies these needs which are beyond a man's ability to supply for himself . . . help to the very poor always secures commendation from all classes, but help to those who do not need it only leaves a doubt in the popular mind, either to our object, or as to our judgment."[24]

Here, George Stuart was making a distinction between the person who only requires the assistance of someone who has a specialized (for example medical) skill, and another, who has the same medical need but has an additional financial need. *True* charity was providing a service, rather than a *free* service, according to Stuart. In using this term, he reflected a view of charity described by Rosemary Stevens as being peculiarly American. The concept, which was developed by the, often Protestant, charitable organization movement that arose in the wake of the Civil War, was referred to as *scientific charity.* Stevens describes the prevailing scientific charitable ethos of America at the turn of the century as including "self-help rather than handouts."[25] In particular, the essence of an act of charity was "giving per se rather than giving to a particular population. An organization that provided useful services, for a fee, to self-reliant individuals could still be recognized as a public charity."[26]

Aside from these general moral arguments, there does not appear to have been any disagreement among medical missionaries about using fees to reinforce other, more specific, moral values. Those who detailed the range of fees they charged obviously expected no argument with the proposition that certain people could be charged, and some quite heavily. Patients were divided into *deserving* and *non-deserving* based on their ailment rather than their ability to pay. For example, according to Kilborn, "rich patients with venereal diseases should be made to pay well for services rendered." Even the poor with venereal disease should "be made to pay something, more than the twenty *cash,* even if it is only 100 *cash* a month."[27] Kilborn's rationalization for making this distinction between patients was unambiguous: not only would they be taught a lesson but also it was easy money for the mission, "the fact of having to pay something will emphasize the doctor's timely warning to avoid such evils in the future. And furthermore it is usually easy to get them to pay, because we are often able to obtain satisfactory results by the appropriate treatment in such cases."[28] A minority argued against overcharging this class of patient. For instance, Jefferys from St Luke's at Shanghai, could "not clearly see the ethics of the physician's quasi attempt at punishing the sins of his patient . . . the natural punishment fully and meetly fits the crime."[29]

Another category of patient who, it was commonly believed, should pay were those with an addiction to opium.[30] Again it was Kilborn who spelt out the case most clearly: "From one class of in-patients I believe it right to demand and receive in every case a fixed fee which shall be large enough to cover cost of food and leave a margin for medicine. I refer to those who come to break off the opium habit. My charge has been 2,000 cash, to be paid in advance, no portion of which shall under any circumstances be returned to the patient."[31]

By contrast, in America, rather than use fees to teach them a lesson, hospital boards tended to adopt policies which refused admission to people suffering from contagious, including venereal, diseases. The Lancaster hospital was one with such an admission policy and the 1906 report contained no mention of venereal cases.[32] In China it was more difficult for mission hospitals to adopt such exclusion policies. Firstly, there was a lack of alternative facilities to which such patients could be referred. Secondly, the primary aim being evangelical meant that no potential convert should be turned away. Lastly, they saw their missionary role as including acting as the moral guardians of their Chinese patients.

MANAGING SUPPLY AND DEMAND

The most pragmatic of the combatants argued for the use of fees to control demand; either in general or for special privileges and consideration. They had also discovered that fees could influence the class of patient who sought treatment. James McCartney at Chongqing found that charging a fee for dispensary visits resulted in a reduction in demand but that it served him well: having fewer patients, he was not so stressed and overworked. As he put it, "having 80–100 patients waiting cause[d] him to behave in any thing but a Christian way."[33]

A universally adopted dispensary procedure was for patients to be seen on a first come first served basis. The demand from those who wanted preferential treatment, such as being seen out of hours or out of turn, could be manipulated by varying the fee. The level of fees charged could also influence demand for home visits. For example, Philip B. Cousland reported that although he had found taking fees "repugnant," his newly instituted fee for all home visits according to the distance ($1 per 3 miles) and for chair hire, regardless of the class of patient, had lessened demand and also had an effect on the class of people who sought treatment. It had proved much better than the old plan of no fee: the number of visits was fewer but the "class of case better." Further, an added moral victory was possible: if a patient was very poor, he could create a "great impression" by returning all or part of the fee.[34] McCartney also reported that, in his experience, once a patient paid a fee he was more likely to return for follow up treatment. This not only increased the chance of a cure but also his opportunity to influence him religiously.[35]

Most missionaries thought that they could achieve the best evangelistic results with patients admitted to hospital and this belief influenced the setting of inpatient fees. Luella Masters, of the MEM at Fuzhou, charged the same five-cent fee for each visit to the dispensary as she did for entry to the hospital wards. Her aim was to encourage women and children to enter hospital where they would get the "attention of the physician; also to teach the doctrine."[36] Others made no charge for a hospital stay, other than for food in some cases, with the same proselytizing purpose in mind.

APPEALING TO CHINESE CUSTOM

Many participants in the debate cited Chinese custom in support of their argument. As has been discussed earlier in chapter 2, there were Chinese charitable medical organizations in existence when the missionaries arrived and some would have been familiar with Chinese practices in relation to charging for services. Sick Chinese in the late Qing had a range of options, the majority relying on "itinerant drug peddlers, mediums, . . . members of religious orders . . . and female practitioners."[37] Wealthy Chinese could engage a series of male physicians to treat them at home for a fee and the poor could visit the free dispensary and, after being examined by a doctor, receive either medicine or a prescription. According to Leung, these dispensaries and clinics shared many characteristics: "they were urban-based institutions where a certain number of doctors served in rotation, and they were financed and supervised by members of the local elite." She cites the regulations of one such institution, at Yangzhou 扬州 (Jiangsu), which paid: "Confucian doctors to take turns treating patients; local pharmacists also prepared and distributed medicines. It was open to outpatients every morning, and those who were seriously ill and without families were accommodated in a sick ward at the rear of the building."[38]

This sounds remarkably like the situation that pertained in most of the medical missionary outfits, which started life as simple dispensaries. It is thus hardly surprising that to Chinese patients, although they may have found the medicine strange, the organization and principle would have been familiar. What becomes clear from a survey of the contemporary record of missionaries is that those who argued against fees cited Chinese benevolent institutions as their model whereas those who argued in favor reinforced their case by looking to the example of the Chinese physician.

After the *pauperizing* argument, the most commonly stated case *for* fees was that the Chinese were accustomed to paying their own doctors. Henry Whitney pointed out that the Chinese "have to pay a reasonable fee to a native doctor" and argued that it would be "an injustice to [those doctors] for foreigners to do such an extensive gratuitous work." He had observed that some "trouble and disaffection [had] arisen, in various parts of China, among native doctors."[39] Luella Masters spelt out her understanding, after ten years experience in China, of the Chinese attitude towards paying for medical treatment: "we have noticed, even in China if a member of a family meets with a serious accident or prolonged illness, that the patient's friends send for the doctor who charges for his services—the physician who charges the highest fee as a rule-and if the case gets well, the physician gets the credit; if he dies, they console themselves with the thought, 'We did all for him that money could do; the best talent was procured that money could procure.'"[40]

Charles Wenyon, with the Wesleyan Missionary Hospital at Foshan 佛山, was another who took his lead from the Chinese payment system. He reported that self-support had been achieved in 1890[41] and described how it had been accomplished: "gratuitous treatment" was provided at the dispensary between six and nine o'clock each morning and thereafter "we receive patients precisely as Chinese doctors do." That meant that a fee—five dollars—was charged for visits to private homes but nothing for "ordinary consultations" at the hospital, for which the doctor merely received "Lai shi (polite offering) which consists of a neat red paper packet containing a few cents worth of cash." Where Wenyon differed significantly from other medical missionaries, and his contemporaries at home, was his early employment of another Chinese custom: "cures by contract" or "Pau I" 包医. He reported that when the missionaries were first asked if they were willing to "Pau I" they felt their professionalism was being compromised and had refused, but had lost patients. According to Wenyon, "the people of Fatshan [Foshan] think it just as natural to get a doctor to contract for a cure of a disease, as it is to get a builder to contract for the repair of their home . . . experience has led us to lay aside our scruples, and to conform to the native custom." He saw several advantages in this system. The patient knew the total cost before commencing treatment—the contract fee was set with regard to the disease and the patient's means—and if the cure was not effected the fee was refunded to either the patient or, if he died, his friends. As well, it matched Chinese customary practice.[42]

McCartney was another to advocate what he called the "Chinese method of contracting the case" if he was called into the city to see a patient "of means." As he reported in 1899: "If the patient is sure to get well, we contract to cure; but if not, we simply contract. If they will not contract we never give any medicine, because in such cases one dose will rarely do any good, and as is the Chinese custom they would call someone else as soon as our backs were turned. If patients are too poor to pay, we make no charge. The custom of contracting the case I believe to be a good one, as in most instances they never call until all Chinese means fail, and in very many instances we are unable to do anything for the patients. If we know we can cure, our reputation is safe, and if we do not, we lose nothing and gain considerable (sic), financially. We generally ask one-half down, and the rest when cured."[43]

Others stressed their understanding of the attitude of the gentry to charity. They said that the gentry preferred to pay, implying that not to expect payment would offend them. For example, McCartney claimed he had found that the "better class *prefer* to pay" and would pay up to five times the ordinary fee if they could be seen out of normal dispensary hours.[44] In America the emphasis seems to have been on providing the facilities for which the rich would pay rather than any concern for their preference for paying. An American-trained Chinese woman doctor, Kang Cheng (Ida Kahn) 康爱德, who ran the Elizabeth Skelton Danforth Memorial Hospital for Women at Jiujiang 九江 in Jiangxi under the auspices of the Methodist Central China Mission with her compatriot, Shi Meiyu 石美玉 (Mary Stone), agreed: "the rich will appreciate more highly the services received" if they paid for them. To support her argument she cited a case where she had seen and prescribed for a sick child without the normal charge. The child's parents administered the medicine "erratically" and subsequently called in a succession of native physicians. She heard later that, in the mother's words, she had "found a fine physician and that the one-thousand-cash doctor was really worth having." Kahn pondered that had she charged her normal—five *tael*—fee the medicine she prescribed might have been given "a fair trial."[45]

Sydney Hodge exemplified those who drew on the Chinese benevolent institutions for guidance to argue against charging fees. Whilst agreeing that there was some validity in the argument in favor of fees, he invoked the example of Chinese philanthropy and pointed out that "in China, where the native gentry support free dispensaries and benevolent halls, it is difficult for us to do differently without suffering by comparison."[46] Another to put forward a similar argument was at pains to distinguish the missionary from the physician in private practice. B. C. Atterbury of the APM, claimed that Chinese benevolent institutions did not charge and that "charging fees for the treatment of the sick when the object is a religious or charitable one is contrary to native ideas as to how such work should be conducted." He thought that charging fees would "occasion remark and suspicion of mixed motives if one whose avowed purpose is to do good puts himself on the same plane with an ordinary practitioner."[47]

Using Chinese custom as the basis for an argument was not always well received; not all agreed that the Chinese had anything they could offer the foreigner by way of example. Whitney, for instance, dismissed Atterbury's case on the basis that "native ideas are no criterion . . . for their ideas are all wrong in this matter" and that any attempt to allay the suspicions "of the heathen" was futile. Neither did he accept the comparison of the medical mission with "native benevolent work [which] would be a disgrace to Christianity." Both Atterbury, who admitted at the beginning of his paper that he "dislike[d] to say anything against the plan [to charge fees]" and put the opposing view "partly for the sake of the discussion," and Hodge were in the minority and were to, eventually, lose the battle.

Mary W. Niles, one of the early women missionary doctors, worked with Kerr and taught obstetrics at Canton.[48] In 1890, she wrote an account of seven years' experience of observing "native midwifery." Of interest in this section is her description of the Chinese practice concerning fees for delivering babies: "The fee for the common classes is $1.00 for a girl and $2.00 for a boy; to the poorest class 50 cents for a girl and $1.00 for a boy."[49] In addition to the Chinese method of contracting for medical care described above, Roderick MacDonald accepted different fees in accord with this particular Chinese custom. He reported that in obstetrical cases he charged $25 for delivering the mother and "if a living female child were born, $5 extra would no doubt willingly be given, but if a son, $10 of course."[50] Atterbury demonstrated that, although he cited Chinese custom to bolster his argument against fees, he did not accept all Chinese custom uncritically.

He commented on a report of a doctor who had agreed with the relatives of a woman in labor that an amount would be added to the fee if a girl was born and a sum of twice that if a boy: "this estimation of one sex being half that of the other may be correct according to Chinese ideas, but if our friend should fall into the hands of some strong-minded women at home, his frankness would cost him a considerable portion of his crop of hair."[51]

The majority of mission hospitals did not charge men and women differently but it was not unknown. Ida Kahn related, "[m]en promise us any amount of money we might see fit to charge if we would only treat them" at their hospital for women and children at Jiujiang. In her view, a part explanation for the relatively low level of fee income at her own hospital, for women and children, was because "the physician who treats both men and women stands a far better chance of accomplishing self-support since the men hold the purse strings, and their own diseases influence the grasp more immediately."[52] George Huntley, of the ABFMS, offered no explanation for charging men forty cash and women twenty to register at his dispensary at Hanyang and, although Hodge had made the case against charging fees in 1891, he reported charging similarly: fifty cash for men and ten for women in 1902.[53]

Chapter Seven
Who Did Pay?

The Chungking Men's Hospital founded by James McCartney of the Methodist Episcopal Church in 1892, serves as an instructive case study of the changing balance, over time, in the source of funds for the operation of an American hospital in China. The reason for this choice is not only prosaic—annual reports are extant for ten of the twenty years (including financial details for nine) from the second report in 1893 through to 1912—but McCartney also proved himself a leader in striving for financial self-sufficiency and the policies he developed set the pattern for those who came later. Whether or not his experience at Chongqing was representative of hospitals in different parts of the country run by different religious denominations will become clear when his record is compared with survey data collected by the CMMA between 1903 and 1910.

McCartney, who had arrived at Chongqing in 1891, started dispensing medicine from rented Chinese premises sometime before establishing the first foreign hospital work in that city in 1892.[1] He described Chongqing in his 1912 report as being of some 400,000 people, located on a rocky promontory, linked by one of the "main rock-paved roads" to the capital of the province, Chengdu 成都 and, thus, "a key to the inner province." He drew his patients from the city and surrounding countryside of "fertile valleys and coal-filled sandstone-hills."[2] In the beginning he provided all medical services gratuitously but within eight years he was able to announce that the hospital had succeeded in achieving the goal of complete self-sufficiency with "the principal support [to come] from the natives themselves" that he had set himself in 1893.[3] He had started in 1891 with $1,000 per annum from the Missionary Society but, "not one cent" in 1899.[4]

EARLY DAYS AT CHUNKING—
FREE TREATMENT BUT STILL THE INCOME FLOWED

In McCartney's first year no fee was asked of people who attended his out-patient clinic but he started his second year with a trial charge of twenty *cash* for the first visit. Because many of his previous patients elected to attend free dispensaries operated by others in the city, the experiment only lasted three months. Since his was the first foreign hospital established in Chongqing we can assume that he was referring to Chinese-run dispensaries which, as we have seen, were common in most large cities in China at the time. However, he did collect *some* money from his patients from the very beginning. He always charged fees for home visits and gave as examples of the type of case (with charges) he could be called out to attend: "500 *cash* for labor, and [for] opium suicides, 1000 *cash* and chair money."[5] In addition, most patients admitted to the hospital covered the cost of their board—two thousand *cash* a month in the public wards and three thousand in private rooms—but not medical treatment. Some inpatients who could not afford to pay for food were accepted but McCartney had adopted the policy of restricting the number of such charity patients to the extent of any excess of receipts over expenditure. In effect, any charity patients were supported by other patients and not by funds from external sources. In 1893 he reported that the total collected from patients' board, sale of medicine, and visits to homes had netted 614.30 *Chongqing taels*.[6] This was spent on "rice, vegetables, meat, and repairs on the hospital" leaving an amount of 124.94 *taels* to be added to endowments, the interest on which provided "support of poor patients who cannot pay their board."[7]

To supplement revenue from patients McCartney supported the hospital substantially by his own efforts. In 1899, he took on the salaried duties of Medical Officer at Chongqing for the Imperial Maritime Customs Office.[8] This provided valuable support for the hospital and its several dispensaries for the following seven years.

CHARGING OUTPATIENTS

Outpatients, who always far outnumbered patients admitted to hospital, were an obvious funding source to be tapped. A small charge fixed on a very large, and growing, number of people could raise a substantial amount. For example, McCartney saw a total of 33,435 patients in his dispensary during 1899, 10,775 of whom were new patients. These outpatients accounted for ninety-seven percent of his patients that year and their number dwarfed the 962 patients admitted into hospital.*

The aborted 1893 trial notwithstanding, McCartney successfully introduced fees for outpatients in 1898—twenty *cash* for the first visit. Although by then there were two foreign free dispensaries in Chongqing, McCartney said he "found no difficulty getting patients." Nevertheless, the numbers of patients did fall by about fifty percent from the 1897 figure. This was partly attributable to the fees but another factor in the fall-off in attendance was the "disturbed condition of the country." He acknowledged that riots, which had been continuous between March 1898 and the beginning of 1899 in the eastern part of Sichuan Province, had arisen in response to his own Mission's persistent efforts to open a branch dispensary and street chapel in the nearby town of Jiangbei 江北. One rented building had been burned down on instructions from the local gentry; another (sublet to them by a Chinese resident) had been sacked, and one of McCartney's Chinese medical students had been murdered. The mission, after receiving compensation for the damage, eventually succeeded in opening a dispensary eight months later in a large compound handed over to them by city officials.

Despite the initial loss of customers, McCartney discovered that charging dispensary fees provided more than money, it gave him "the satisfaction of knowing that those who applied for treatment really had something the matter with them." Return visits trebled. Previously, when no fee was charged, the majority never returned. He was particularly pleased with a new fee—one hundred *cash*—introduced for out-of-hours consultation that had worked "splendidly [and brought in] nearly as much as the dispensary."

McCartney was one of the few doctors who, once they had established a reasonably sized hospital, still managed to find time for itinerating (traveling into the countryside to see patients) and disseminating religious literature. The dispensing fees he charged these patients did not contribute to the hospital's upkeep but covered his expenses. He reported a successful trip, taken during 1899, when he raised 13,000 *cash* in just three or four days by charging twenty *cash* per patient. He collected additional funds from the sale of religious books.[9]

McCartney's financial reporting was not consistent throughout the period under review until 1908 (when a more-or-less standard format was adopted) which makes a longitudinal analysis of dispensary fee income difficult. Because I have been unable to isolate those funds derived solely from

*see charts at www.michellerenshaw.com

outpatients I have, instead, collated all fees identified as being from Chinese patients, excluding payments for board.

These included, variously, fees for visits to patients in their homes (from the beginning in 1893), dispensary visits (from 1899 onward), funds character-ized in two of the reports as being for "medical" and "dental" treatment, and receipts from the sale of medicines (identified separately in two of the reports). The picture emerges of erratic and relatively low levels of income in the early years, gradually rising until 1908 when income stabilizes at just over $2,000 Mex. per annum before rising substantially again in 1912 to over $3,000 Mex.[10] When payments for board are included, the income from Chinese pa-tients exceeded $5,000 per annum from 1912 onward. (see Figure 2)

In the dispensary McCartney continued to treat the very poor without charge but now they had to wait until everyone else had been dealt with. Along with the new practice of charging patients heavily if they wanted to be seen out-of-turn or out-of-hours, McCartney abandoned any pretence of equality of access.

PRIVATE PATIENTS' FEES

Whilst, like their counterparts in America, most foreigners in China and wealthy Chinese preferred to be treated at home, McCartney's hospital

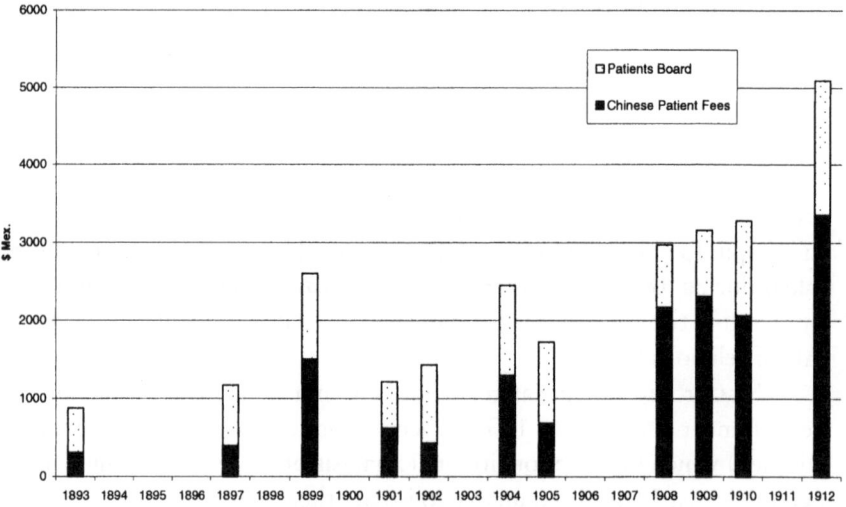

Figure 2. Total Income from Chinese Patients, Chungking Hospital, 1893–1912.

Source: Extracted from financial data included in Annual Reports, Chungking Hospital, 1893–1912

provided a minimum of private accommodation. But, instead of relying on this small number of private patients to support the hospital, he charged the ordinary patient in the ward for his board. When appealing for donations of the $15.00 per year he estimated to be the annual cost of financing a free bed, McCartney pointed out to potential supporters that, according to the report of a large hospital in America where beds cost $500 per year to support, "nine-tenths of the inpatients during the year received free treatment." This was "by far a larger proportion than our mission hospital can do in a heathen land. We daily turn away many needing hospital treatment who are too poor, and we have not the means to supply their food."[11]

Thus, philosophically, he saw his hospital and his role as being more properly comparable to a public hospital catering for the poor in America, than to the more prolific proprietary or voluntary hospitals with their emphasis on private patients. Had his hospital been in America, however, it would have certainly been classified as a religious voluntary hospital on the basis that it was run under the auspices of a religious organization, it was funded substantially from donations and subscriptions, and it charged patients fees.

COMMERCIAL ACTIVITIES

1899 was a busy and significant year for the hospital. As well as fully implementing the dispensary fee policy, McCartney ventured into commerce; first targeting the foreign resident population of Chongqing but also competing with Chinese drug merchants. He entered into an arrangement with a British firm in Bristol (Ferris and Co.) from whom he could buy drugs at wholesale prices at ten to fifteen percent discount to the English prices. He then opened, what he called, a "foreign drug store" to "supply drugs and druggists' sundries to foreigners in West China." (see Plate 19) As well, it gave "the natives the chance to get pure drugs at a moderate price [because] the prices charged by natives selling foreign drugs are exorbitant."[12] All profits were to be available for running the hospital but he appears to have applied them to building up inventory until 1905 when stock was purported to be valued at more than $17,000 Mex. From 1908, the store became a regular, reliable, and increasing source of funds; turning over in excess of 8,000 *taels* ($11,400 Mex.) in 1902[13] and $33,400 Mex. in 1912 and contributing some $1,385[14] and $3,960[15] respectively to hospital running costs. He steadily diversified the stock to include such items as soap, of which they sold "300 cases" in 1901. McCartney noted wryly that it had not yet made "any appreciable difference in the general appearance" of the potential 65,000,000 people in China but he lived in hope that the "300 may soon increase to 3000."[16] The hospital would arrange for postcards to be sent to "people at home for $1.00"[17] and when an aerated water plant was installed in 1905 they sold "several hundred dollars worth of waters."[18] By 1912, McCartney was referring to it as both a drug store and "partial grocery supply depot."[19]

His contemporaries did not necessarily applaud his entry into business. The relationship between the missionary enterprise and commerce was the subject of continuing debate in the pages of missionary journals and English language newspapers.[20] Merchants wrote that those who were critical of missionaries should instead see their presence as encouraging trade. For example, an advantage could be gained from the "curiosity of the Chinese" and the clothing worn and watch or pocket knife carried by

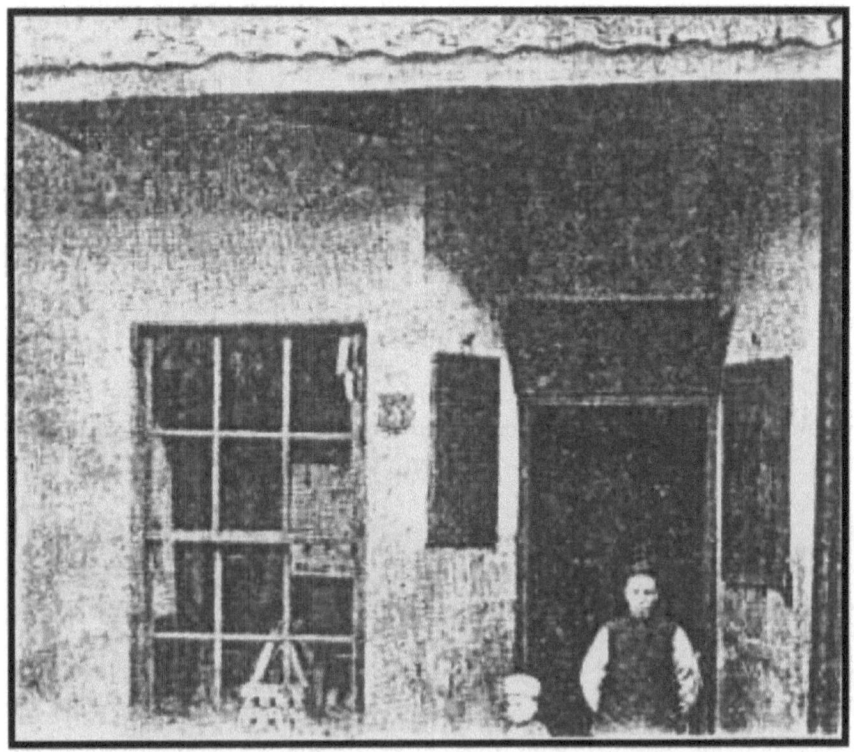

Plate 19. The "American Dispensary" at MEM(S) Chungking Hospital, 1899

Source: James McCartney, *The 12th (1902) Annual Report of Chungking General Hospital of the Methodist Episcopal Church.* (1903): 6.

Courtesy of the Burke Library, Union Theological College, New York

traveling missionaries could "prepare the way for the influx of foreign goods by and by." Similarly, when Chinese visited missionary establishments they would be exposed to foreign goods such as glass for windows (to replace paper or oyster shell), stoves, 'superior' Californian flour and foreign salt that might all find a market in China.[21] Missionary correspondents were at pains to emphasize that they did not "reap any personal profit" but some did acknowledge that their work had become "one of the most effective agents of modern commerce."[22] A supporter of missionary work, Isabella Bird, endorsed comments by "Consuls Carles and Clement Allen" that missionaries "unconsciously help British trade by introducing articles for their own use, which commend themselves to the Chinese."[23] Not all missionary correspondents agreed that this was a good thing and Thomas Gillison represented those who warned that money was a hindrance to spreading the gospel. He spoke of the dangers inherent in charging for medicines and turning the hospital into a business.[24] In McCartney's opinion, the issue was a simple one; the Chinese who patronized his store appreciated the "one price store" where there was no haggling.[25] In addition, he had found that the "middle and better classes" preferred to buy their medicine than get it free, just as they preferred to pay for medical treatment.[26]

Another commercial venture was the optical department, which yielded "good revenue." For example, in 1898 the hospital spent 68 *taels* on spectacles that were sold for 113 *taels*. One more of his enterprises, referred to as "Drawn Work," involved women patients being provided with materials from which they sewed small items for sale—whilst being read Bible stories—with any profit going to the hospital.[27] Henry Fowler's emphasis was not so much on making money or bible reading as providing employment for his long-term patients. He reported that he had set the patients in the "Leper Home" attached to his mission to making "women's silk hairnets and fishing nets which [were] eagerly sought-after" once they had been disinfected.[28]

Charles Ewing, at Tianjin, pursued one commercial avenue that was not explored by McCartney. Ewing explained how it was the argument that it was "Chinese custom" that had persuaded him to adopt the idea of investing in real estate to provide a flow of rents for mission use. "It seems most natural for [the Chinese], when they have any money for the church, instead of using it at once, to invest it, preferably in land for rent, using the proceeds for the church from year to year."[29] Ewing's experience was not a happy one, however, and, he complained about having to spend time going around the countryside collecting rents. He thought the *only* benefit was financial and that it diminished the church to the level of a "financial corporation."

In addition, he had found owning land to be "the most serious obstacle" to the mission work because the "money from rents . . . goes to the local church and puts a damper on their self-support."[30]

APPEAL TO CHINESE PHILANTHROPY

Alongside his other initiatives, McCartney continued the practice of soliciting funds in the form of donations—in money and kind—and subscriptions from his supporters at home and from the Chinese gentry and officials of Chongqing. The proportion of American donations and subscriptions was reasonably consistent and averaged twenty-eight percent of current expenses between 1893 and 1912.[31] McCartney received his most constant support from a number of branches of the Epworth League, a youth organization of the Methodist Episcopal Church founded in Ohio in 1889.[32] Chinese donations, on the other hand, averaged closer to twelve percent of current expenses over the same period. [33] The 1901 list of donations includes sums of 140 *taels* and 100 *taels* from the Governor of Sichuan and the Tao-tai respectively.[34] In 1902 these were joined by the provincial treasurer (50 *taels*), *Foo* (35 *taels*), *Tsentai* (10 *taels*) and *Pahsien* (50 *taels*) and a number of individual members of the gentry. However, in September 1911 when all but three missionaries, of whom McCartney was one, were ordered to leave the province and go to Shanghai following an "anti-dynastic uprising . . . in Chengtu," there were no official donations and a mere $10 Mex. was received from a Chinese individual. The American consular staff ordered the evacuation but McCartney recorded that the "revolution in the Chungking district has been noted for the quietness and lack of bloodshed with which it has taken place." He had expected a large number of wounded but "considering the amount of gunpowder that has been set off we have had very few indeed."[35] Despite all his efforts to encourage donations, the funds he collected from patients (with one minor exception in 1899[36]) always exceeded any he was able to coax out of local officials and the gentry.[37]

McCartney explored every available avenue to secure his hospital's viability and the extent to which he succeeded in these various endeavors is illustrated in the accompanying graph, which shows the changing blend of sources of funds between 1893 and 1912.[38] (see Figure 3) He attributed the fall in donations from America in 1912 to a perceived "fear that the revolution in China would upset things so badly that we would not be able to make use of the money." He described the year as having begun "under a rather shaky form of Republican government" but reassured his readers that "our" government was stable and his work was "prosperous."[39] What is clear from figure 3 is that the funds for the hospital were increasingly locally sourced—particularly from patients.

In McCartney's hospital, where only five percent of rooms were for private patients, the Chinese patients' contribution ranged from 31.6 percent of operating expenses in 1897 to 63.0 percent in 1912, with an average of 43.2 percent for the period.[40] This contrasted with the Lancaster Hospital, with 57 percent of its patient area devoted to private rooms, which sourced only 34.5 percent of its running costs directly from patients in 1905–1906.[41] Except for the two years of most active hospital construction (1901 and 1902), the Chinese always provided the major part of the funds required to run the hospital. In fact, in five of the ten years for which data is available, the total Chinese component of the income—patients' fees, board, purchases, and donations—more than covered the current expenses.[42] In summary, at Chongqing the Chinese paid fees for dispensary as well as home visits; they paid for their board in hospital and for their medicines; they bought drugs and other imported goods from the drug store; they subscribed annually, and donated to building funds. These Chinese patients, though, were not the equivalent of the middle class *private* patient who sustained the hospital

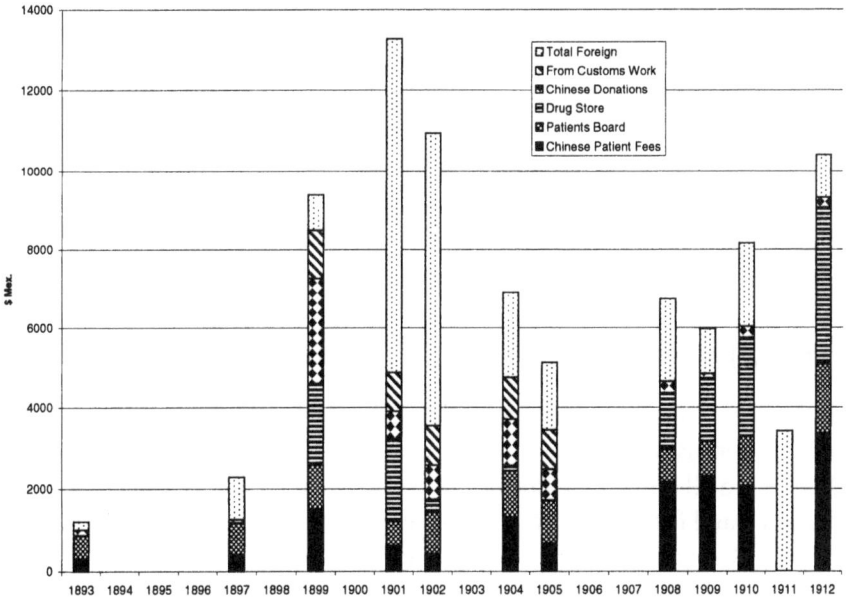

Figure 3: **Mix of Sources of All Funds, Chungking Hospital, 1893–1912**

Source: Extracted from financial data included in Annual Reports, Chungking Hospital, 1897–1912.

in America. In his second annual report, McCartney provided details of 445 of the 447 men and 48 women admitted to hospital (that is, excluding the 4,324 new patients who were seen as outpatients in the dispensary) in terms of their occupations. What emerges is a cross-section of ordinary Chinese. The two largest groups were farmers (79) and coolies (74) followed by 27 merchants, 25 housewives and 25 classified as *gentlemen;* there was an un-known number of beggars, 4 opium shopkeepers, 8 shoemakers, 16 street vendors, 13 cooks, the same number of both tailors and *yamen* runners and smaller numbers of wood carvers, barbers, butchers, millers, bakers, along with inn-keepers, a fortune teller, a coffin maker, and a mechanic.[43] The many thousands who made use of hospital outpatient services were even less likely to be of the upper and middle-income groups but they contributed substantially to the costs of the hospital through their registration and at-tendance fees along with their purchases from the drug store.

In conclusion, in a number of financial respects McCartney's hospi-tal differed fundamentally from its counterpart at home. It was not sim-ply transplanted but was adapted to suit a different economic and cultural environment. Not only did a greater proportion and a different class of patients pay fees but also they did so for a wider range of services. Despite the Chinese reputation for philanthropy in respect of their own benevolent institutions and McCartney's best efforts to encourage the Chongqing offi-cials and gentry to support the hospital, the proportion from this source was never substantial. Between 1893 and 1912, funds from Chinese donors only once matched that from patients (1899) when both contributed approxi-mately $2,600 Mex. Otherwise, between 1901–1905 Chinese donations hovered between forty-four and fifty-eight percent of that from patients and in 1908 the proportion dropped to less than ten percent and, in1912, to less than five percent.[44]

THE WIDER PICTURE

How representative, then, was McCartney's hospital? The CMMA con-ducted censuses of foreign hospitals in China by sending out "statistical blanks" to all known missionary hospitals and we have the results from one hundred and fifty two hospitals that replied at least once between 1903 and 1910.[45] Unfortunately, there are some inevitable problems with the data. Firstly, the coverage of hospitals was incomplete. The Editor of the *CMMJ,* J. B. Neal, was concerned that the forty-seven 1903 returns represented "not more than half" of the hospitals and dispensaries in China. He named the de-linquents, mainly from the larger centers, who failed to respond in an effort to shame them into participation.[46] Secondly, the information provided by hospitals was incomplete. Detailed financial information did not feature at all in the first survey report although obviously some was collected because a summary attached to the report stated that of the forty-seven hospitals and dispensaries listed only six required no fees or charges at all and that four of these accepted donations.[47] In the 1904, 1905, and 1906 surveys hospitals were asked about their policies relating to fees for dispensary visits, home calls, medicines, and hospital stays as well as income from sales and from foreign and "native" contributions.[48] Although the majority did, not all hospitals responded to the questions relating to finance. In 1907 publishing any financial details was abandoned and, from 1910 on, only a financial summary was included in the table of results.[49]

A third problem was that the data were not necessarily comparable across institutions or time. Any interpretation of the statistics contained within these returns, or the financial statements in annual reports that presumably formed their basis, must be undertaken with caution. The hospitals did not employ specialist administrative staff and it was the doctors, or their wives, neither of whom had any training in up-to-date account keeping practice, who kept the records and compiled the reports. But standardized accounting was still a future phenomenon in the West. In America in 1887, two unconnected but related events occurred that should have had a defining impact on the practice of accounting: the American Association of Public Accountants was incorporated and the Commerce Commission Act, which provided for federal regulation of railroads, was passed.[50] The Accountants Association, with no paid staff and run by volunteers, by 1892 still had only thirty-five members and their "technical meetings," designed to develop "uniformity in practice" and model forms of reporting, apparently came to little.[51] Despite the Commerce Act requiring a uniform accounting system, at the turn of the century "there was no uniform adherence to standards of auditing or of account maintenance throughout the United States."[52] The term "generally accepted accounting principles" was used for the first time only after the stock market crash in 1929.[53] The difficulties associated with comparing financial information in China is further exacerbated because hospitals in the various parts of China, sometimes depending on their national origins, reported in different currencies. These included *Taels,* "real *cash,*" "*cash,*" "small *cash,*" Mexican dollars, cents, £ Sterling and $ Gold. *Taels* were not coins but a weight in silver of a certain degree of fineness. They were used for accounting purposes only and were not necessarily consistent in weight, touch, or value. Particular *taels* though, for example, the *Huiguan* (used to account for customs levies) and the *Kuping* (used by treasury for all government taxes) were, in theory, uniform throughout the country. Although the charges were calculated and accounted for in terms of *taels* they were paid in the local currency. There were more than ten kinds of Chinese dollars in circulation at the turn of the century but, because they were most highly valued in the province which minted them and at a discount elsewhere, they were not popular. Various foreign currencies circulated throughout the country; the most commonly used being the Mexican dollar, which members of the Missionary Association used most frequently for reporting. Chinese silver coins—five, ten and twenty-cent pieces—were available but, like the dollars, varied widely against the *tael*. The common currency of the people was "copper *cash*," minted in ten and one *cash* denominations. Theoretically there were 1000 *cash* to the *tael* but this was not consistent over time; for example between 1905 and 1912 the exchange rate decreased from 1100–1200 to 1700–1800 *cash* to the Shanghai *tael*.[54] The editors of the *CMMJ* were aware of the shortcomings of the reports they published. In 1907, instead of their usual appeal for members to furnish statistical returns and chastising those who had failed in the past, they complained about the standard of reporting and the difficulty in comparing results as "there seems to be as many ways of making statistical returns as there are doctors and hospitals." In their view, "fallacies occur all along the line [and it was] difficult to get such returns as are worth getting." They noted, for example, that the calculated cost per bed could be misleading. The reason for this was that in some hospitals patients dealt directly with a cook who was not an employee of the hospital. Any monies paid by patients, or expenditure by the cook, did not pass through the doctor's hands or records. Recorded operating costs in these hospitals necessarily appeared low. In the hospitals that employed a cook, and provided meals, all costs were included in the expenditure statement and produced apparently higher running costs.[55]

The problems of comparability and accuracy persisted and as late as 1915 the editor of the *CMJ*, responding to an article in *The Modern Hospital*, urged the adoption of "truth" in financial reporting and "uniformity in accounts and balance sheets in all our hospitals." In particular, he drew the reader's attention to the fact that there was no common definition of terms such as "total cost" which to the "average missionary physician, thinking in terms of money grants from the Home Boards or gifts from sympathizing supporters, the total cost of running the institution is often unconsciously the result of a subtraction sum, viz. gross expenditure minus local receipts in fees, etc."[56]

Any survey of hospital annual reports for the period reveals the wide variation of forms in which financial information was conveyed. Rarely

were separate balance sheets and income and expenditure statements prepared and, consequently, purchases of capital items such as land, buildings,
furniture and fittings were included along with current expenses such as
food, coal, wages, and medical supplies. The format and terms used in statements not only varied between institutions but also varied within the set
of annual accounts of the same institution. Despite these limitations, the
surveys contain much useful information.

Ninety-six hospitals answered the question about fees at least once
between 1904 and 1906 and seventy-one of these (that is, 74 percent)
reported that they charged outpatients. The charges made for dispensary
visits were mainly reported in *cash* and ranged from as low as two *cash,*
charged by the Rhenish Mission[57] at Dongwan 东莞 in Guangdong, to
one hundred *cash,* by the Danforth Memorial Hospital at Jiujiang and the
Wuhu General Hospital in Anhui, both run by Methodist Episcopalians.
Although the majority of dispensary fees lay in a reasonably narrow
range—twenty to sixty *cash*—there was some variety in the method of
application. It would appear that by far the majority charged a flat fee per
visit—eighty-five percent in 1904 and even more, ninety-one percent, in
1906.[58] Others charged a fee for a set number of visits or for a set time.
For example, the Yangzhou 扬州 Baptist Hospital in Jiangsu charged eighty
cash for three visits and at the American Baptist Hanyang 汉阳 Hospital
in Hubei a forty *cash* charge covered two weeks attendance. Still others
charged one fee for the first visit and a lesser fee for subsequent visits: St
James Hospital at Anqing 安庆 in Anhui charged forty *cash* for the first
visit and twenty thereafter. One—the MEM hospital at Suzhou—recorded
that they divided patients into first and second class and charged accordingly—fifty-six and twenty-eight *cash* respectively. There, the foreign physician attended first class patients and "a native graduate with the foreign
physician as consultant" attended the second-class patients.[59] The rationale for adopting these variable methods of charging lay in a perception
shared by many missionary physicians. They had observed the Chinese
custom of 'doctor shopping' in the sense that patients routinely consulted
a number of Chinese doctors, or other healers, in succession until they
found one they considered sufficiently skilled in their particular disorder.
This meant that patients would expect the initial treatment to work and,
if it did not, would not return a second time. Charging a lower, or no, fee
for subsequent visits or a set fee to cover a number of visits, or weeks, was
an attempt to encourage patients to return. For Omar Kilborn, a strong
advocate of self-support, the reasoning was more pragmatic: his patients
could not afford to pay for ongoing treatment. He wrote in 1901 that the

"vast majority of out-patients after the payment of twenty *cash* registration fee, should not be asked for anything further, even though they come for a month or more, for the simple reason that they are too poor to pay.[60] In 1906, according to his response to the surveys, he had varied his 1905 charge of twenty-five *cash* for the first visit and nothing after, to thirty *cash* for one month's attendance. The survey returns reveal that the strategy of varying subsequent fees was implemented by only a tiny minority of hospitals (declining slightly between 1904 and 1906) but whether this was because they thought it would be ineffective or would involve too much of an administrative burden is not clear.

Some idea of the level of impost of these fees on the ordinary Chinese patient, particularly if they were in the majority charged for each and every visit, can be gauged from the comment made in 1905 by Dr Francis Tucker. At his hospital in a village in Shandong they had raised the dispensary registration fee from "thirty *cash* (1 cent)" to fifty, which was an "average half day's wage."[61] It is unlikely that poor Chinese would have paid so much out of mere curiosity. It is more likely an indication of the value placed by the Chinese on the medical service they received from the dispensary that so many were willing to pay so handsomely.

A relatively common tactic that served to increase income while accommodating the preferences of some patients and influencing the behavior of others was to charge heavily in certain circumstances. Most dispensaries were organized according to the principle of 'first come, first served' and a number of the early hospital reports described in some detail their strategy for ensuring the system was fair. Inevitably, among the patients there were those who did not want to wait their turn to be seen. Kilborn advised bluntly, "see them at once and charge them 100 *cash*." For those who came on "non-dispensary days, or out-of-hours on dispensary days ... charge them 300 *cash*."[62] Many did. George Cox, of the CIM at Zhenjiang 镇江 in Jiangsu, where they charged sixty *cash* to register with the dispensary, reported that those who came "out of hours and cannot wait their turn pay 50 cents."[63] Another advised that at his dispensary anyone who came before noon paid the full price for their medicine, which meant "a few will come then who would never enter with the crowd of poor people."[64]

An analysis of these statistical returns provides evidence that missionaries adapted the financing in response to their environment.[65] As regards fees for outpatient services, hospitals in China had more in common with each other than they had with their counterparts at home, whether in Britain or America. Of the British missions that provided financial information, the 74 percent that charged fees (twenty-eight of thirty-eight hospitals) was comparable to the 79 percent of American hospitals (forty-two of fifty-three hospitals) that charged fees.*[66] Based on this limited sample, it seems that the British were just as likely to charge fees as were their American counterparts, whereas charging for hospital care was more prevalent in America than it was in Britain. The policy of fee charging was not closely correlated, either, with the length of time the hospital had been in existence.[67] Whilst most hospitals waited until they had established rapport with the Chinese before introducing fees, some had still not introduced fees many years after their founding. For example, in 1905 there were four early American hospitals (established before 1890), each with a minimum of fifteen year's experience, which still provided free dispensary consultations and treatment.

However, there does appear to be some correspondence between the charging of fees and the denomination of the missionary society sponsoring the hospital. Baptist Missions were the least likely to charge fees and interdenominational and Methodist missions, the most likely.[68] Of the twelve hospitals under the auspices of American Baptists, none charged fees in 1904 and six still provided free treatment in 1906 whereas of the five American Board (ABCFM) hospitals four charged fees in each of the years. The four CIM (international, but mainly British) hospitals all charged fees as did the fourteen Methodist-run hospitals—eleven American Methodist Episcopalian, two British and one Canadian.[69] All but one of the twelve of the London Missionary Society (LMS) hospitals charged fees. Presbyterian missions, which were the most numerous (twenty-nine of the ninety-two British or American hospitals), displayed the most variability in fee policy. American Presbyterians, both North and South,[70] with fifteen hospitals, had eleven that charged fees and four that did not. Of the twelve British Presbyterian hospitals,[71] six charged and six did not. These figures would suggest that some missions (for example the CIM, the American Baptists, the LMS and the American Methodists) decided policy centrally. The CIM, established by Dr. Hudson Taylor who had been inspired by the work of the German born missionary to China with the Netherlands Missionary Society Karl Gützlaff, was the only society with its headquarters in China. It was the most aggressive when it came to moving into the interior of the country and one of the principles laid down by Taylor is particularly pertinent to this discussion: it must "never go into debt: nor . . . solicit donations or subscriptions: nor . . . publish the names of its supporters." Others, most markedly the Presbyterians—both British and American—appear to have set policy locally and according to local conditions.*

*see www.michellerenshaw.com

The foregoing analysis of fee income from outpatients highlights the most striking divergence of practice in China from that in either contemporary America or Britain. Rosenberg describes free outpatient treatment, for those too poor to hire their own physician, as having been an enduring feature of American hospitals since the late eighteenth century. Gratuitous treatment was the distinguishing characteristic of the American outpatient department but the needs of the patient was not its only raison d'être. The department's usefulness accrued equally to the hospital and its professional staff as to the patient: outpatients were a good source from which to select inpatients as the subjects of clinical training for doctors and nurses.[72] Stevens describes the American turn-of-the-century outpatient department as being "in theory at least, for those [patients] too poor (or ignorant) for private practice." Hospitals and dispensaries adopted different, local, definitions of poverty, often qualified by terms such as *deserving, honest* or *worthy,* to justify access to free treatment and the rare hospital that charged a fee did so in order to propel those they deemed able to pay in the direction of the private physician.[73] The outpatient department was never considered, as it was in China, to be a source of funds for hospital operations. Outpatient departments in China differed markedly from the institutions with the same name in America in another respect. Although they, too, functioned as feeders to the hospital-proper and as providers of clinical material for teaching and research, in China they had a different, more important primary purpose, evangelism. Or, as Dr Robert Beebe expressed it in an address to the Ecumenical Conference in New York in 1900: "When we consider that medical missions are undertaken and conducted by societies of the church whose one great purpose is the evangelization of the world, whose revenues are secured on that plea and whose life and energies are due solely to that great vitalizing idea, it is evident that medical missions have this great purpose also . . ."[74]

The greater the number of patients they saw, the greater their potential evangelizing influence—the goal of medical missionaries was not so much to restrict access as to maximize it. At the same time, they were just as concerned about abuse of a free system by those who could afford to pay but, in contrast with their counterparts in America, they had more interest in diverting patients from, rather than to, private practice. First there were no, or very very few, foreign private practitioners of Western medicine in other than the largest and oldest treaty ports. The only alternative—Chinese private practitioners—practiced either the Chinese traditional medicine or the sorcery that the missionaries were trying their best to replace. Medical missionaries were faced with the problems of balancing a complex set of competing aims: essential fund-raising, maximum contact with Chinese, avoidance of pauperization, and demonstration of their Christian charity, and the 'superiority' of Western medicine. For most of them, the solution was to set an affordable fee for the majority, allow free treatment for the destitute, and charge the rich, and those deemed morally degenerate, heavily.

CHARGES FOR MEDICINE

In America it was common practice for the gratuitous treatment given in outpatient departments to include the supply of medicine.[75] The system in China varied only marginally. According to the 1906 survey, fifty-nine (of a possible eighty) hospitals responded with information about charges they made for medicines in either the hospital, or the dispensary. Of these, a third made no charge, another third replied that they did charge but gave no details, and the remainder responded that they charged only for a few drugs. The selection of medicines identified as attracting a fee was more indicative of the attitude of the prescribing physician than of its intrinsic cost: *potassium iodide,* commonly used with mercury, for the treatment of syphilis[76] and *santonin sulphur*[77] for worms.[78] Revenue from medicine sales was not a significant contributor to hospital funds other than for a few, like McCartney, who set up American style drug stores selling patent medicines and other requisites.

PRIVATE PATIENTS

Since hospital historians regard the paying patient as one of the most significant characteristics of American hospitals of the period, it is important to examine this aspect of the American hospital in China. Unfortunately, it is not possible to isolate funds collected from private patients in the published statistical returns. Information relating to private patients was not specifically sought but eighty of ninety-six hospitals surveyed answered a question about inpatient fees. Regrettably, there was no uniformity at all in the manner of reporting the level of fees: some hospitals specified a sum per day, others an amount per week or month, still others just stated an amount with no further detail. Only ten (12.5 percent) stated clearly that they charged no fee at all. Only four specifically mentioned private patients: St Luke's in Shanghai charged first class patients $2.00 Mex. and fourth class 12 cents per day and a private room at Suzhou could be had for between $3 and $5 per day whilst ward patients paid 10 cents. The difficulty in interpreting the data in relation to private patients is exemplified by McCartney's response to the survey. It is clear from his annual reports, from 1893 onward, that both Chinese and foreign patients were accommodated in private rooms for a higher fee than he charged ordinary patients. When he built a new, one hundred-bed hospital in 1901 he included eight private rooms: five for Chinese and three for foreigners. Yet this aspect of his operation was not reflected in the survey results.[79]

In the absence of specific information, an insight into the relative place that private patients played in hospitals in China and America can be gained by comparing plans for new buildings. The technical journal, the *Modern Hospital,* ran an architectural design competition for a small hospital in America in 1923. The rules stipulated that fifty percent of the accommodation should be in private or semi-private (single or double) rooms.[80] The private accommodation in the Lancaster hospital, built in 1905, was already in line with this requirement.[81] The Highland Hospital in Fall River, Massachusetts, established in 1905 by a group of private practitioners, consisted solely of private rooms.[82] By comparison, the five percent of beds for Chinese private patients in McCartney's hospital is negligible. Those who wrote about hospital construction in China generally advised that some provision be made for private patients who are "used at home to retirement, and fret at being with the common herd. Private wards should be arranged for these, and are much appreciated and may be a good source of revenue to the hospital, as they are willingly paid for."[83]

However, the numbers of private patients were always comparatively low and they never contributed disproportionately to hospital finances. For example, the plan of St. Agatha's at Pingyin shows only two private rooms compared to accommodation for twenty-eight in three wards.[84] One of the highest private-to-ward bed ratios was to be found in the ABM Hospital at Shaoxing in Zhejiang where the seven private beds still represented only seventeen percent of the total.[85] Although almost all missionary hospitals had some private rooms available, none, among the more than three hundred I have been able to identify, relied to any extent on Chinese private patient fees for its conduct. Many hospitals make mention of their provision for any foreigners who could not be treated at home. For example, Richard Wolfendale, when describing the London Missionary Society's hospital at Beijing, explains that the four small rooms are "special private wards for foreigners and the bluejackets of H.M.S. navy."[86] Foreigners everywhere were accommodated privately but this was a very minor aspect of a hospital's work and was not seen as a potential financial bonanza, as it would have been in America.

In conclusion, the ordinary Chinese patient, whether in hospital or using outpatient services, certainly was a paying, but not necessarily a private, patient. Many, like those in McCartney's hospital, paid for visits to the dispensary; medicines or, at least, medicine containers; admission to hospital; their food and, if they were unfortunate enough to suffer from a venereal disease or were addicted to opium, an additional amount. Compared with hospitals in America, the American hospital in China depended more on patients for its operation and those patients were amongst the poorest in the society rather than the better off. In many respects, it would appear that Western hospitals in China, whatever their national or denominational origin, probably had more in common with each other than they had with their respective counterparts in Britain or America. McCartney's hospital at Chongqing, at least in matters financial, represented the norm. Looked at from the perspective of finances, then, the Western hospital in China had a unique identity.

Section IV
The Patient's Experience

In the home lands, hospitals, old and new, large and small, are clean . . .
many of the patients when brought to the hospital are from dirty homes,
and are as filthy as the most filthy Chinaman. But before they enter the
hospital ward, they must be bathed and made clean, and why cannot
this be done here?

—Editor, *CMMJ* 1901

How would the experience of a patient entering a missionary-run hospital
in China compare with one entering a small to medium sized hospital in
America? For the American experience, I employ secondary sources supplemented by annual reports of a number of private, city, state, voluntary, and
religious hospitals. Not being able to find first-hand accounts by Chinese
patients of their encounter with a Western hospital, I rely on and draw in-
ferences from accounts by missionaries and other witnesses of the various
policies, practices, and physical conditions in a large number of hospitals.
Although this method cannot capture fully the subjective experience, there is
sufficient objective detail available to draw meaningful comparisons.

One could argue that any differences between the experience of a
patient entering an American mission hospital in China and a hospital in
America in the last decade of the nineteenth or the first decade of the twentieth century were merely differences due to an accident of timing. It might
be assumed that the late nineteenth-century Western hospital in China was
simply somewhat less developed than its counterpart in America, that the
two hospitals shared a common history and would share a common future
when the hospital in China 'caught up.' Section IV tests this assumption, in
particular, from the point of view of a patient.

The conditions in China, both physical and in terms of personnel,
would have been adequate for the practice of Western medicine had the
medicine the missionaries brought with them been the essentially palliative

care provided in the hospital's immediate forerunners—the almshouse and asylum. However, the introduction of the hospital, as a concept and a reality, into China coincided with a revolution in the theory and practice of Western medicine and, in particular, in the role of hospitals. At the end of the nineteenth century, what the missionaries offered was the curative, increasingly 'scientific,' medicine that was developing out of an appreciation of the ramifications of the germ theory. The use of anesthesia and aseptic surgery encouraged adventures into previously dangerous waters. Diagnosis, treatment and monitoring were aided by technological developments—the microscope (from the 1840s), the medical thermometer (from the 1880s), the X-Ray machine (1896)—all of which medical missionaries were able to acquire if they could raise the necessary funds.[1] Medical missionaries were attempting to practice medical intervention on a similar scale and extent as they would had they been in America but, as we have seen in the earlier chapters on their hospital buildings, many were operating under conditions which could, by comparison, be called medieval. Stevens has described the best of American early twentieth-century hospitals as 'models of cleanliness, efficiency, and expertise. Where only twenty or thirty years before there had been noise, dirt, and disarray, there was now control and organization: the rustle of the nurses' uniform, the bell of the telegraph, the rattle of the hydraulic elevator, the hiss of steam. . . . '[2] In China at the same time it was rare to have running, far less hot, water; there was no electricity and machines, such as the X-ray, had to be powered by batteries, and lighting provided by oil lamps.[3] In addition, there was a lack of trained staff, especially nurses, who had made such a difference to the safety of hospitals in America and Britain. Although there can be no 'typical' patient or hospital, it is possible to speculate on how a person may have experienced hospitalization at the turn of the twentieth century in an American hospital in China. The timing of the arrival of medical missionaries, economics, the Chinese setting and patients, the lack of opportunities available to women physicians in America, and the evangelistic ambitions of the physicians all combined to create a unique institution, quite distinct from its counterpart in America.

Chapter Eight
Entering a Hospital

> When the hospital evangelist steps upon the little platform and reads a portion of scripture there is never any opposition, there may be indifference, and perchance silent contempt for the foreign doctrines, but there is, at least, outward respect.
>
> —Omar Kilburn 1910[1]

An American patient would be likely to have entered a hospital through the agency of a private medical practitioner who had admitting rights in a particular hospital rather than via a public dispensary. In contrast, it would be most unusual for a Chinese person to enter the hospital as an inpatient other than by first attending a dispensary, probably situated within the hospital compound.[2]

Public dispensaries had arisen in America in the late eighteenth century and were staffed by unpaid, part-time, aspiring specialist practitioners. Their principal purpose was to provide primary health care for the very poor who could not afford to consult a private practitioner but also to supply, so-called, *clinical material* for teaching and research. In China, dispensary patients were also considered the best method to 'feed' the hospital but the emphasis was less on the quality of them as clinical material than on the need to diminish the Chinese patients' fear of, or antagonism towards, foreigners and their medicine. In America, ordinary (general practice) physicians viewed free dispensaries as a threat to their income and campaigned against them. But, rather than drawing attention to their own interests, they used the twin arguments that free medical care pauperized the recipients and encouraged abuse of the system by those who could afford to pay.[3] As Paul Starr points out, had the nineteenth-century public dispensary in America made the transition from treating only the "sick poor ... [to] ... serving society as a whole" it, rather than the hospital, may have emerged as the "nucleus for community medical services."[4] In fact, the stand-alone dispensary disappeared and was preserved only in the form of the outpatient department of a hospital.

In China on the other hand, the dispensary was a familiar and long established component of the traditional medical market place. As we saw in chapter 1, public dispensaries, where doctors saw patients, prescribed remedies, supplied medicines, and performed simple procedures, had existed in China since at least the Song dynasty. There were many operating in Chinese towns when the American medical missionaries arrived in the nineteenth century. There is no evidence to show that the medical missionary chose the dispensary model *because* it was acceptable, or familiar, to the Chinese, let alone that it was a conscious decision to adopt a Chinese approach. Rather, it was a matter of economics and practicality. A large number of patients could be catered for at little cost and work could start almost immediately upon the missionary's arrival. Once the physician had acquired sufficient of the local language, the only physical necessities were a room (or sometimes a courtyard) in which patients could congregate, a supply of the most basic drugs, a table, and a stool.[5]

It would seem that the choice was fortuitous in that the model of a physician sitting in a room, examining and questioning a patient, and prescribing medicine was very familiar to Chinese people throughout the country.

SIT AND WAIT

If it was the initial visit to the mission dispensary patients would first be registered, which usually entailed an assistant, or gatekeeper, recording their name, address, occupation, and age and, where appropriate, collecting any fee. Each patient would receive a registration number, sometimes written on a piece of paper to be used as a ticket for future visits. George Huntley's hints on how to improve a dispensary service included encouraging the patient to remember his ticket number, "it being a Chinese superstition to destroy the ticket when the disease is well, as a retention of it would cause a return of the trouble."[6] Along with the ticket the patient would be handed an identically numbered "prescription sheet" on which the physician, or their assistant if they had one, would record the date, case notes, and details of the medicine to be collected from the pharmacy. (see Plate 20) The hospital would retain these prescription sheets as part of the patient's record.

Most dispensaries had adopted some system so that patients could be seen by the physician on a 'first come first served' basis.[7] The most common

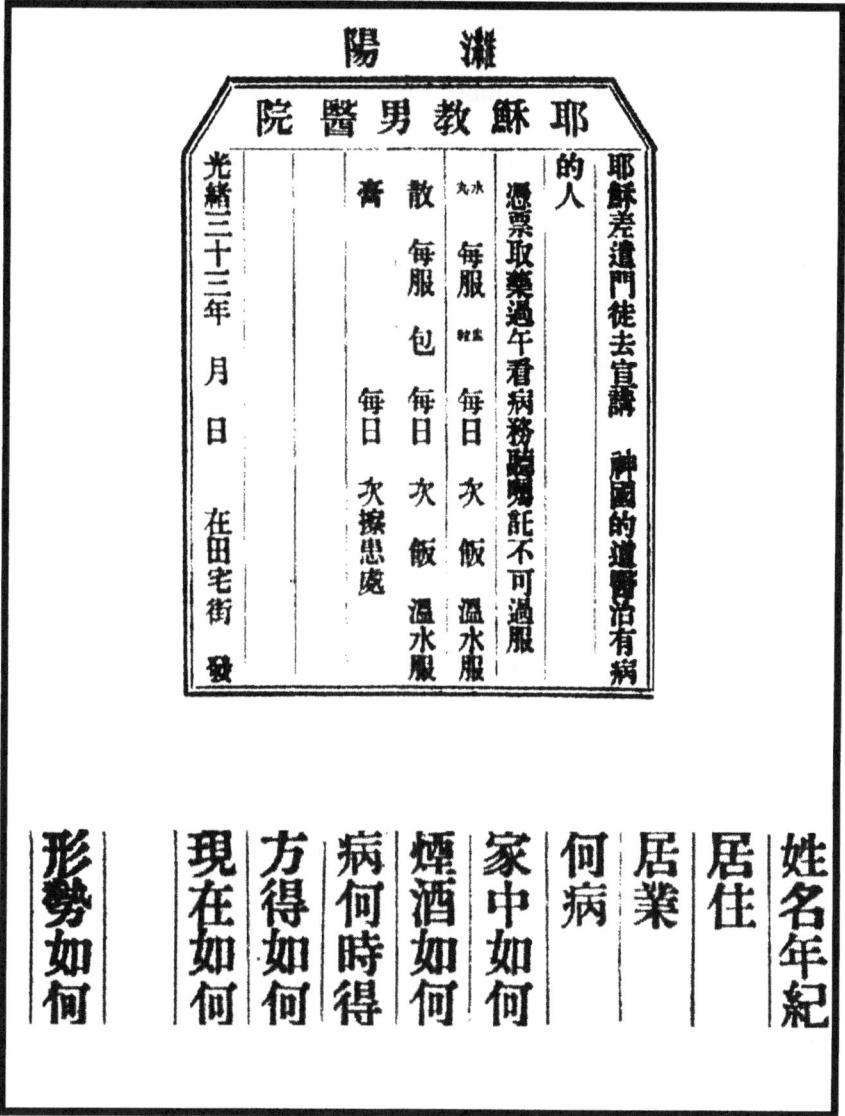

Plate 20. **Prescription Sheet and Patient Record wood type block recommended by Charles Roys**

Source: Charles K. Roys "Some Dispensary Methods." *CMMJ* 21, no. 3 (1907): 112, 114.

method was to hand out consecutively numbered bamboo strips to patients as they arrived. George Hadden, at Hengzhoufu 衡州府, Hunan, praised the efficacy of the "humble bamboo tab" which he described, in 1917, as still being "the universal auxiliary of all." He had modified the system using color: black for new patients, red for returnees, and red with a blue cap for a "privileged repeater, usually a daily dressing, who is entitled to be admitted as soon as he arrives irrespective of his order." This coding would give the treating doctor valuable information about the patient and, added to the lined-up collection on the desk after the consultation "is rather impressive to the patients, a minor effect not altogether without its value."[8]

Patients at Duncan Main's CMS hospital at Hangzhou, say, would then sit and wait in a "large, clean, airy, well ventilated [room] provided with very *comfortable* seats" which gave Main the perfect opportunity to engage in what he called *button-hole* theology.[9] Isabella Bird, who visited Dr Main in 1896, described the outpatients' waiting room and the attempt he had made to appeal to his Chinese visitors and patients as "large and handsome, decorated with scripture pictures, in which patriarchs and apostles appear in queues and Chinese dress."[10]

It would be while waiting to see the physician in China that an American patient would be most acutely aware that she was not at home. If the hospital was one that catered for both sexes she would most likely have entered by a separate gate or door and been directed to the women's waiting room or, at least, the women's side of the waiting room. A Chinese patient in an American hospital might have been quite discomfited by having to wait to see the doctor amongst patients of the opposite sex. In his summary of the collected wisdom on hospital construction in China, Jefferys recommended that a model dispensary should include either two waiting rooms—one for women and the other for men—or a larger single room divided by a railing: men on one side, women on the other.[11] The competition rules for the design of a small (thirty- to forty-bed) hospital in America made no mention of segregating men and women while they waited nor did any of the twenty published plans make any such allowance. The Lancaster General Hospital, according to the floor plans, had but one "reception" room. In contrast, I have rarely encountered a design or description of a hospital or dispensary in China that did not have provision for some segregation of the sexes in waiting rooms. Most chose the option of separate rooms. For instance, in 1907 when the new ACM dispensary was opened at the St James' Hospital (at Anqing), special note was made that the separation of the sexes in the dispensary was now 'complete.'[12] This had not been the case in the original St James, built in 1903. In that hospital, according to the floor plan, women waited in a separate room but entered a common consulting room, albeit through a separate door.[13] Claude Lee's hospital at Wuxi, on the other hand, included a "large waiting room divided by a railing for men and women, each division opening into treatment rooms separated by a central drug room."[14]

American patients arriving at a hospital waiting room in China would be further reminded that they were not in America because the hospital could be more realistically described as an evangelical tool than a medical facility: they would be harangued, often by an enthusiastic Chinese preacher. At Jinan, they had found that Chinese Christians were wanting to address the patients for "an hour to two hours." This did not seem to the missionaries there to be "an ideal way of attracting men or women who, after all, had not come with any primary intention of listening to the Gospel" so they introduced a system to limit preaching to half an hour and those who did not wish to attend could "remain outside."[15] The preaching was not necessarily confined to the period before the clinic opened. T. W. Ayers, with the Southern Baptists at Huangxian 黄县 in Shantung, reported that "during the clinic there is constant preaching in the waiting room."[16] Kilborn, whose comments head this chapter, was not alone in being under no illusion about the effect of such preaching; nor was the irony of what they were attempting lost on them. For example, the editor of the *CMMJ* in 1893 could not resist imagining "the immigration of a band of Chinese missionaries to rural England, and the reception they may meet with at the hands of our gentle country folk."[17]

Some warned their fellow missionaries of the inadvisability of preaching by disparaging Confucianism: "to undertake to substitute for that code (the code of ethics Chinese have lived by since before Christ) even the more ennobling ethics embodied in the Sermon on the Mount by attacking the former is a great error." The writer likened speaking against Confucianism to denigrating the great thinkers of Europe to Christians and he reminded his readers that Christ had respected the opinions and prejudices of those to whom he spoke and had used persuasion rather than dogmatism.[18]

EXAMINED

The sheer numbers of patients, the absence of nurses, and the impulse to influence as many patients as possible left many physicians unhappy with the level of medical service they were able provide in the dispensary. In 1906, A. F. Cole vividly described his professional dilemma: "The range of cases seen is very wide: one has to treat every manner of complaint: without a foreign colleague and without any nurses, we confess that lack of time for study tends to make one superficial and almost a quack: one almost necessarily becomes a mechanical instrument for inserting so much medicine into so many mouths; it is true that surgery occasionally lifts us out of the realm of quackery."[19]

This was Cole's first year at the CMS Men's and Women's Hospitals at Ningbo during which, with three "native assistants," he treated a total of 6,624 outpatients (in twice weekly sessions) and a further 256 on visits made to nearby towns.[20] At the same time, he had charge of both hospitals through which over 500 patients (316 men and 187 women) passed; performed 126 operations under general (chloroform) and 21 under local (cocaine and eucaine) anesthetic; carried out 180 "minor" operations; and extracted 181 teeth.[21]

When their turn came, a patient would enter a separate examination area sometimes partitioned off but often remaining in full view. This arrangement was commonly adopted so that Chinese who were waiting, and any friends or relatives who had accompanied the patient, could see what the doctor was doing. They hoped that this would inspire confidence, allay fears, and prevent rumors from arising. Kilborn's approach to this problem was to invite patients into his consulting room in groups of ten at a time. They would sit on a bench while he called them individually to a chair next to his desk to be examined.[22] Although the large numbers of patients could cause difficulties, Elizabeth Reifsnyder stressed that the medical aims were at least equally important as the evangelical. She asked, "Are we justified in having dispensaries with the two-fold object in view—the dispensing of that which *we* deem the most important, the healing balm for their souls, and yet slightingly care for their bodies which the Chinese consider of vastly more significance?"[23] When it came to examining patients, for instance, Reifsnyder agreed with Jos. Thomson, who wrote articles about Chinese medical practice for the missionary's journal. He advised physicians to adopt a Chinese approach and "always listen to both pulses."[24] As she expressed it, "questions must be asked, answers must be gotten, the tongue ought to be looked at, and to ease the mind of the patient, as well as for one's own gratification, the pulses must be felt."[25] Edward Hume, who had learnt much about traditional procedures of diagnosis from the first Chinese doctor appointed to the staff of the *Hsiangya* hospital, Dr Hou Kung-hsiao, made a habit of feeling both pulses.[26]

George Cox drew even more on the expectations of the Chinese as a guide how best to examine patients: approach them on their own terms, he advised. He thought that if he took both right and left pulses, listened to the story of the cause of their problem, told them how wonderful the medicine was, and how it would restore equilibrium patients would have confidence in him.[27] Charles Roys was another concerned with Chinese sensibilities. He was seeking a way to "handle dispensary cases to secure rapidity and thoroughness, combined with the utmost possible deference to the laws of Chinese etiquette"[28] He postulated a fundamental principle: "that every pa-tient who comes to us should be met and treated as nearly as possible as a Chinese guest would be treated by a Chinese host." He recognized that this would mean operating quite differently from at home where an assembly line style had meant that they could "go over rank after rank of patients . . . with ease and rapidity." Although they could teach Chinese assistants, he felt that the medical work would "lose a very large proportion of its influ-ence" if they delegated "all the courteous observances which take such a prominent a place in Chinese life" to assistants. In his dispensary at Weixian 卫县 (in Shandong) he had made the consulting room, in orientation and furnishing, as close as possible to a Chinese guest room with "an entrance door in the centre of the southern side, table and two chairs opposite the door on the northern side of the room." The patient, who had been given a "tally-card" by the evangelist in the waiting room, should be met at the door by the physician and shown to the "seat of honour" on the doctor's left. He should then be politely asked questions as to "honourable name, venerable age and exalted residence" followed by a standard set of questions about his disease in such a way as to elicit yes/no answers. The physician should spend at least five minutes with a new patient and an assistant, furnished with a copy of the questions, should take down the answers unobtrusively. For this purpose, Roys had had a list "cut upon a wooden type-block of a size to fit the heading of the pages of an ordinary Chinese account-book, ruled with red lines."[29] (see Plate 20)

ADMITTED

The number of Chinese who had contact with Western medicine through the dispensary was many times greater than those who experienced a stay in hospital. In 1906 for example, about half of the 166 hospitals and 241 dispensaries in China responded to the statistical survey conducted by the CMMA. They reported that of the 913,200 new and returning patients treated (in hospitals, dispensaries, while itinerating and in peoples' homes) a mere 34,000 (3.7 percent) were admitted as inpatients.[30] Hospitals did not occupy a very significant place in the range of medical alternatives in America either. In 1910, it was estimated that only between seven and eleven percent of sickness in New York City resulted in hospital admittance, the great majority was cared for at home unless major surgery was necessary.[31]

In both America and China, it was in the outpatient department that the potential inpatient would be categorized and dealt with in terms of his or her disease. Anyone suffering from venereal disease, contagious disease, or a chronic condition would be unlikely to be admitted to a contemporary voluntary hospital in America. No person with an infectious or contagious disease was to be accepted without special permission according to the rules of the Lancaster General Hospital.[32] Similarly, Auburn City Hospital ruled, "cases of pulmonary tuberculosis and venereal diseases are not to be received."[33] St John's Hospital, St Louis, went further and disallowed patients "suffering from mental aberration and alcoholics."[34] Such patients would have been referred to municipal hospitals that could not refuse them. There were no rules for admission included in the 1908 annual report of the Pennsylvania Hospital and a survey of the medical statistics for that year reveals that they did indeed accept patients suffering from infectious diseases: over five hundred cases of typhoid and twenty-seven of pulmonary tuberculosis, for example. Patients with venereal diseases were treated in short-term "receiving wards," in the medical and surgical outpatient departments, and in the gynecological department.[35]

Missionaries in China, on the other hand, did not have the luxury of choosing their patients. There was nowhere to refer them and a patient who was refused admittance represented a loss of a chance for religious influence. Their overriding aim was to reach as many as possible and sinners, even more so. If it were true, as experienced medical missionaries Jefferys and Maxwell asserted in their *Diseases of China,* that "syphilis is exceedingly prevalent among all classes" no one could have afforded to send so many patients away. Jefferys and Maxwell also reported that syphilis was, "on the whole, mild in type—superficial—and usually responsive to rational and aggressive treatment." So the hospitals took them in and, as has been discussed earlier, commonly charged them "a double fee or more because of the troublesomeness of their treatment, the necessity for extra precautions, and perhaps partly, because of the deliberate circumstances of their acquirement of the disease."[36]

Patients with other contagious diseases did not evince a debate about morals and appropriate fees. The issue was merely one of practicality—how could doctors protect their other patients? One built "a small ward enclosed in glass, adapted for a few consumptive patients . . . and at either end of the third floor, rooms which can be shut off from the rest for contagious diseases."[37] Another, the APM (S) hospital at Qingjiangpu 清江浦 in Jiangsu, relied on the arrangement of buildings: "The buildings are all Chinese style, one story, built around courts, with foreign windows and doors. The arrangement is similar to the pavilion plan now so much in favor in Western lands, and lends itself readily to thorough ventilation, sanitation, and if necessary to isolation."[38]

It is rare to find any direct reference in hospital reports to the exclusion of a class of patients. Given that an important function of these reports was to encourage support from benefactors it was probably not in the interest of the writers to draw attention to any people being refused treatment and, the desired, exposure to Christianity. That some discrimination was practiced by some hospitals is revealed in an article about a matter that was of concern to the women in charge of the Tooker Memorial Hospital at Suzhou. One of their patients was a young girl who had been sold into a "life of shame" by her father. She was not the first and they were concerned that they might not be able to cope with the escalation in this aspect of the work. They attributed the increase to a number of factors: the obvious success of their treatment, their "proximity to the *Moh Lu,* where such dens of iniquity abound" and, significantly, the fact that the other hospital in town "does not take such patients." They did not appear to consider following suit; rather, they observed, "many things make it undesirable to admit these patients to the general wards, but with our present accommodations no other plan seems possible." In the meantime, they were praying for guidance.[39] Obviously, policies on admission of patients were not uniform throughout the mission field but it is equally clear that patients in an American hospital in China would have come in contact with a greater range of contagious diseases than they would have had they been in a hospital in America. Whether this made the hospital in China a more dangerous place for patients, either physically or morally, is a moot point.

ADMISSION PROCEDURES

One of the most hotly debated issues surrounding patients entering hospitals was whether a bath should be compulsory. The majority, whatever their preference, did not implement the practice. Some simply lacked basic facilities but others argued that, as Chinese did not customarily bathe, especially in winter, insisting on it would act as an unnecessary deterrent to patients. Claude Lee went so far as to identify being allowed to "refrain from admission baths" as a draw card for patients to enter his old hospital when he built a new one in 1913. He hoped "they will in time appreciate the advantages of baths, clean clothes belonging to the hospital, clean white beds with fresh sheets, and other ordinary hospital customs" but he was resigned to it taking a long time. As he saw it: "It is not likely that a conservative people like the Chinese who have for uncounted generations regarded a bath in winter as fatal will rush unadvisedly and lightly into a bathtub at the behest of a 'foreign devil.'"[40] Cole, by 1910, had still not convinced his patients to bathe on admission: a bath "purchased some seven years ago . . . has since been used for keeping our supplies of sawdust!"[41]

Doctors James McCartney, at Chongqing, and Duncan Main, at Hangzhou, were two physicians who rejected the argument that the Chinese would not accept it and insisted on patients being given a bath on admission. McCartney claimed he had been told that the "Chinese would not take a bath or keep themselves clean, that they would not wear our clean cotton shirts" but he had found that his experiment with both had "proved a huge success."[42] Main might have insisted on an admission bath but, in 1909, he complained, "[a]s to the *daily bath* we can only say that this state of hygienic perfection is not yet attained to in our hospitals, except in summer, but we aim for it, and in time hope to have it where foreign nurses can superintend the male patients."[43]

Butchart, in 1901, recommended a "shower bath" which, he said, had been adopted universally by institutions at home. It was economical, clean and "entirely feasible." He added that a stove should be used to warm the room and that the provision of another small room where "they can sit and drink tea and cool off before going out will be a benefit and suit the Chinaman's ideas."[44] Balme, almost ten years later, wanted to "lay to rest . . . that time-honoured bogey, 'the patients will not stand it,'" He was sure that patients would comply "provided it is introduced with patience and tact by someone who thoroughly believes in it himself. But of course no patient, in any country, likes to be offered a shallow, tepid bath in an unheated room, with the outside temperature at zero!"[45] In America, by comparison, by the end of the nineteenth century standard hospital admission procedures included "a compulsory bath and, in many institutions, delousing."[46]

Another common admission strategy adopted was to require all patients to have a "middleman" who could act as an intermediary and, when necessary, on their behalf. For example, if the patient himself was incapable, the middleman could give the consent for an operation which medical missionaries had required since Peter Parker at Canton in the 1830s. He could also guarantee any unpaid fees. At Main's hospital in Hangzhou, having an intermediary was insisted upon and his role included taking care of the patient's clothing when the patient was given hospital garments.[47] The CMS Hospital at Ningbo made an exception only for emergency cases but all other patients were "expected to find a local man to go surety for them, otherwise, if they die, no one may come and claim the body, or if they steal, we have no means of recovering our property, for the police are of little use."[48]

The practice was common but not universal; some advocated merely asking for a substantial deposit from any one admitted to the wards and only requiring a guarantor if the patient could not pay.[49] Most often, the middleman would be a relative, a man on behalf of his wife or children for example, but not necessarily. The requirement would not have struck Chinese patients as odd because it was common, in a society based on reciprocal relationships, for transactions to be effected through 'contacts.' All medical missionaries would have had to become familiar with, and adept at, dealing with the Chinese through intermediaries in relation to their own need to rent or buy land, for instance, and as Christie commented, "the settlement of quarrels by middlemen . . . is universal."[50] Thus, the needs of the hospital for financial and legal certainty were met within the boundaries of Chinese custom.

FELLOW PATIENTS

In China, as elsewhere in the world, the pattern and nature of hospital admissions, and hence one's fellow patients, varied depending on the geographical location, the presence of various epidemics, time of the year, and the weather. In addition, in China at that time there were other, more political, factors at work. Most hospital reports, whatever the year, made mention of the political conditions prevailing in their locality. When the situation was not described as *quiet* it was characterized as *unsettled* which could mean anything from riots, looting, banditry, and arson, which were sometimes, though not necessarily, directed against foreigners in general and missionaries in particular. At these times, unless they were attacked and forced to closedown completely, the attendance at clinics could falter, but just as often, hospitals could be inundated with injured combatants or victims; for example, robbers and pirates were said to be active around Ningbo during 1911 when many of the wounded were treated at the CMS hospital.[51] The introduction of foreign machinery and weapons into the country also led to an increase in the number of accidents.[52]

Hospitals in the countryside were particularly prey to the vagaries of the agricultural cycle. As William Wilson (reporting on the commencement of work at Suidingfu 绥定府 in Sichuan) pointed out, the autumn harvest affected the rate of admissions: the hospital emptied when the harvest started and filled up again when it had been brought in.[53] The hospital for women run by the Irish Presbyterian Mission (IPM) at Jinzhou 锦州 in Liaoning experienced a dramatic drop in the number of outpatients in 1900. This was due not, as one might have expected, to Boxer activity but "mostly [to] robber and *wolf* scares of four months in the summer."[54]

CLASS

The hospital population was more diverse than might be imagined—as we have seen in reference to McCartney's hospital at Chongqing. The MEM Women's hospital at Zhenjiang 镇江 (in Jiangsu) reported that their patients were "principally from the middle and lower classes, with a sprinkling of ladies from the higher."[55] Slave girls, brought "by wealthy owners, willing and able to pay for treatment [were a] large and important part of in-patient and out-patient practice" in the Church of Scotland hospital at Yichang 宜昌 (Hubei)[56] and Lucy Saville (LMS Women's Hospital, Peking) reported that they had treated "several wealthy Mohommedan girls this year; such delightful girls, the daintiest of little ladies."[57] A.W. Douthwaite described his inpatients at the CIM hospital at Chefoo (Yantai 烟台, Shandong) as being "of a higher class than those who attend the dispensary, most . . . being naval and military officers and tradesmen." His other patients could not be admitted to hospital as they were "too poor to contribute to their support" and he had no funds to supply food for them.[58] The physician in charge of the dispensary and hospital at Chengdu associated with the West China Medical Mission of the MEC reported that the number of patients from the official classes was increasing and that the sight of "the provincial treasurer . . . riding in his official chair, and accompanied by his tens of lictors bearing fasces, umbrellas, and lanterns . . . [coming] for treatment" had a reassuring effect on the "common people."[59] The hospital population in Ayers' Warren Memorial Hospital, at Huangxian in Shandong, came "largely from the middle and upper classes." Although they did admit the very poor at no charge, a "very small percent.of our attendance is from this class . . . we constantly feel that we are keeping from us many of the very poor whom we would be glad to treat."[60]

In the early days, rich patients who consulted the medical missionary would expect the physician to attend them in their home. With the introduction of more complex surgery that required hospitalization and private rooms for paying patients, class differences among patients in hospital became more visible. As early as 1888, St Luke's reported that the new Women's Branch had a few private rooms for those patients who could afford to pay and a "separate structure is provided for the treatment of pauper sufferers, with whom it is found that the other classes of Chinese decline to mix."[61]

GENDER

According to Rosenberg, at the turn of the century in America "men far outnumbered women" as hospital patients.[62] He provides no data for this claim and, while it may be true for the American hospital population as a whole, a small sample of seven hospital reports covering the years from 1887 to 1915 casts doubt on the universal applicability of the assertion. Each of the hospitals catered for both men and women, they varied in size from large (Pennsylvania[63]) to small (Auburn City[64]), and include examples of each of Rosemary Stevens' categories: public, private charitable, and proprietary. In only two of the hospitals were there significantly more men than there were women; in three hospitals, the number of women admitted matched the number of men and, in the last two women predominated.[65] Taken as a whole, in the seven hospitals, the ratio of the average occupancy rate of men to women was approximately 1:1.*

The situation in China was very different. Although the published statistics from 1903 onwards listed the total number of beds available in the various hospitals, it was not until 1910 that the CMMA published information about the number of hospital beds available for men as opposed to those for women.[66] Of the 99 hospitals that provided data on the number of beds in 1910, it would appear that 31 catered exclusively for men, 13 for women (and children), and 55 for both men and women, "although not as a rule in the same building."[67] The smallest of these, run by Wesleyans (WMMS) at Daye 大冶 in Hubei, had but two beds, both for men. The largest was the oldest, the Canton Missionary Hospital started by Peter Parker in 1835, which had beds for 200 men and 120 women. In all, the 99 hospitals reported having 4,268 beds for men and just less than half that, 2,024, for women: that is, a ratio of two male beds to each female bed.[68] When one compares the number of patients admitted, however, a different picture emerges: the number of inpatients admitted to these 99 hospitals in 1910 was reportedly 37,589 men and 13,532 women; that is, a ratio closer to three to one.*[69] In other words, medical missionaries provided a disproportionate number of beds for women. Either women stayed longer in hospital or the occupancy rate of women's beds was less than that of men's beds. The statistical returns, and most annual reports, provide insufficient information

*see www.michellerenshaw.com

about occupancy rates or lengths of stay for men compared with women to make a proper judgment as to the extent to which these affected the total number of women admitted to hospital.

Thus, whereas an inpatient in the American hospitals surveyed above was as likely to be a woman as a man, in China patients in Western hospitals were three times more likely to be men. There were at least two forces at work: the reluctance of Chinese women to consult a male physician in certain circumstances and, when there *were* female physicians, problems associated with entering an institution for a period. Certainly, many women physicians commented on the difficulties they faced persuading Chinese women to enter a hospital as inpatients. According to a report on the hospital for women operated by the SPG at Peking in 1900,[70] it was "still an exception for Chinese women to consent to life in a foreign compound, and if there is any possibility of recovery in their own homes they very much prefer the dirt and squalor there, with painful cart journeys to and from the dispensary to becoming in-patients." According to the writer the "excuses are manifold" but they read as though they could equally have been enunciated by the great majority of women anywhere until very recently: "There is no one to look after my house. I have two or three small children, whom I cannot possibly leave. My husband will not let me go away from home. I will come as often as you like, but I cannot live there."[71]

Dr Margaret Polk, of the MEM (S) hospital at Suzhou, was one of the relatively few *women* who contributed regularly to the *CMMJ* and spoke at medical conferences. At a meeting of the Shanghai Medical Missionary Association in January 1901, she outlined wide-ranging concerns about the state of women's medical work. In relation to the difficulties she had faced in persuading the more wealthy Chinese women to accept treatment she explained that the "woman will often be surrounded by people whose unreason will prevent her yielding. [I had to reason with] the father-in-law, the mother-in-law, two or three of the older sisters-in-law, the woman's own family, and last but no means least in a Chinese family, the servants."[72] In her experience, even if she could persuade a woman to enter the hospital she would not stay long: young wives were not allowed out at all, and wives of officials were more restricted than others; poor women were needed at home; and some feared that their husbands would take a new wife if they were away too long. Dr Mary Fulton, the woman "in charge of the largest medical work for women in China,"[73] described similar difficulties still being experienced twelve years later: "It is not easy for a Chinese mother to leave her home duties. Then she controls no money, and the husband gives only grudgingly. The women are afraid to stay as long as their needs require. One said she must hurry home, or her husband would bring back another wife during her absence. The men go where and when they please, and carry all the money with them. They stay in a hospital as long as they wish."[74] Mary Brown had observed that, "the elderly women are less particular, but the younger women are very much hedged about by custom and prejudice."[75]

The restrictions noted by these physicians were common but not universal. For example, H. T. Whitney of the ABCFM explained why they had few problems attracting women to their dispensary at Fuzhou. There was "a large class of 'field women,' large-footed, who work in the fields with men, bear heavy burdens, carry produce to market, go about boldly on the streets, and mix freely with the crowds, so that they would naturally come to a free dispensary . . . it may further be stated in this connection that in later years a fair number of the better class of women, 'bound-footed,' annually visited our dispensaries."[76] Dr Kate Woodhull, with the same Board and also at Fuzhou, reinforced this insight. She wrote of the independence of "field women" whom she thought were the happiest women in China. She described them as privileged in that they could "walk whenever and wherever they like, go to the stores and make purchases, etc." and they could be said "socially, to be almost emancipated."[77] Regardless of the concerns of many medical men and women, increasing numbers of Chinese women did enter hospitals as patients and many more visited dispensaries. Graham, in her study of American Protestant schools, concluded that missionaries "used the schools, both boys and girls, to challenge the Chinese attitude towards gender and women's place in society." There is less evidence that *medical* missionaries challenged Chinese norms in relation to women. They more often tried to make their hospitals attractive to women by conforming to Chinese custom and extending the segregation of the sexes in dispensaries to the hospital-proper. Inpatients were separated, according to sex, to a greater extent in China than in America. For example, the Church of Scotland hospital at Yichang reported that it had "been found necessary this year to fall in with the demands of Chinese etiquette and have the women's ward in a separate building from the men."[78] Jeffreys, whose experience had been mainly in relatively cosmopolitan Shanghai, argued that separate institutions for women, *staffed by women* (my emphasis) were unnecessary. He agreed, however, that hospitals could "meet the utmost of Chinese needs of good taste"—one could organize common administrative areas but a "properly guarded barrier" should separate wards. He also suggested "a double entrance, for men and women."[79] The rigorous separation of the sexes in the Wuchang General has been discussed earlier: although the amount of accommodation for men roughly equaled that for women and children, Hussey allowed for complete duplication of all facilities so that the sexes could not mix. The original hospital, built in 1883 for the MEM at Suzhou, was another that exemplified this approach: two hospitals, one for men and another for women, had occupied adjacent compounds. They were completely separate both physically and in their management.[80]

THE TREATING PHYSICIAN

If women patients were in the minority it was not because of a lack of women physicians.[81] In stark contrast with the situation in America, a patient in an American hospital in China at the turn of the century would have been at least five or six times more likely to have been treated by a female physician. The first female foreign medical missionary in China, Dr Lucinda Combs, arrived in 1873 and went to Peking with the MEM.[82] A steady stream of women followed her: many were stationed in the treaty ports but others ventured into the interior and established new medical work.[83]

It has been well documented that in America—and in Britain even more so—opportunities for women to pursue careers in medicine were limited.[84] One of the early women missionary physicians to go to China, Anne Houston-Patterson, wrote, in an autobiographical piece for the *Medical Woman's Journal* in 1887, that in her home state of Virginia there was "not one woman doctor."[85] Medical schools were not open to American women before 1890 when Johns Hopkins, after a woman offered them a large donation with the stipulation that they should admit women under the same conditions as men, became the first. In 1891, Houston-Patterson, like all her sisters who sought medical careers, graduated from one of the women-only colleges started by and for women: the Women's Medical College of Baltimore. Other schools followed Johns Hopkins' lead "usually after a bitter and protracted battle"[86] but, paradoxically, this had the effect of further limiting women's options. A number of the seventeen women's medical schools established during the latter half of the nineteenth century closed.[87] At the same time, opposition from men meant those medical schools that did open their doors imposed quotas on women—about five percent from 1910 and for the next fifty years (other than in wartime). In fact, there were fewer women studying medicine in 1909 than there had been in 1894: down from 1419 to 921.[88]

Moreover, having graduated in medicine did not guarantee that a woman physician would find acceptance. In 1887, Charlotte in North Carolina "had the distinction of possessing one [woman doctor] but the Doctors Club of that city would not allow her to join!"[89] Estimates in the secondary sources of the number of female physicians practicing in America at the turn of the century vary somewhat but there is general agreement that the percentage was very low. Starr states that in the twenty years between 1880[90] and 1900 the percentage of women doctors in America doubled from 2.8 to 5.6 percent.[91] Marrett cautions that even this small percentage may be misleading because the total numbers included the comparatively larger proportion of women who practiced as homeopaths.[92] She provides data for ten cities, taken between 1892 and 1898, which show that female "regular" (that is allopathic) practitioners contributed between two and seven percent of all regular physicians in those cities.[93]

Paul Varg described the young American male missionaries as not necessarily "typical or religious aesthetes [but rather driven by the] normal excitement over an unusual career in an unusual corner of the world, free from the more prosaic patterns of the ministry, or a position in business at home."[94] If this description is valid, it is probable that this would have been even more the case for women physicians. In middle to late nineteenth-century America, there were few openings for those women physicians in "existing medical clinics, dispensaries, hospitals and institutions"[95] and so they were forced to establish hospitals, exclusively for women and children, where they could practice and where trainee women doctors and nurses could gain clinical experience. The missionary enterprise offered adventurous women the opportunity to practice a far wider range of skills than at home.[96] They were more likely to be able to work as equals with men, performing mainstream medical work, rather than as handmaidens.[97] Houston-Patterson was one such woman. The daughter of a Presbyterian minister, with an aunt who was a missionary in Mexico, she had wanted to be a foreign missionary since she was six years old. She arrived in China in September 1891, three months after graduating from a course that lasted only two and a half years. She had had "no internship" and, although she had been required to be present during operations, she had had no opportunity to practice surgery. Her daunting task was to "open up in China with no consultants, no nurses, 'no nothing.'"[98] Many like her were attracted to the role and were eagerly sought by missionary societies who believed that women were better suited to work among—and influence—the women of China than men were.[99]

Mary Davidson voiced the most common reason for welcoming women physicians: "the very strong objection raised by many ladies in China to being attended by one of the other sex."[100] As early as 1899, in a paper read to the West China Conference, she noted that, ironically, in America where medical women had made such apparent progress in education and patients did not object to male physicians, women were less able to use their training than in China. In China, women could enter as equals into the medical and surgical professions where men have "so long enjoyed exclusive rights and privileges."[101] She urged that the "voice of this conference may be clear and strong in emphasizing the great need for many more qualified women, who may hear the call and quickly respond to it." The conference did pass a resolution (proposed by Dr Richard Wolfendale, seconded by James McCartney) indicating "hearty sympathy with medical work amongst women by women; and its belief that there is much scope for many fully-qualified medical women than are at present working in these western provinces."[102]

The extent to which missions succeeded, and women responded, is illustrated in Figure 4, which compares the rate of men and women physicians arriving in China from 1869, when at least forty-seven male physicians had already arrived, to 1905 (when the *CMMJ* ceased reporting arrivals) Although the rate of arrival was always less than that of the men, the percentage gap between the number of medical men and women, declined steadily from one hundred percent in 1872 to under forty percent in 1905.*[103] By the time that Johns Hopkins first accepted women, more than twenty percent of all missionary physicians in China were women. The percentage steadily increased until, by 1906, fully one third were women.[104]

This picture is dramatically different from what could be found in America during the comparable period. A sample of reports from American hospitals will serve to demonstrate the point. In 1887, the seventy-bed Maine General Hospital had no women medical staff, either resident or consulting.[105] At the Lancaster General (Pennsylvania) in 1906, the only women on the staff were the chief nurse, the matron, and the bookkeeper.[106] Similarly, the medical and surgical staff of the Pennsylvania Hospital in 1908 was exclusively male.[107] The Auburn City Hospital, New York, was unique among this selection in that all the members of its Board of Managers were women. Nevertheless, not one woman was employed amongst the resident staff nor were there any women among the visiting (or consultant) medical, surgical, homeopathic, obstetric, or pathology staff.[108] By 1915, of the ten medical staff at the private Highland Hospital at Fall River, Massachusetts, only two—the pathologist and anesthetist—were women.[109] Even as late as 1925, there were only two women members of a medical staff numbering twenty-two at the Bloomingdale (Psychiatric) Hospital at White Plains, New York.[110] One might have expected that the Babies Post-Graduate Hospital in New York would have female medical staff but, in 1917, there were none

*see www.michellerenshaw.com

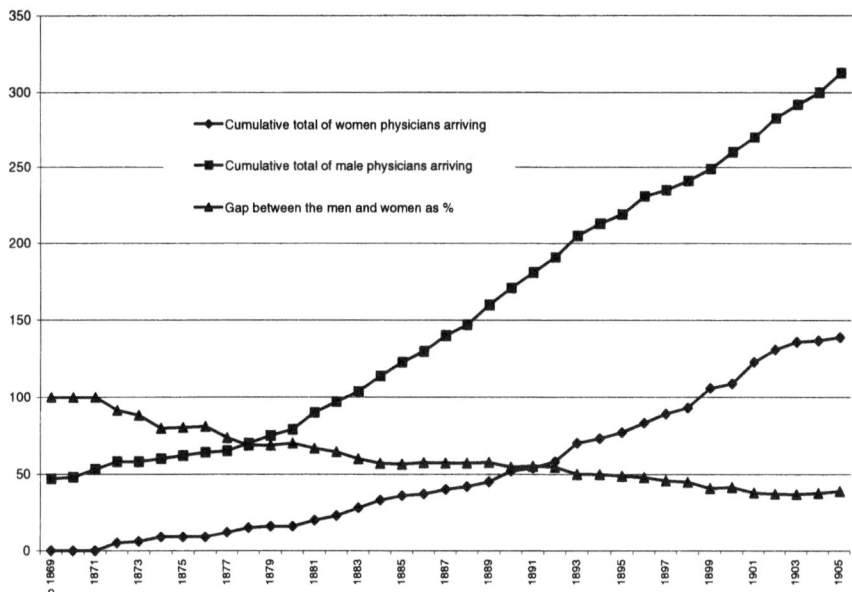

Figure 4: **Comparison of the rate of arrival of male and female physicians to China, 1860–1905.**

Sources: Figure constructed from a count of newly arriving physicians in *CMMJ* (1865–1912)

among the twenty-six visiting, and two resident, physicians or surgeons.[111] Not that American hospitals of this era were devoid of feminine influence: all had matrons, nurses, and active women's auxiliaries. In China, on the other hand, hospitals had male assistants, no auxiliaries, and no matrons but did have women physicians. They were most prevalent in American-based mission hospitals: at least thirty-six percent of all American physicians working in China were women in 1906. There were fewer women doctors in the hospitals of British mission societies—eighteen percent—but they were still far more common than in Britain.[112] A woman medical practitioner in England, in a letter to the *Lancet* in 1873, the year the first woman physician arrived in China, had referred to "the four ladies now practising in England"[113] and, according to Starr, there were still only a mere 258 female physicians in the whole of Britain at the turn of the century.[114]

Of the women who responded to the call to "send us a lady physician,"[115] many confined their practice to women and children as did the majority of their sisters who stayed in America.[116] An exception was Dr Susan Tallmon, who arrived in Linqingzhou 臨清州 in late 1905 to re-establish the medical work at the ABCFM hospital which had been abandoned during the Boxer rebellion. In February 1908, she opened a "general dispensary, private examining room and drug room" in a single room in the court where the missionaries lived. (see Plate 21) She worked alone except for the help of an "empirically trained man"—presumably in Chinese medicine.[117] She saw both men and women and, for the four months between November 1, 1909 and March 1, 1910, the number of men and boys (632) treated at the dispensary was greater than the number of women and girls (512).[118]

The first hospital run by women, for women and children, was at Fuzhou. In 1875 Dr Sigourney Trask, of the Women's Foreign Missionary Society (WFMS) of the MEM, built a hospital, later to be named the Magaw Memorial.[119] Another was the Tooker Hospital for Women at Suzhou, established by the APM (N) in 1900, where two women referred to as *Miss* Mary A. Ayer and *Miss* Frances F. Cattell, despite them both being doctors "trained and graduated from Woman's Medical College Pennsylvania," were in charge of all the medical work.[120] These 'women only' hospitals faced their own peculiar problems. For example, what were they to do with men? Elizabeth Reifsnyder raised the issue in 1887. As she said, "at home the woman is a free moral agent, so far as going to the dispensary is concerned," whereas in China men accompanied their wives, mothers, and daughters. If these men needed medical attention, she would treat them but her real dilemma arose when it became obvious that there was nothing wrong with the women who came to her demanding "attention for their men folk."[121]

As distinct from the men, the women who worked as medical missionaries were overwhelmingly young and single.[122] Of the 132 medical women who arrived before 1905, 116 (87.8 percent) were single. By comparison, of the 208 men (for whom I have been able to determine marital status) only 72 (34.6 percent) were single. The rest of the men were either already married—many with young children—or married very soon after arriving.[123] This disparity between the marital status of men and women inevitably meant that the women had to become even more independent and resourceful than would have been necessary at home. They often worked alone and, whilst they usually had no family to care for, they had no 'wives' to provide the kind of supportive work that Mrs. Maxwell took on for her husband at Yongchun 永春 in Fujian. Dr Maxwell was grateful and described the extent of her responsibilities: "She has charge of the kitchen, oversees the collection of money by the students, and makes it pay its way well . . . she also takes charge of the operating theatre for me."[124]

If these single professional women were a novelty in their homelands, they would have been even more extraordinary in China where women were

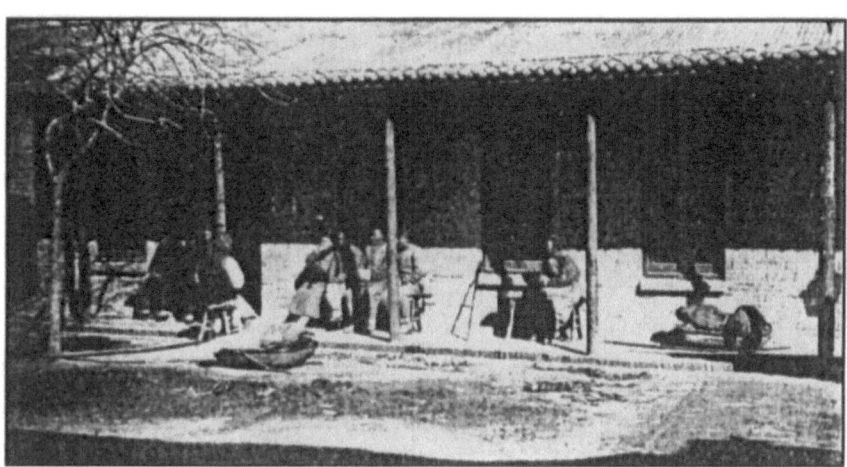

Plate 21. "Preaching to Patients Waiting for the Dispensary to Open" at the ABCFM Hospital, Linqingzhou, 1905
Source: Susan B. Tallmon, *Glimpses of Lintsingchow Hospital: A.B.C.F.M.*, 1910: 5.
Courtesy of the Burke Library, Union Theological College, New York

seldom formally educated. A rare mention of Chinese women doctors (as opposed to midwives or Chinese women trained in a foreign institution) was made by Margaret Polk who reported that she had come across three: one taught by her physician husband; another old woman who came to the hospital and a third, thirty-five years old, from "an official family." She admired the last of these and noted that "the family treated her with marked respect." She was sure that if she had come across three there must be others, which meant "there was no foundation for the belief that the education of Chinese women in medicine is an innovation, or for the oft repeated statement that China is not ready for women physicians."[125]

As an aspect of the missionary intention to see hospital work devolve to Chinese control, many women missionaries did indeed encourage Chinese girls who had been educated in mission schools to take up medicine as a career. Mary Brown made a plea for the training of Chinese women as physicians to the Shandong Missionary Conference in 1898. Nonetheless, she did see a number of potential problems with such a scheme. Firstly, in her experience, Chinese were characteristically unwilling "to perform disagreeable offices for one another." She attributed this to "a remnant of the selfishness of heathenism [which] medical training does not always eradicate." Secondly, the custom of early marriage also militated against requiring trainee doctors to be single so she accepted some married students. They had to pay their own way, help with dispensary work, their parent or guardian had to promise they would stay for four years, and they had to have "unbound feet."[126]

It was not long before some young Chinese women were traveling to America to train as physicians. The first of these was Jin Yamei 金韵梅 (1864–1934) from Ningbo who went to New York in 1881. She opened dispensaries in Xiamen, Chengdu and other locations when she returned to China in 1888.[127] Another, Hü Jinying 胡金英, supported by Sigourney Trask, became, in 1883, the "first Chinese Methodist medical doctor."[128] Gertrude Howe, educated at Michigan University, arrived in central China in 1872 to open a school. She adopted four Chinese girls, including Kang Cheng, known as Ida Kahn, and Shi Meiyu, (Mary Stone) and taught them English and science to prepare them for medical training at Michigan.[129] In 1901, they took charge of a new women's hospital for the Methodist Central China Mission at Jiujiang in Jiangxi: the Elizabeth Skelton Danforth Hospital.[130] These Chinese women physicians, as will become obvious later, brought a singular perspective to hospital work in China.

The fact that the missionary field was a hospitable arena did not mean that professional women were exempt from some of the limitations placed on their sisters at home. Margaret Polk spelled out some of the difficulties women physicians faced. When she spoke, before a mostly (if not entirely) male audience, she described a medical woman's typical experience: being patronized by men, attempting to rebel, and finally succumbing to either marriage or playing the role of nurse to the male physician. She thought that a woman physician felt that she "dare not take the initiative in anything, since by doing so she 'loses her womanliness.'" Physical restrictions on women, she thought, also meant they found it difficult to get out among the people and become familiar with the "thoughts, the customs, the superstitions, and the emotions that dominate the people for whom [they] would work."[131] Being a woman, though, did not mean that Susan Tallmon was sequestered within the mission compound. In a letter home, she described the type of conveyances furnished by patients who called her to see them at home. In the city, it was usually a sedan chair carried by two men but in the country, it was more commonly a cart drawn by "mule or pony or both" and on one occasion a cart pulled by a "little red cow." (see Plate 22).[132] Whatever the boundaries being a woman imposed, it would seem from their hospital reports that the great majority overcame them and that the practice they carried on was as diverse as any man's.

There is debate in the literature as to the extent to which a female presence among the medical staff influenced the workings of a late nineteenth-

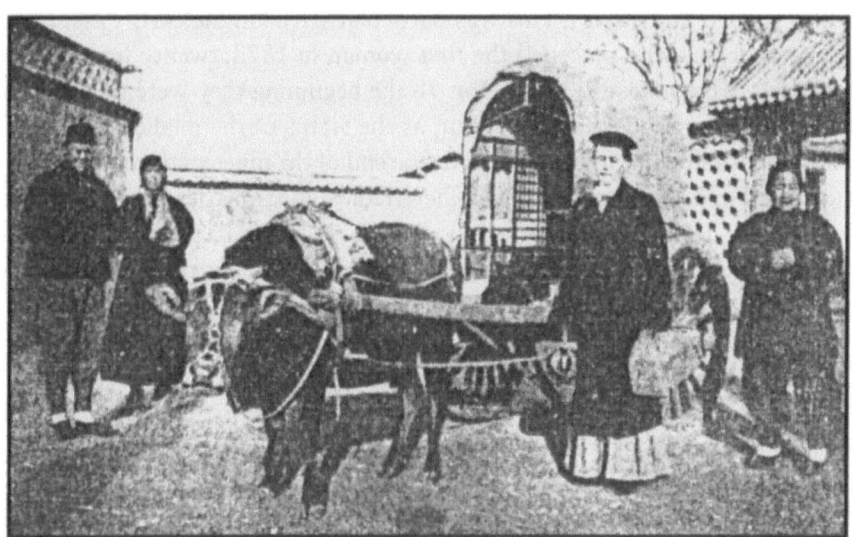

Plate 22. Susan Tallmon of the ABCFM at Linqingzhou
Source: Susan B. Tallmon, *Glimpses of Lintsingchow Hospital: A.B.C.F.M.*, 1910: 14.
Courtesy of the Burke Library, Union Theological College, New York

century American hospital. The notion that women were specially suited to working with women and children was commonly believed and promoted by women, and is assumed by scholars such as Mary Roth Walsh.[133] But, as Morantz and Zschoche have demonstrated, concrete evidence that women treated obstetric patients significantly differently from their male counterparts is, at best, inconclusive. For example, they found no appreciable difference between men and women in the willingness to intervene technologically in a birth. The medical outcome for patients did vary with the sex of the physician, but "only to a small extent and only in an indirect manner." They concluded: "women physicians probably exhibited a different orientation to patient care. Thus men and women doctors acted alike in most therapeutic situations, but for very different reasons and with different meanings, different both to themselves and to their patients."[134] So, although it is beyond dispute that the American hospital in China was very different from its equivalent in America, in terms of the professional staff gender profile, it is less clear what effect this would have had on the style, or type, of treatment offered to patients.

Another aspect of the professional staff profile in which the hospital in China differed from its counterpart at home was that a significant proportion of male physicians who, in addition to being trained in medicine, were also trained in theology. This was particularly true in the early days: of the 54 physicians who preceded the first woman in 1873, twenty-four, or 44.4 percent, were ministers of religion. In the beginning they were missionaries first and physicians second.[135] But, as the status of the medical profession rose in Britain and America towards the end of the nineteenth century things changed in China as well as at home. Medical missionaries were caught between the demands of two worldly masters: they had to meet the standards set by their professional associations whilst still being responsible to the missionary associations that employed them. The early days saw clergymen, untrained in medicine, dispensing simple remedies, especially as a means to secure a hearing where prejudice prevailed. McCartney, in his usual blunt way, attacked the practice: "It is said that a missionary naturally is more able to heal disease than a Chinese quack. This may be so, but for my part I can see no difference between an Anglo-Saxon quack and a Chinese quack."[136] Robert Beebe also disapproved of clergymen doing medical work except for looking after their own families when professional help was not available. He thought it potentially dangerous to the patients and to the reputation of the mission.[137] Similarly, the Editor of the *CMJ*, after praising the "faithful men who have trodden this difficult path [Christian ministry]" went on to state, "that of all classes of professional men, the average minister is the very least fitted to practice the science of medicine."[138] Eventually the medical profession prevailed over the clergy and the proportion of purely medical men increased so that, between 1873 and 1905, all but 39 of the 259 men (85 percent) who arrived were physicians only.[139]

SIZE OF HOSPITAL

Another factor, which would have affected the patient's experience of hospital, was its size. There was pressure to increase the number of beds to cope with increasing demand but any expansion was limited by the availability of staff and, to a lesser extent, of funds. In addition, if any staff became available the various missionary societies adopted different policies as regards the priority they put on expanding existing facilities or opening up new fields of influence.

Missionary hospitals in China came in all sizes.[140] Of those replying to the 1910 CMMA statistical survey, a hospital with between thirty and forty beds was the most common (modal size) and the median hospital had between fifty and sixty beds.[141] This picture, though, is somewhat misleading because those hospitals that reported having both male and female beds were generally in effect two separate hospitals: separate buildings in separate compounds. When this feature of hospitals in China is taken into account, it emerges that women's hospitals tended to be small: the majority having between 10 and 30 beds.[142] Men's hospitals, on the other hand, were more often medium sized: the majority having between 20 and 60 beds.[143]* Presumably, smaller hospitals, while meaning fewer people came under the influence of the 'physician as evangelist,' did enable a closer relationship between them and their Chinese patients.

So, whilst the extent to which local custom was taken into account would have affected the ease, or anxiety, with which the patient approached the foreign institution, administrative procedures, arrangement of physical spaces, and staffing would have also had an impact on a patient's experience in the hospital. Admission policies, for example, not only determine whether or not a patient himself is admitted, but also affect the nature of one's fellow patients. It was a conjunction of the situation in America as regards opportunities for women with the reticence of Chinese women to be attended by a man, that determined that relatively more patients in China would be treated by a female physician than in America. While the size of the hospital and the ratio of beds provided for men and women would have had some influence on patients, there are other aspects of life in hospital that had a more direct impact. Apart from the nature of medical treatment, these include the arrangements made for sleeping, eating, and nursing; the extent of enforcement of rules and regulations on the ward; how long the patient stayed in hospital; and how dying and death were dealt with, all of which would have colored the patient's experience.

*see www.michellerenshaw.com

Chapter Nine
Life on the Ward

Certainly it is difficult to keep patients from expectorating on the floor and from storing food, articles of clothing, and tobacco and pipes in the bed.

—John Kerr, 1873[1]

Patients in China would have experienced a wide range in the general appearance and amenity of hospitals at the turn of the century. S. R. Hodge's rhetorical question provides a glimpse into what they might have encountered in the 1890s. He was perhaps being more optimistic than practical when he asked: "Why should a Mission hospital be a series of sheds with hard boards to lie on, and with barest of furniture in its wards? Why should we not make them as comfortable as the hospitals for our poor at home, providing such things as water beds, air-pillows and invalid chairs?"[2]

What Hodge did not include was an account of the difficulty many missionaries faced achieving the most basic of requirements—cleanliness. According to the editor of the *CMMJ* in 1901, it was a "sad fact [that] wards of too many of our mission hospitals too nearly approach the condition of the homes of the inmates."[3] Incidentally, the belief that Chinese homes were dirty was not universal among Western medical men and women. When Dr Arthur Stanley, the Health Officer in Shanghai, wrote an article about Chinese hygiene, W. Hamilton Jefferys agreed with him that "as far as natural hygiene goes Chinese hygiene is in some important respects superior to that in both the large cities and in the country districts of Europe and America . . . London, Philadelphia, Naples especially, and Italy in general."[4] Jefferys added his own experience in Philadelphia of "finding [a] child in a garret room approached by a narrow ladder-like staircase, one of eight people in a room ten by twelve feet, two minute windows nailed down, so that neither of them could be opened . . . The room crowded with old clothes, vermin and other live stock, stale food and urine standing, and the air literally rotten."[5] A number of the correspondents who took issue with Stanley disagreed with his claim that prostitution and drunkenness was less prevalent than at home but no one challenged his opinion about Chinese hygiene.

Nevertheless, many mission hospitals struggled to achieve the sanitary conditions advocated by hospital reformers at home. The Jieyang 揭扬 Hospital in Guangdong reported, in 1904, that, "from the point of view of an enlightened physician of the twentieth century [their hospital was] unhygienic, unsanitary and dirty, in spite of strenuous and united efforts to make it otherwise."[6] Even as late as 1919, another was to write, "no more can be tolerated wards which are dirty and disorderly, patients who are clad in their own 'questionably clean garments' and cared for by their own 'questionably capable' friends or hirelings."[7]

In contrast, Main's hospital at Hangzhou clearly impressed Isabella Bird when she visited in 1896. She described it as, "abreast of our best hospitals in lighting, ventilation, general sanitation, arrangement and organisation . . . the purity of the walls, floors, and bedding is so great as to make one long for a speck of comfortable dirt."[8] She waxed even more effusive in her praise for the large ward in the women's hospital with its, "highly varnished floor, flowers, pictures, tables, chairs, and harmonium [like a] pleasant double drawing-room in a large English mansion."[9]

FURNISHING AND BEDDING

In America, the idea that the hospital setting could be intimidating is obvious from the many references in annual reports to the trouble they took to make the rooms 'homelike.' The Sisters of Mercy described how they had taken "special care . . . to the proper furnishing of the private rooms . . . all tastes and likings, the simplest as well as the most fastidious can be satisfied." Their concern also extended to the wards, where the "the comfort and convenience of patients have been carefully considered" in the design and furnishing.[10] The Lancaster Hospital 1906 report included a photograph of a private room, "handsomely furnished by friends," with its pristine white sheets, dressing table and washstand with mirrors, chair for a visitor, and curtained windows, which was typical of what American hospital administrators considered 'homelike.'*

In China, too, hospitals considered the effect that furnishings might have on their patients. After all, if it had proved difficult to persuade patients

---

*see www.michellerenshaw.com

to enter a foreign compound how much more difficult would it be to persuade them to actually live there? L. G. Thacker of the Quanzhoufu 泉州府 Women's Hospital in Fujian, considered it imperative to take a patient's physical comfort seriously because, as he said, "they hardly know they have souls, but they know they have bodies."[11]

A. Marston, of the SPG Hospital at Peking, on the other hand, thought: "We have to repress our desires for wards and hospital nursing until the people are more ready to appreciate them." In her view, hospital accommodation in China was "sufficient" for their present needs.[12]

Economic considerations, though, were just as important as concern for Chinese comfort when it came to furnishing mission hospitals. The choice of beds in particular was a major concern. Whenever a report of the opening of a new hospital appeared, mention was made of the type of beds: the most pride was expressed in beds of American or English manufacture with iron frames."[13] Apparently, not all of the CMS patients at Ningbo fully appreciated these 'luxuries.' Although the hospital was "furnished with iron spring bedsteads, and as a rule these are greatly appreciated, and patients strongly object to being removed to the hard beds in the ward for septic cases. On the other hand, we have walked into wards at night, and have been surprised to see several patients sleeping on the floor, the reason given being that the floor was more comfortable."[14]

Cost often meant that a minority of Chinese patients experienced the foreign bed. For example, at the Soochow Hospital in 1914, Dr Park reported that although a small ward of twelve beds, to be used for the most important surgical work, was "fitted with Lawson Tait beds and with bedding and clothing as a hospital should have, it is the only part of our hospital which is so equipped."[15] In 1919, when Balme conducted his survey, only forty-five percent of the hospitals had *any* foreign beds. However, not all agreed that expensive foreign beds were necessary or, even, desirable.

Charles Lewis, who, as we have seen earlier, favored building in the Chinese style because he believed this would make patients feel more at home, carried this philosophy through to the provision of beds: his were "boards on trestles such as the patients were used to sleeping on at home."[16] Another early hospital, at Funing 福甯 in North China, described their wards as being off a courtyard, "very simply arranged and furnished . . . with tiled floors, trestles for beds and lumps of firewood for pillows. But it is the best we can do and the people are satisfied."[17]

When it came to bedding, some followed Richard Wolfendale's advice—he advocated that missionaries, rather than imitating the home hospital, should look to indigenous custom. In his prescription for the ideal mission hospital, he argued that bedding and clothing need not be foreign: "blankets, foreign sheets, and pyjamas are not really required. We are not come out to China to make the Chinese British or Americans. The cotton vests, etc., worn by them is all that one desires, provided they be kept white and clean. Then the *pukai* [cotton wool quilt] can be kept absolutely clean by changing the outside covering."[18] A photograph taken in a ward at the APM *An-ting* Hospital for Men in Beijing gives some idea of the ward conditions. (see Plate 23) In Luella Masters' MEM hospital at Fuzhou, the problem of indigenous versus foreign bedding was avoided as patients not only paid for their board but also provided their own "fuel, food and bedding" and the hospital stepped in only if the patient's was "too dirty or not suitable." In such cases, the hospital rented bedding to patients, or, if they were very poor, provided it at no cost.[19] As far as the *type* of bedding was concerned, straw mattresses in removable cotton covers were considered ideal: "by emptying and burning the straw, boiling the mattress and pillow covers and washing iron frames and wire springs the beds can be effectively cleansed and vermin exterminated."[20] Balme's 1919 call for hospitals to provide clean bedding and clothing gives some indication of the conditions prevalent in many hospitals: "It is quite useless to spend soap and water on a dirty patient if he is to pass his time sleeping in dirty clothes or on verminous bedding . . . and it as well to remember that private patients, who gladly pay for private rooms, are often the dirtiest of all." [21]

Some of those who were early into the field, especially in the north of the country, fully embraced traditional Chinese sleeping arrangements in their hospitals. Douthwaite, who established the hospital for the CIM at Yantai (Chefoo), explained that his guiding principle was to arrange his hospital "in accordance with the tastes and habits of the people, as far as can be consistent with cleanliness. We have a few beds for surgical cases, but most of the patients prefer the brick k'ang to which they are accustomed." In his hospital, the *kang* 炕 was a brick platform with a top composed of stone slabs plastered with clay, which was heated by burning grass, or other fuel. In summer, it was covered with straw matting and, in cold weather, padded quilts. His patients preferred "these hard, comfortless beds [to the] spring mattresses which are provided for those who desire them [and would] lie or sit for weeks, quite happy and contented."[22] Peck described the *kang* common in Chinese homes in Shandong as being built, in autumn, of mud bricks and warmed, mainly, by the waste heat from the food-kettle. In spring the *kang* were dismantled and, with the valuable soot, spread as fertilizer on the fields: wooden beds were used in summer. Peck wondered aloud whether he should "adopt some modification of this plan, or confine them to beds

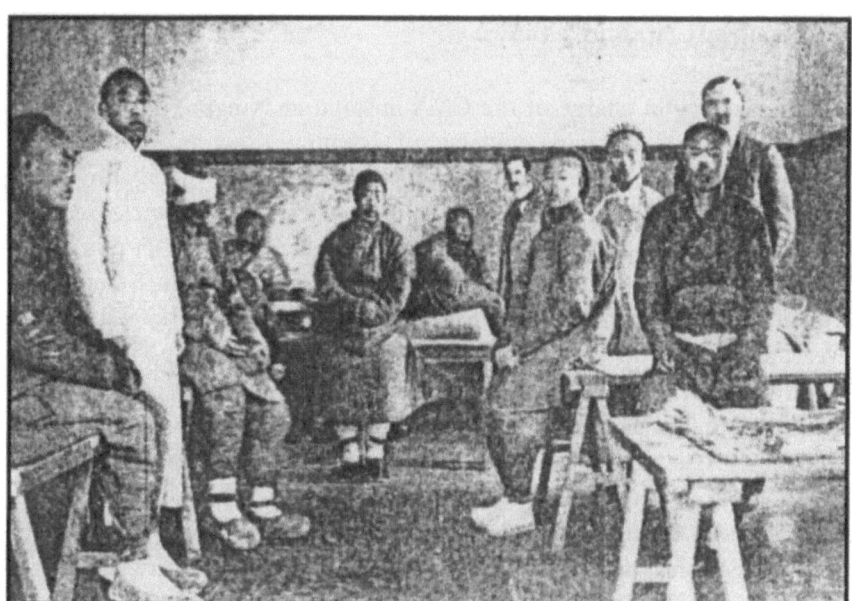

Plate 23. **A ward in the APM An-ting Hospital for Men (APM), Peking**
Source: *Hospitals in China. Medical Mission Series.* 1912: 11.
Courtesy of the Burke Library, Union Theological College, New York

and try and warm the beds during the cold weather . . . the latter plan most consonant with our foreign ideas, is most at variance with the habits of the people." He noted that Mackenzie, at Tianjin, had opted to provide foreign beds but his was the only "testimony [he knew] of, as to experience in this latitude."[23] He decided to retain the *kang,* whether driven by the desires of his patients or lack of funds, he does not say but, in 1902, he provided his patients with only "a spot on a brick bed big enough to sleep on . . . to be shared perhaps with a dozen others. . . ."[24]

An interesting example of the use of the *kang* was to be found in the LMS hospital at Qizhou 祁州 in Shanxi. There, the women's ward comprised "one long k'ang capable of accommodating 15 patients comfortably." This was in contrast with the men's ward, which was "larger, and possesses 25 separate k'angs for as many patients." They offered no explanation as to the reasoning behind this distinction but no doubt, it was a considerable advance on having to resort to, "stowing away patients in the coal cellar for lack of accommodation."[25] This brings us to another common feature of hospitals in China—overcrowding.

OVERCROWDING

The missionary in charge of the CMS hospital at Ningbo, described how they coped when a "raging epidemic of dysentery" saw an influx of boys into hospital from a Christian orphanage in 1910. They had "allowed 27 patients to occupy a 17 bed ward; our floor being so infinitely cleaner than some of their own beds, and no difficulty at all was found in putting up 'extras' on the planks."[26] But periodic outbreaks of disease such as this one were not the only causes of overcrowding in hospitals: sometimes it was the everyday demand that was simply overwhelming. The LMS at Xiaogan 孝感 in Hubei started in 1900 with only six beds but they immediately received so many patients that they had to turn all the available rooms into wards: "the patients slept anywhere—on forms or tables, and *under* them, on the bare floor, even in the yard outside. For weeks it was unsafe to move about the dispensary at night without a light. One was pretty sure to kick some patient's legs or tread on him. We had only a small native house, but within four and a half months 197 patients had managed to come and go."[27]

Although physicians grumbled about inadequate accommodation in annual reports aimed at potential donors, many appeared to think that the Chinese were not so concerned. Josephine Bixby observed, at her American Baptist hospital at Jieyang in Guangdong, where patients "have often to sleep two—not to say three—in a bed . . . being crowded into narrow quarters [it] never has an adverse influence upon the temper of the Chinese." She cited a couple of typical situations: "A crying baby in a ward containing a dozen or twenty other patients calls forth no comment unless questions are asked as to how the little one rests . . . another patient with a foul-smelling disease is quietly endured as one of the conditions of receiving hospital privileges."[28]

A feature peculiar to mission hospitals elsewhere further exacerbated overcrowding in hospitals. In America, under certain circumstances at St John's, for example, when a patient in a private room was "dangerously ill" the hospital allowed a friend, relative, or nurse to accompany them.[29] The situation in China was similar to that faced by a doctor in charge of a Western hospital in Japan in the 1870s, who commented: "we would have no patients had we not accepted their families."[30] In China, it was, firstly, a matter of cultural sensitivities. As Balme explained, it had been "neither easy nor polite to induce patients to come into the hospital unless they were allowed to bring their friends to live with them." John A. Anderson, who was working in Western Yunnan, agreed: he "rather liked his patients to bring their friends or servants with them. It helped to keep the patients from being homesick, and it brought more people under the influence of the gospel."[31] Secondly, it was a matter of necessity. Few hospitals, especially in the early days, had nursing staff.[32] Those they did have were mostly men, more properly described as orderlies. If patients in China needed nursing care they had to provide their own. "Two or three servants" frequently accompanied private patients[33] and family members—husbands, sons, daughters, sisters, fathers or mothers—attended patients in wards. By 1920, Balme acknowledged that the psychological necessity for patients to be attended by family had diminished, but the lack of nurses and orderlies remained. This meant that thirty-seven percent of the hospitals in his survey reported that *all* patients brought friends to stay with them in the wards, and a further fifty-one percent allowed them to do so. In other words, as late as 1920, eighty-eight percent of hospitals had to accommodate friends and family—who often slept on the floor next to the patient "for want of a spare bed."[34] Lucy Saville's hospital for women at Beijing was one of the exceptions. In preparation for introducing clinical training for Chinese nurses, she reported (in 1906) that she had "almost entirely abolished the heretofore prevalent practice of allowing mothers and friends to live with the patient in the hospital."[35] Josephine Bixby, on the other hand, described a situation of having three women in a small room. It becomes obvious that the three patients were not alone in this room—when the attendant of one patient had to leave, the attendants of the other two took over all her duties—there had been at least six people in the room "scarcely large enough for two."[36]

HOSPITAL FOOD

Nursing, reassurance, and company, important as they were, were not the only things relatives and friends provided. In many hospitals, they were also responsible for patients' nutrition. They collected fuel and brought, prepared, and cooked patients' meals. Peck painted a grim picture of what little he was able to offer his patients in the way of physical amenities, and the consequences: "we have not money to feed you. You must bring your own grain or be able to buy your food . . . we cannot supply you with clean bedding. You must bring your own. So our patients are often enveloped in garments saturated with indescribable filth . . . we have no staff of nurses; if you are going to need attendance, you must bring some one from your home; thus there are two or more persons to feed instead of one. We cannot even furnish fuel for cooking the food."[37]

In Chinese hospitals, the management of the culinary department, when it was present, was also distinctive. Whereas American hospitals included a cook on the staff, many hospitals in China did not employ a cook directly. For example, Duncan Main's hospital arranged with a "head cook" who engaged four others to help. The terms of the contract allowed a payment of twelve cents per day, or $3.60 per month, on behalf of each patient, "whether on a special diet or not."[38]

Most Chinese hospitals provided somewhere for cooking, usually a lean-to or shed in the compound away from the hospital-proper. Family and friends cooked on a "native stove" using every variety of fuel, "from coal balls to bamboo sticks."[39] Dr Mary Latimer James described her early days with the American Church hospital at Wuchang, where they were, "forced to cook in a dark shed-like structure, wedged into the angle of a building, and I am not infrequently put to it to cheer up the cook and provide warm food for the patients and nurses, when snow swirls around his neck, or heavy rains wash away not merely his fire, but also his primitive brick stove."[40]

A minority of hospitals did institute their own culinary department. Josephine Bixby reported, in 1905, that three years previously they had abandoned the system of requiring patients to bring charcoal and cooking utensils with them. Instead, they charged them 100 *cash* a day for meals prepared by a general cook. The new system had "met with much opposition in the start, for it was not their 'custom,' but it is now in such general favor that no one would wish to go back to the old plan."[41] It is hardly surprising that Bixby welcomed having control over a kitchen. Her American training and experience would have led her to expect to be operating under a set of rules such as those in place at the Lancaster General or Auburn City Hospitals. Visitors to private patients at Auburn were forbidden to bring in "wine, liquors, food or delicacies of any kind . . . without the permission of the Superintendent or attending physician."[42] Similarly, at the Lancaster General, in addition to the same prohibition, patients were not "permitted the use of any diet other than that which may be ordered by the proper officers."[43] Bixby, who clearly had a low opinion of her patients' behavior, could now regulate their diet. As she saw it, this was a "very important thing with people who are so prone to over-eat, under-eat, to eat dead or half decayed food rather than see it thrown out, and to eat at any and all hours of the day or night."[44] It was not until 1919 that the Soochow Hospital abandoned the "farming out method" and had its own kitchen, which, although more expensive, they thought afforded them more control over the quality of the patients' food. They congratulated themselves that, despite the cholera epidemic that year, no case of cholera had arisen within the hospital.[45]

Writing in 1919, Balme thought that the kitchen was "admittedly the weakest spot in the majority of mission hospitals of to-day." He was here referring mainly to physical conditions, such as lack of screening from flies, inadequate removal of fumes and smoke from dirty stoves, and too many "hiding-places for stale food." On the subject of food, he was less prescriptive and referred simply to the need for "a controlled dietary."[46] However, and possibly luckily for the patients, many medical missionaries were unable to exercise any control over diet because their patients were being provided for individually by friends and relatives.

DIET

It would seem from the literature that most historians of the hospital in America and Britain have considered the question of patients' diet to be of only passing interest.[47] Mention of food is usually restricted to noting that nineteenth-century hospitals, seeking to attract private patients, used the 'daintiness' of the food as a selling point. Contemporary American hospital financial reports also shed little light on the subject because expenditure on foodstuffs is subsumed, more often than not, under the headings; 'provisions' or 'table bills.' An indication of what constituted 'regular fare' at Lancaster General in 1905 cannot be deduced from the long lists of donations from its many active women's auxiliaries: from puddings and jams to fruit and vegetables, cereals and cooking oils, to ducks, chickens and eggs. The lists of donations 'in kind' served the same purpose as the list of financial contributions—to thank those who gave, and encourage others. The hospital made no specific requests for types of foods nor, it would seem, did they refuse any donations, so it is not possible to deduce their policy on patients' diet. Auburn City Hospital Thanksgiving and Christmas dinners of 1909 appear to have been lavish affairs, with donations of turkeys, chickens, gallons of oysters and ice cream, plates of "macaroons and lady fingers," and fruit, including apples, bananas, grapes, oranges, figs, and dates listed as being donated.[48] "Special diets" were available for some patients, at additional cost, but as to their composition, no information is given.[49] If the hospital followed the dictates of contemporary literature as to what constituted 'invalid' food, one can only imagine that these special diets were unappetizing. While a popular contemporary manual for medical practitioners emphasized the therapeutic value of a nourishing diet, stressing it should be "bland [and] non-irritating."[50] The only condiment allowed was common salt, and that, in strict moderation. Certain stimulants were allowable in cases where "the appetite for food is almost wanting"; these included "wine, ale, and porter [because] previous habits must be attended to, and the drunkard must be supplied with his accustomed stimulant."[51] A household encyclopedia aimed at women, published in 1900, suggested feeding a patient various forms of gruel, meat broths, and jellies. All were prepared by boiling the main ingredient—cornmeal, oatmeal, beef, chicken, mutton or rice—in water for several hours. The writer described them as containing "little nutritional matter," and made no suggestion as to how to make them more palatable.[52] It seems that Cecil Davenport with the LMS at Wuchang in 1899 was following this regimen but he despaired of his Chinese patients who "almost invariably . . . refuse to take beef tea, or milk, or chicken broth. They have not come to the stage of knowledge that would lead them to honor the great physician who had it put on his tombstone that "he fed fevers." They prefer nothing, or peanuts, or raw pears, or pig's stomach, and all sorts of sweetmeats—and smuggle them in and eat them."[53]

DIETETICS IN CHINA

Most medical missionaries took little interest in the details of their patients' diet. From a survey of the scant supply of articles and correspondence, it seems that most of the men were more concerned about the practicalities of providing food than the nature of the food itself. In the main, it was a few women physicians who commented on diet. A notable exception was Fred Judd who wrote a letter to the editor of the *CMMJ* in 1906 calling on "senior medical people" to contribute their experience of "dieting patients on native food." He had observed that, in comparison with America, "in this land [diet] seems to occupy an even more important place, at any rate in the minds and habits of our Chinese patients. One of the commonest questions they ask is 'what foods shall I abstain from?'" He thought that, although many Chinese ideas may be "fanciful or even ridiculous," they *were* based on experience and, "in some cases we may even be able to learn a lesson from them."[54] His call apparently went largely unheeded since he was still asking the 1911 Conference to deal with "practical topics . . . such as the role of Chinese diet in disease."[55] Judd seems to have been one of the few medical missionaries who took seriously the fact that dietetics had always been an integral part of Chinese traditional medicine.

The idea of regulating diet as a way of preventing or curing disease was not confined to China. Ancient Greek and Roman medicine attended to diet but in the West, according to Ackerknecht (who included a history of dietetics in his history of therapeutics), prescribing diet for illness steadily declined throughout the eighteenth century.[56] In America the 'diet kitchen' did not form part of the normal hospital until after the Civil War in the mid-nineteenth century whereas in China during the Zhou dynasty (1121–249

B.C.E.) the imperial "department of dietetics even preceded that of medicine in order of priority."[57] In all societies, including the missionaries' home countries, there was a considerable body of folklore relating to the efficacy of various foods and medicinal herbs but in China the common wisdom surrounding food and diet belonged to a far more coherent, 'rational' system. Dietetics was a distinct but integral component of the traditional medical system.

Chinese medicine, a complex system woven from three parallel traditions—demonology, Confucianism and Taoism—is grounded in the same *yin-yang* 阴阳 polarity, *wuxing* 五行 (Five Phases), and *qi* 气 metaphysics that underpins all Chinese traditional thought about science and nature.[58] Illness indicates disharmony, and disharmony is the result of imbalances such as too little (depletion) or too much (repletion) of *yin* or *yang*. Harmony, and thus health, is indicated by the free and smooth flow of *qi*. Ideally, illness should be prevented rather than cured but when treatment is called for it is to restore the balance of *yin* and *yang*. As well as the drugs (vegetable, animal, and mineral) described within the various pharmacopoeia published throughout Chinese history, all foods were classified within the same cosmological system and could be prescribed according to their supposed interaction with the person, his disease, his temperament, the season,and so forth. For example, foods, classified on a continuum ranging from hot (or heating) to cold (or cooling), could be used to counteract the effects of diseases whose symptoms were similarly classified. Thus, 'warming' foods may be used to compensate for problems classified as 'cool' and, *vice versa,* 'cool' foods help to reduce heat symptoms.[59] There was not necessarily consistency throughout the country as to which foods belonged to which category but the theory that internal balance should be aimed for by giving the appropriate foods was universally understood.

LAY KNOWLEDGE OF DIETETICS

Knowledge of the role of diet in the treatment of disease and recuperation was not confined to medical practitioners but was widespread among all classes of the society. Anderson says, "almost all traditional Chinese families had someone who knew a good deal about traditional nutrition, and everybody had someone in the neighborhood who knew a lot."[60] As well as wisdom handed down from generation to generation, the explosion of popular publishing, which occurred in late Ming and early Qing China, increased people's knowledge. A feature of the popular literature, which included "household encyclopedias, guides to everyday etiquette and family ritual ... medical and prescription handbooks, morality books, almanacs, and manuals of geomancy"[61] was their "close connection with everyday activities."[62] According to a conservative estimate made at Hankou, fifty percent of their adult patients could read public health notices "readily"[63] which meant that the literate and semi-literate had access to medical knowledge, which included dietetic theories.

Just as the patients' friends and relatives would have among them experts in diet, so a hospital cook, left to his own devices, would have brought dietary knowledge and beliefs with him.

THE HOSPITAL COOK

Such was the situation in McCartney's hospital at Chongqing. In this institution, in 1893, the "bill of fare provided [was] two kinds of vegetables and rice three times a day, with beef on Wednesdays and pork on Saturdays."[64] McCartney usually did not itemize food within his financial statements but in 1908 he was on furlough and his colleague included some details in *his* report. The proportion of expenditure on the various classes of food was: 64 percent on rice, 16 percent on vegetable, 11 percent on meat, 4.8 percent on salt, and 4.4 percent on lard.[65] This, when compared with the expenditure by mill workers in Shanghai in 1920 (53 percent on rice, 8.5 percent on vegetables and legumes, 11.4 percent on meat, fish and seafood), would indicate that patients at Chongqing were being fed a reasonably typical Chinese diet.[66] McCartney was apparently happy with the arrangement he had with his cook but, as the American-trained Chinese physician, Shi Mei-yu, pointed out, "so often the kitchen is given to the entire charge of the cook who takes his squeezes and gives the patients very poor food—poor as to food value."[67] It is noteworthy that it was a Chinese woman doctor, albeit trained in America, who wrote the only substantial article dealing with diet published before 1916 in the journal read by most medical missionaries. Because "nourishing food," with sunlight and fresh air, were "such an important part of the cure," Shi Mei-yu advocated taking charge of the kitchen and paying close attention to "the study of dietetics." She did not use typical Chinese cosmological language but, rather, the Western scientific terminology familiar to her audience. She advised them to follow Chinese custom in the preparation of food; to focus on the foods that they liked; and to take account of differences between the normal diet of the rich and the poor. Both classes ate rice and vegetables—the rich added meat and the poor, meat-substitutes. In particular, they used "varieties of beans and modifications of beans" which were plentiful and cheap as were eggs and fish. The examples she gave of meals provided at her hospital attest to the variety. Morning, noon, and evening meals were based on rice supplemented, in the morning, with "beans, bean curd, fresh vegetable, and a little dried turnip or squash." At noon she added "one kind of meat, some form of beans, two kinds of vegetables" and in the evening "some form of bean curd, eggs, and two kinds of vegetables." She promoted the use of ripe fruit but discouraged the use of "salt vegetables, salted meats, and peppers" while acknowledging that small quantities acted as "appetizers and may be allowed." She understood that her patients did not take kindly to some foods, such as "straight meat broth," a common feature of American invalid food, so she suggested flavoring them with vegetables "like turnip, arrowroot, celery, dried dates, onions, or a handful of rice." She thought that convalescents, or those with "weak digestion" and consequently on a restricted diet, could still have variety: she used "soft rice, arrowroot flour, lily bulb flour, bean curd cheese, vermicelli, eggs, vegetables, or light meats cooked very tender, scraped beef, and cooked fruit." To make milk more palatable for Chinese, who had "never tasted it," she had found that "giving a bite of ginger" took the taste away. She considered that it was impractical to prepare complex menus for each meal and recommended allowing for patients' idiosyncrasies by preparing all food according to the rules of a "wholesome diet" from which the patient may choose because, "obviously in regard to particulars, each patient must be a law unto himself."[68]

Anderson has demonstrated, in relation to the boat people of Castle Peak Bay, Hong Kong, whom he claims are "not very different from other Chinese," that "in practice, essentially all illnesses—other than broken bones and the like—were first treated by diet modification . . . the eldest woman in the household was normally the chief caregiver; others acted under her orders."[69] In determining what foods to feed to a patient in hospital, Anderson makes the point that "diet therapy had to be tailored to the individual. People differ in their response to food . . . often a food that was "cool" for most people was experienced as "heating" by some . . . individual experience over time, and the immediate environmental context, both affected nutritional therapy. Any caregiver would take these factors into account."[70] Thus, from a patient's point of view, given that the majority were being fed by friends and relatives or a Chinese cook, we can assume that local dietary customs would have been very evident in the hospital. The majority of patients of missionary hospitals were poor, the food they could afford would have been limited to rice, and a little vegetable but it is most unlikely, given that they were steeped in the tradition, that anyone would have fed the patient food that was contra-indicated.

It is beyond the scope of this book to make any assessment or judgment as to whether Chinese patients would have been better or worse off than their counterparts in the West, as far as diet was concerned. The Health Officer at Shanghai, though, did write: "Concerning the quality of the Chinese food a European would generally say there is no 'stamina' in it. Diseases, however, like rickets and gout, which are attributed to disordered metabolism, are conspicuous by their absence among the Chinese. Functional disease of the stomach and alimentary tract are less common than among Europeans, and the teeth of the Chinese are admitted by all to be exceptionally beautiful and good."[71]

In one hospital, some patients definitely did suffer from the effects of a rule not to accept patients who would not agree to "our diets and stick to them." Anne Fearn acknowledged that it was her "desire for cleanliness, and in our anxiety to provide only the best foods [that] inadvertently were responsible for bringing two dread diseases into the compound, tuberculosis and beriberi." By providing (the more expensive) polished rice the hospital had "unknowingly taken away the very vitamins they needed because, aside from their *san woen van* (three bowls of rice), they ate little else save a flavouring of cabbage, pork, chicken, or fish. First one girl and then another was sent home to die."[72]

It is unlikely that such a tragedy would have occurred had friends and relatives been providing the girls' food. As well, the advantage to the patient's psychological health is self-evident. As Anderson puts it, "when they could do nothing else—as was all too often the case—they could at least make the patient feel that family, neighbors, and community cared and were acting to help."[73]

It would seem that, rather than a conscious decision to accommodate Chinese preferences, a coincidence of factors—the Chinese custom of relatives being responsible for the care for the sick; the importance of diet in the Chinese medical system; and the missionaries' lack of resources—combined to create an indigenous institution, so far as 'hospital food' was concerned. It is doubtful that medical missionaries would have had much success controlling their patients' diets, even if they had had the resources, as will become clear when we examine their attempts to regulate patients' and their family's behavior.

CONTROL OF PATIENTS

The change from mid-nineteenth century almshouse to early twentieth-century American medical facility was accompanied by an increasing emphasis on control of patients. The efficiency that was the mark of a well-run ward required that patients' demands not be allowed to prevail. Rosenberg's portrayal of life on the American hospital ward in the 1870s, which had not changed significantly since the beginning of the century, in many ways could have been of life in a mission hospital in China well into the twentieth century. During this period American patients had, according to Rosenberg, "hoped and expected to find relatives and friends a source of emotional support in strange and threatening surroundings ... been reluctant to take baths and change out of their own clothes; slept in wooden beds on straw-filled mattresses and ... used the hot flues for spittoons and emptied their urinals into the sink." Their visitors had smuggled in food and drink and paid little attention to stipulated visiting hours, and vermin—"lice, bedbugs, flies, and even rats [were] tenacious realities of hospital life."[74] In other words, the chaotic circumstances were similar to those existing in many mission hospitals in China in the late Qing. On the other hand, by 1910 in America the transformation of the hospital was complete and "the average patient's experience had become something very different." The social organization of the hospital had also changed and, in particular, "appropriate discipline" was to be imposed on patients, who were considered to be "exacting and, in some cases, querulous."[75] It was not that nineteenth-century hospitals had lacked rules, but now the rules were more likely to be enforced. All hospitals established and published a set of rules of behavior for patients, and often, their visitors. Patients at the Lancaster General were supposed to "conduct themselves with decorum towards each other, the officers of the hospital, and the nurses and servants; they shall not use profane or indecent language, become intoxicated, or behave rudely or indecently; they shall not smoke tobacco or play at any game of chance in the hospital."[76]

They were also forbidden to leave the hospital without permission, read in bed at night, or eat any food not ordered for them. Charity patients were expected to work for their keep by helping with nursing, or other duties. Visiting was restricted to two hours per day (in the afternoon) and visitors were forbidden to bring in foodstuffs or medicines for patients.[77] The Auburn City Hospital operated under a similar regime but included a proscription on bringing more than "one change of underclothing [or] any piece of baggage larger than a hand bag" into the hospital. Private patients could have visitors anytime between 11 A.M. and 8.30 P.M. but they were asked to visit only their "own friends and to leave the Hospital quietly without loitering in the hallways or on the stairs."[78] Sometimes more indirect methods of control were employed; staff could distance themselves from patients using, not only the barrier of the uniform which set them apart, but also the manner in which they addressed or treated them. Rosenberg gives the example of nurses being encouraged to control patients by withdrawing "little privileges she has been enjoying—by passing her with a curt 'Good Morning' and so on, until she realizes she must obey the general law."[79]

Hospitals in China, too, had rules: "We find that the Chinese like discipline (providing it is not strict)," McCartney said in 1893, and "have endeavored to have all the rules obeyed which were made when the hospital was established."[80] He adopted a peculiarly Chinese avenue to disseminate his rules, a calendar. Since the Zhou dynasty, astrological and calendrical calculations had been the exclusive prerogative of the state and the resulting calendars were distributed only among officials. However, during the Tang, to counter the proliferation of illegal versions spawned by the invention and spread of printing, the state started to publish special editions for sale to the public.[81] During the Qing about 2,340,000 were printed each year, and after distribution to officials, surplus copies sold "to an eager public."[82] As well as basic calendrical information such as the phases of the moon, the year's solar divisions, times of sunrise and sunset and so on, they provided monthly guidance as to agriculture, meteorology, and auspicious days and times for various ritual and mundane activities. The latter included such things as "bathing and grooming, cutting out clothes, household cleaning and decoration, establishing a new bed. . . ."*[83] A popular derivative of the calendar, the privately published almanacs were, according to the Rev. A. P. Parker, "perhaps the most universally circulated book in China."[84] They were cheap and extremely useful tools for daily life, providing advice on "family life, food, etiquette, travel . . ." and, by the late nineteenth and early twentieth centuries, "had become conduits for new information on recent educational and political changes, modern science and technology . . ."[85] McCartney, capitalizing on the Chinese fondness for such literature, produced his own calendar in which were printed "plain instructions about itch, small-pox, tuberculosis and the like" as well as the "rules and regulations of the hospital."[86] He distributed over fifteen thousand of them, without charge, to his clinic patients in 1908.[87] Others also discovered the value of the calendar and missionary societies started producing them in large numbers. According to the U.S. Consular Service in China, "no form of advertising is more popular with the Chinese than an attractive calendar issued toward the Chinese New Year."[88] But they were not without their own inherent dangers; missionaries wanting to produce them were advised to take care that

*see www.michellerenshaw.com

the information was accurate because giving the "hour of eclipses" wrongly was "very prejudicial to the reputation of Christianity."[89]

Not all physicians were as keen on rules as McCartney. The Chinese were viewed, by some, "as not only ignorant but conceited and self-willed, and sickness does not render them any more amenable to laws and regulations. The key to successful work amongst them lies in unfailing good-humour and inexhaustible patience . . . and the combined exercise of gentle firmness and persuasive love. . . ."[90] W. Hamilton Jefferys advised medical missionaries that they would save themselves "endless trouble" and their patients "endless ingenuity" if they were to limit their "rules to the bare necessities and extend [their] elasticity to the utmost degree short of, and sometimes past, the breaking point." In his own hospital, St Luke's Hospital at Shanghai, the rules were restricted to forbidding gambling, and cooking or heating water, "except on the stove provided." Patients who refused treatment were required to leave. He advised breaking any rule that patients needed permission to leave the ward, and his guiding principle was "to say yes unless [there was a] good reason not to." His patients "may smoke and talk all night" and friends could come and go, or not go, as they pleased. They often slept on the floor next to the patient and ate hospital food, as long as they paid for it. He cited times when a patient had had as many as fifteen visitors at one time.[91] The central role of evangelism in a mission hospital goes some way to explain the reason for such advice and was enunciated by Miss G. L. Thacker, who wrote in 1912, "*Hospital Rules* are, of course, necessary, but any rule the obeying of which seriously detracts from a patient's idea of comfort may make him or her less receptive to the Gospel."[92]

Jefferys deftly summed up the essential difference between hospitals in China and those in America, from the point of view of the control over patients' behavior, when he wrote, "the hospital is far more homey and far more human than eleven-tenths of our rule-trodden institutions in the dear homeland, and it suits the Chinese patients very well indeed."[93]

LENGTH OF STAY—THE EVANGELISTS' DILEMMA

The desire to influence patients religiously played a role in the length of time a patient would stay in a hospital in China. Patients were more likely to be encouraged to stay longer than they would have had they been in America. Many factors affect the average time a patient spends in hospital, whether in America or China, which makes simple comparisons risky. These factors include, the mix of patients in terms of medical and surgical cases or, if mainly medical, the ratio of acute to chronic conditions; the type of treatment regimen in use, which can be related to the level and type of technology or staff available; seasonal conditions which affect the types of diseases encountered; and the presence of epidemic, or famine, in the locality. Less directly, where the patient lives,, the level of support they have in the neighborhood of the hospital, and cultural beliefs all have an effect.

In America, a general decrease in the length of a hospital stay coincided with the emphasis, in the newly established hospitals, on catering for acute rather than the chronic cases that had predominated in the earlier almshouse-type institution. In an effort to restrain rising costs associated with new technologies and improved facilities for private patients, hospital administrators attempted to shorten hospital stays. They succeeded to the extent that between 1870 and 1900 the average stay dropped from "roughly six weeks to one closer to three."[94]

In China, most medical missionaries concentrated more on the practice of surgery than in America. There were a number of reasons for the surgical focus: Western therapeutics at the time were not demonstrably more efficacious than Chinese except for "inoculation for smallpox; quinine therapy for malaria . . .; a certain number of medicinal plants not employed by Chinese doctors, such as digitalis; analgesia (e.g. using opium) and anesthesia; and even before anesthesia and antisepsis, a range of surgery including control of bleeding. . . ." In addition, around the turn of the century, "Chinese medicine . . . had a greater base of recorded effective drugs than Western medicine."[95]

Although China had a rich history of famous—probably legendary—surgeons performing 'amazing' operations stretching back to the sixth century B.C.E., surgery was never a major component of traditional medicine. In Qing China, the practice of waike 外科, which included, but was not confined to, surgery, was limited to acupuncture; counter-irritation measures, such as pinching the skin, application of plasters (blisters), and moxa; simple operations, including for harelip and entropion; and castration.[96] Western surgery, in particular of the eye and the removal of cumbersome, disfiguring tumors, provided a dramatic demonstration of the medical missionary's skill. The missionaries hoped, in addition, it would be seen as evidence of their technological superiority, which they believed to be a consequence of 'Christian civilization.' Kilborn noted that his practice was comprised of markedly more surgical than medical cases partly, he thought, "because the superiority of scientific surgery [was] more easily demonstrated to the Chinese than that of scientific medicine."[97]

The ratio of surgical to medical cases in a hospital affects the average length of a hospital stay, but few hospitals in China during the period under review reported their medical and surgical patients separately. The great majority gave total patient numbers, often divided into male and female, with a list of operations undertaken.[98] Most reports noted that surgical cases predominated but the few reports where data are available illustrate the difficulty of making generalizations. For example, in 1916 at the *Hua Mei* Hospital run by American Baptists at Ningbo the ratio of medical to surgical cases was 1: 1.53.[99] This figure is much lower than that provided by Park for the hospital run by the MEM at Suzhou, where the ratio (in 1914) was 1:2.63.[100] In Shanghai, at St Luke's Hospital for the Chinese, one of the oldest hospitals in a city with a long and extensive contact with foreigners, the situation seems to have been different from the rest of the country. Here, in 1904, the number of medical cases admitted to hospital was roughly equal to surgical, 398 to 468, or (1:1.18). The author of the report noted that every year they had witnessed a "marked increase in the quantity and severity of the accidental surgery ... due to the growing shipping and manufacturing interests of fast-growing Shanghai." He lays the blame for these dangers firmly at the feet of foreigners but, equally, attributes the "confidence of the natives in Western scientific methods [which] increases in leaps and bounds" to the efficacy of foreign surgical methods.[101]

In choosing to accept patients for surgery rather than those suffering from chronic conditions, for whom they could do little, missionaries faced a dilemma. Their principal and guiding purpose was evangelical and the longer a patient stayed with them in the hospital the better their chance of influencing them to accept Christianity. As the founder of the China Inland Mission, Hudson Taylor, had remarked to John Anderson, "chronic diseases are God's way of bringing people to himself, and that although from a medical point of view they are rather hopeless, they are very hopeful from the preacher's standpoint."[102]

Cole expressed the sentiments of many of his counterparts when he valued his female patients at Ningbo who were "under treatment for three or four months, which gives us a good opportunity for teaching them."[103] A number of patients appear to have taken up almost permanent residence in hospitals. Eliza Wells spoke, in 1904, of "a girl who has been an inmate of the hospital for several years ... she knows the gospel well, having heard it many, many times."[104] If, on the other hand, they took in long-term patients the number of people who would come under their influence was diminished. It was the perennial question of quantity versus quality, with the answer depending on whether the medical or religious imperative was paramount. In this dilemma were echoes of that other quandary medical missionaries found themselves in: was it more desirable to treat large numbers in the dispensary; spread the word widely whilst itinerating in the countryside;

or spend more time with fewer in hospital? The missionaries wanted it both ways—greater numbers and longer exposure. The tension created between these twin aims required a balancing act. They took in a mix of patients, surgical and medical, and encouraged them to stay long enough for the fullest recovery and most religious influence, but not so long as to take up beds sought after by potential patients and possible converts. The author of the first annual report of the Philander Smith Memorial Hospital at Nanjing, noted that they looked to inpatients, rather than outpatients, for results of religious work. They had observed that: "Many will accept the Gospel much as they take their medicine, seeming to think it is the way to do it at a foreign hospital, and that it will please us and gain favors. Others are probably honest in their desire to know the truth and take some pains to learn. A few other (sic) again, are not willing to hear, and will roll themselves up in their bed and cover their head when a service is held in the ward."[105]

As Francis Tucker commented: "results are most marked with the inpatients, those who stay in the hospital from several days to several months." So, during 1904, the hospital's "512 inpatients were urged to stay as long as they would that they might get the more physical and spiritual benefit." This policy had resulted in much overcrowding but little extra expense (for dressings and medicine only) since patients furnished their own food and bedding.[106] One of the earliest hospitals in which the shift of imperative from religious to medical was observable was the Hospital for Chinese at Shanghai, established by the LMS in 1844. In 1905, when hospitals in the interior were still young and endeavoring to gain acceptance, this hospital was fifty years old and a familiar part of the Shanghai medical scene. It adopted a policy of limiting admission to those who absolutely needed hospital treatment and reported, "for instance, 454 of the native police force were warded during 1904. During the year [1905] only 152 were warded, the rest being treated as out-patients, getting well just as soon, and probably getting back on duty the sooner." [107]

Without the religious imperative, hospitals in America had a simpler problem; they could concentrate on making efficiencies in hospital administration and control the type of patient they admitted, and thus reduce the length of time spent in hospital. The Auburn City Hospital 1910 annual report provides useful relevant data covering a number of years. In 1906, for example, there were 1.8 surgical cases to each medical case and the average stay was 18.5 days.[108] In China, McCartney was one of the few medical missionaries who regularly reported the number of "hospital days." In each year between 1904 and 1910 patients in the Auburn City Hospital spent fewer days in hospital on average than patients in McCartney's hospital at

Chongqing. At Auburn, the average length of stay gradually declined from twenty to a little over sixteen and a half.[109] At Chongqing between 1901 and 1911, on the other hand, the average length of stay was more consistent, hovering around twenty-five days.*[110] This figure was very close to that reported by the LMS Men's Hospital at Hankou in 1904—twenty-five and a half days.[111] As hospitals became more sophisticated, and shifted their emphasis from religious to professional, the time people spent in hospital decreased, more in line with their counterparts in America. For example, in 1917 when the Soochow Hospital had a number of specialist departments and classes of accommodation, the average stay for all patients was a mere 12.5 days. This increased to 14 days if those who stayed one or two days are removed from the calculation. The patients who stayed longest were those being treated for opium addiction; the length of stay also varied with the class of patient—third class patients staying the longest.[112]

SPECIALIZATION

There were neither enough medical people nor hospitals anywhere in China at the turn of the century to allow for the specialization, within the one institution or between institutions, such as was occurring in America and Britain. Other than isolated instances of establishments for a particular class of patient—an insane asylum (by Kerr at Canton[113]); a leper hospital (by Kuhne at Dongwan 东莞[114]) or a sanatorium for tuberculosis sufferers (by Main at Hangzhou[115])—the majority of hospitals still had only a single medical missionary, assisted by any Chinese he or she was able to train. This did not mean that all hospitals dealt with the same range of medical problems, however.

A survey of the lists of operations undertaken by various hospitals reveals that some degree of specialization did occur, and it seems to have had as much to do with the reputation of the physician as with any particular location or peculiar timing. Thus the Canton Hospital, which was made famous by Peter Parker for the number of bladder stone operations, continued to enjoy its reputation under Kerr, who, it was said, had performed more "stone operations [than any] other known surgeon, barring one."[116] Similarly, in 1904, one third of Samuel Cochran's sixty-five hospital patients at Huaiyuan 怀远 in Anhui were operated on for the same complaint. This increased to thirty-six the following year and to forty in the eight months to April 1906.[117] Cochran had "discovered and exploited a similarly profitable

*see www.michellerenshaw.com

field [as Kerr]."[118] In his 1910 work, Jefferys noted that *vesical calculus* (bladder stone) was "found pretty much all over China" and most hospitals would meet between one and ten cases each year. It was particularly prevalent in Guangdong and Anhui. As his information was based on reports from physicians, rather than any epidemiological survey, he cannot have known whether there were in fact more bladder stones in a particular population or simply that people sought out the doctors who had a reputation for expertise in this specialty.

Throughout the primary literature, there are many stories of hospitals successfully treating one patient for a particular complaint and subsequently being approached by others (often from the patient's hometown) with the same complaint. Also, many doctors reported the considerable distances traveled by some patients to get to the hospital. It would seem that a specialty arose, not so much out of training or conscious intent, but from the interaction of demand created by reputation, with the doctor's expertise. Increased practice of a particular operation would improve the doctor's performance, and hence his or her reputation, and demand would rise correspondingly, establishing a cycle that was beneficial to doctor and patient alike. By comparison, specialty practice in America had developed, throughout the nineteenth century, from being considered a "style of quackery" to a lucrative business based on post-graduate training, often undertaken in Germany or France.[119]

The pattern observed in China seems to have more in common with what Chang Che-Chia, who outlined the role and place of traditional physicians in Qing society, has described. In particular, he canvassed the role played by a doctor's "reputation" in traditional Chinese medical practice.[120] Physicians could be informally classified on a continuum from the most respected, "famous physicians" (*mingyi* 名医), through "literati physician" (*ruyi* 儒医) to "ordinary" (*shiyi* 时医). Another class, hereditary physicians (*zuchuan shiyi* 祖传世医) practiced healing on the strength of inherited, secret prescriptions. These classifications were not exclusive: while all *mingyi* were also *ruyi*, in that they were Confucian scholars who also studied medicine, not all *ruyi* were *mingyi*. Famous doctors could charge higher fees, but relying on reputation made them more vulnerable when they failed. The skills of *shiyi* were generally considered "not outstanding" and a label of "hereditary physician" was descriptive only and did not imply any particular level of expertise. The Qing government had abandoned earlier systems of examining medical practitioners and, although the labels "more or less graded the quality of the physician," they were not assigned under any defined criteria. As far as competence within a class was concerned, people had to find other ways to judge a doctor. Doctors as a group were not generally highly regarded in Qing society and the main concern of people, and government, was how to recognize a "quack"—of whom there were many. Chang describes the strategies the people adopted to discriminate between physicians. First, they learnt as much as they could about medicine so that they could question and effectively test the doctor. This option of "knowing medicine" would not have been available to potential Chinese patients of missionaries as they lacked access to Western medical knowledge. Another technique was to hide their symptoms from a doctor and assess his competence according to whether he could identify their problem, and lastly they could rely on the recommendation of friends and family. This last method "solved the conflict between the necessity to test the doctor's ability and the importance of trusting a doctor."[121] One can assume Chinese people would have carried this aspect of Chinese medical culture into their dealings with medical missionaries. That this was the case seems to be borne out in an observation by Barton, of the CMS Hospital at Ningbo, "The particular branch of medicine in which the foreign physician individually excels becomes speedily known among the Chinese. Probably there is no country where a man's reputation spreads faster than in China. This is easily demonstrated by a comparative scrutiny of the surgical procedures in different hospitals where there is a predominance of certain operations." His own practice that year had been dominated, on the medical side, by cases of "tuberculosis, syphilis, dysentery, and intestinal parasitic infections."[122]

As well as the lists of operations, further evidence of the role that reputation played in the specialty is evident in the many descriptions of people traveling excessive distances to consult particular doctors. The medical missionaries, with whom we are principally concerned in this study, were rarely trained specialists in any particular field of medicine. China afforded them an opportunity, often denied them in America, to undertake a practice limited only by their confidence. Physicians in America may have performed simple surgical procedures but when they got to China many of these same doctors, often alone and isolated from their peers, could undertake heroic operations. Not all of them became specialists in China, but a significant number did. It is possible to attribute this directly to their being away from home, but also to Chinese customary behavior in relation to medical practitioners. Cole acknowledged the role reputation played in his practice when he described most Chinese as being unwilling to consult him without a recommendation from someone who has "been in and *actually come out of it again* without having lost a liver or eyes or some other personal property at the hands of the foreigner."[123]

DAY SURGERY—AN INNOVATIVE SOLUTION

As is obvious to anyone who has lived in China, Chinese who have to travel prefer to do so, if possible, "safe within [their] net of relationships."[124] The traveler is handed from one relative, friend, or "friend of a friend," to another who, as locals, can organize accommodation and anything else he may need. There is ample evidence that many Chinese traveled long distances for treatment in the missionary dispensaries and hospitals. The report of the Methodist New Connection Mission (MNCM) at Leling 乐陵 for 1892 described patients coming "from 521 different towns and villages, covering the large area of 17,000 square miles."[125] Similarly, A. Lyall reported that in the course of a year at Swatow they had patients "coming from 1,600 to 1,800 different towns and villages."[126] Cecil Davenport referred to patients who had regularly "come scores, or may be hundreds of miles." In 1905 he had had twenty-six "scholars from a city 100 miles west" who came to break their opium habit.[127] Another, William Wilson, who reported using his 'cure for the opium habit' as a lure to attract patients who would not come into hospital in the interior, had patients who came from "cities and towns up to 120 miles away."[128]

Such a patient, who had to move away from his familiar surroundings, would seek out, through his contacts, people who could ease his passage through unfamiliar territory and who could look out for him or act on his behalf when he reached his destination. If his medical problem was not severe enough to demand hospitalization, he might be lucky enough to have somewhere in the hospital town where he could live while visiting the dispensary for treatment. If he was less fortunate he may have to spend time in a local hotel and, failing that, he may have to be admitted to the hospital.

This phenomenon, coupled with the overcrowding and poor physical conditions in many hospitals, gave rise to a distinctive phenomenon, which sounds modern today: the notions of 'day surgery' and 'hostel' accommodation. The Tuckers, one week in 1912, had their largest ever number of inpatients, nearly twice as many as they had room for: "some sleep in their carts, others on the floor of an old building, well propped with timbers to keep it from falling, and many on the hospital porches." Other patients "complain that the rooms, with their broken brick floors and decrepit roofs, are not suitable to live in." The solution was for patients to "hire quarters away from our dilapidated buildings."[129] Samual Cochran at Huaiyuan, writing in 1905, bemoaned the fact that his buildings were so unsuitable that his patients also had to stay in neighboring inns. This meant he lost the opportunity to give "close medical attention and the influence of daily instruction in the Christian truth."[130]

In some places, enterprising Chinese established hotels or inns near hospitals to provide familiar-style accommodation for wary patients. Charles Lewis at Baodingfu, describes one such establishment near his hospital: "A man runs an inn, which is called the "Hygiene Hotel" (*weisheng tien*) ... many as soon as they are able to leave the hospital, go there to live and come to the hospital for dressings. The inn can probably accommodate thirty patients. It is filled mainly with discharged patients from our hospital."[131] The medical missionaries saw some considerable benefit in this arrangement and at least one, Arthur Peill at Cangzhou 滄州 in Hebei, reported in 1904 that during the past year he had built a "commodious and very convenient inn, which [was] also a food-shop for the patients and an annexe to the wards."[132]

In America, where the availability of medical care was considerably greater and clinics within easier reach of the majority, people did not need to be admitted to hospital but could attend the dispensary, or outpatients clinic, on a regular basis for ongoing monitoring, treatment or dressing. Snell asserted that in China somewhere between fifty and seventy-five percent of all inpatients were in fact suffering from minor ailments that could be adequately treated in the dispensary. The problem was that many traveled considerable distances to visit the sparsely situated hospitals and, if they had no friends or relatives with whom to stay, had to be admitted to hospital. Snell suggested that, as new hospitals were built the old buildings be retained as hostels: "Why not provide a good but an inexpensive building where this ambulatory patient can pass the time. Provide for him entertainment, religious and general instruction. His disease is not so severe but that he can take in a little instruction and [we can] continue to care for them about as we have been" he asked. Those who did need a major operation could still enter the hospital "the day before operation [but be released in a] week or ten days and kept in the hostel for a few days longer before returning home." This would leave the new, modern hospital for "those saturated with disease" who would have the "constant attention of skilled, faithful, loving nurses and the expert attentions of competent doctors. Many more of this class will then be sent home well and happy instead of in coffins."[133] This brings us to how dying patients were catered for in the missionary hospital.

DYING AND DEATH

From the earliest days, medical missionaries were concerned about how best to deal with death in the hospital. It was commonly agreed among medical missionaries that it would be ideal if there were no hospital deaths. This was obviously impossible, since more often than not, the people who came to them only did so after their own doctors, folk healers, or priests had failed. The best they could do, therefore, was to make every effort to minimize the risk. The missionaries were concerned for their own reputation, safety, and legal position but most often couched descriptions of the strategies they adopted in terms of Chinese beliefs, and what they called *superstition*. The first tactic, to avoid deaths during or following surgery, was to try to dissuade anyone who did not have an excellent prognosis from going ahead with an operation. If they were not able to convince the patient, his friends and relatives would be brought into the discussion to add weight to the argument. If they still decided to proceed: "We make it 'sine qua non' that there shall be one or more friends present at the operation, in order to see fair play. The plan works splendidly. There is afterwards no suspicion that we have plucked out an eye or mysteriously extracted blood or 'virtue' or what not. The Chinese are wonderfully suspicious and inventive and we need on that account to do everything quite openly."[134] This plan, which had been introduced for their own protection, had proved successful at the LMS hospital at Xiaogan 孝感 and, "a thing not by any means to be despised in China, the good name and 'luck' of the hospital has been maintained."[135] In the event that death appeared imminent, this hospital, in common with most others, "kept in mind the desire of every Chinese to die in his own home and have frankly told the man and his friends the condition of affairs. Acting in this way we have never heard a word of reproach when the patient was removed or after his decease."[136]

Most hospitals reported low inpatient death rates. For example, only eight of the 503 inpatients who passed through Cole's hospital in 1906 died in hospital but "many others were taken out by relatives on point of death, because of superstitious fears."[137] Cole elaborated in 1909, "Chinese dread, as a rule, that their relatives should die outside their own homes, fearing that their spirits would become wanderers."[138] As James Watson has explained, Chinese and European beliefs about the meaning of death differed. Whereas in Europe, it was thought the body and spirit parted company at the moment of death, in China, separation of the spirit from the body too early "before the ritualised expulsion from the community was thought to bring disaster." The spirit was easily disorientated, particularly by movement, and might become separated from the body. Keeping it and body together was "one of the primary goals of Chinese funeral rites."[139] Susan Naquin's description of the circumstances surrounding death in North China in the nineteenth and early twentieth century (1870–1940) may also shed light on why the Chinese did not want to die away from home. She explains that it was considered unlucky to die "on the communal *k'ang*." At the last opportunity, the dying person would be transferred, on a flat board, to a special room where the family would gather and the "formal expression of grief" would begin with the dying person's last breath.[140] Thus, if the person died away from home, not only might the spirit be prematurely separated from the body, but also, the family might not have been able to carry out their duties to the dead person. Hence, removing patients before death would have served both the interests of the hospital and those of Chinese patients and their families.

How to cope in the unfortunate instances when a death did happen within the hospital exercised the minds of all medical missionaries. Although before 1916 autopsy and dissection were illegal in China, Butchart recommended that hospitals include a morgue in their plans.[141] A body could be "locked up in a secure way, so that it cannot by any possibility be mutilated and hence spread an evil report." He advised that the "dead room" should be placed so that "the body can easily be removed through a back gate in as quiet a manner as possible." This would have the dual purpose of protecting the hospital's reputation and being sensitive to the Chinese, whom he described as having "a great prejudice to its being removed by the front way."[142] A survey of the plans of hospitals that provided such a room reveals that most took this advice. For example, McCartney described the "kitchens, wash house, dead house and servants dining room, [as being] in the rear with back doors opening on the city wall."[143]

Butchart was assuming that there would be someone to whom bodies could be given for burial but when this was not the case it raised another level of concern for many missionaries. Charles Lewis of Jinan suggested, in a letter to the editor of the *CMMJ*, that hospitals try to get "the Governor (who has some reasonableness) to issue some sort of grant . . . putting them on a par with temples as regards the disposal of bodies having died in them."[144] This would also enable him to take in "this miserable class of patients whom we pity and do not have the heart to turn away to die with no attention at all." It would make it compulsory for the *Ti-pao* (local constable) to take the bodies and dispose of them and if relatives turned up they could be referred to him. Lewis' Chinese assistants, and other Chinese with whom he had discussed this solution, had considered it "a feasible plan." The editor disagreed: "we would hardly like to be thought of by the people as being in any sense in the same category as temples" but he acknowledged that others may think differently and invited discussion.[145]

Despite their anxieties, few hospitals reported that they had experienced significant repercussions from death in hospital. Somerville's experience in his LMS hospital at Wuchang seems to have been typical. A death had caused "not only no trouble, the others did not stampede, those waiting to come in did not lessen and none refused to be operated on. It was like a hospital at home."[146]

In medieval times in Europe, it had been considered lucky to die in the monastic hospital among people who would pray for your soul.[147] In America, too, death was a common feature of life on the ward until, coinciding with change in the patient population to include more members of the middle class, dying patients were routinely removed from the ward in case the sight of them upset the new, largely paying, patients.[148]

In a number of respects, patients' experience of hospital in China would have been much the same as that of their counterparts in America. In both, patients had to tolerate being the objects of observation and experimentation. As the century wore on and hospitals in China became more organized and more highly staffed, they introduced standardized methods of recording cases that could be used for statistical analysis and epidemiological investigation.[149] But, it would seem the similarities were fewer than the differences. In China, segregation of the sexes was absolute; friends and relatives stood in for nurses, cooks and launderers; beds could be communal; quilts took the place of sheets and blankets; lumps of wood replaced pillows; the number of men outnumbered women patients to a far greater degree; patients, who were more likely to be treated by a woman physician, also tended to stay longer; and preaching and Bible reading were ubiquitous.[150] These dissimilarities cannot be explained by recourse to a simple cause. Firstly, they were the result of the interweaving of a number of factors, which would have arisen out of operating a medical mission in any foreign country: lack of funds and staff and the primacy of the evangelical imperative while, at the same time, attempting to adhere to contemporary Western notions of best practice. Secondly, distinctiveness, for example the feminization of hospitals, could arise from an interaction of several influences: sexual discrimination at home, the opportunity afforded by necessity, and a desire to attract Chinese women patients. Thirdly, it is clear that, to a substantial degree, certain differences were due to the missionaries' response to Chinese patients' preferences, cultural practices, and beliefs. These included the arrangements made for meals, the laxness of hospital rules, and the number and types of people resident in the hospital in addition to patients. All these determined the nature of the American hospital in China and distinguished it clearly from its America template.

Conclusion
The New Chinese Hospital

While the motive of the Chinese in opening these dispensaries may have been a questionable one of opposition, they could in no way have more perfectly demonstrated their appreciation of the same work done by foreigners [than by the] imitation of the plan pursued in the Mission dispensary: preaching rooms attached where patients are harangued on the sacred edict while waiting for medicines.

—Eleanor Chestnut, 1900[1]

If the Chinese were going to establish their own hospitals modeled on a foreign example then it would have been to the modified, sinicized, hospital that they would have looked and not the hospital as it existed in America.

However, before proceeding to examine the evidence for the extent to which the Chinese hospital is a direct successor of the introduced, albeit adapted, hospital it is necessary to summarize what we know about the character of any indigenous models available to them. As we have seen in chapters 1 and 2, the idea of a place where sick people could be cared for away from their own home was not unknown in China. There had existed in China, throughout much of her history, institutions and systems for the provision of medical care which, had they existed in Europe, would have been included in the history of the hospital as precursors to the modern hospital. In the Tang dynasty (618–906 C.E.) Buddhist monasteries had fulfilled a similar function to that of Christian monasteries and hostels that had existed from the fourth century in Western and Eastern Europe. A state-run welfare system, which had included institutions with medical staff, had operated during the Song (960–1279 C.E.) and Yüan (1279–1368) dynasties. This system had given way, in the Ming (1368–1644) and Qing (1644–1911), to institutionalized care provided by voluntary charitable organizations established, principally, by the gentry. Institutionalized care in China never became as highly 'medicalized' as in the West but, then, neither was the hospital in the West until the state of medicine demanded it. Physicians had not been included on the staff of hospitals in Europe until the thirteenth century, and it was not until the eighteenth century that the defining characteristic of a person entering a hospital in Europe was sickness requiring, specifically, medical care.[2]

When the missionaries arrived, there were Chinese welfare and medical institutions in existence, admittedly offering a different form of medicine premised on a different view of disease, in many of the towns and cities where the missionaries established themselves. The missionaries were entering a medical market place with a wide variety of providers of healing services, some of which included institutionalized medical care. It was not vacant territory. So, missionaries had to find a *niche* for themselves; they did so, largely, using their knowledge of surgery, which did not form part of the Chinese medical system.

The other ingredients considered essential for the development of a hospital, a motive and the means, were both present in China. For example, the alleged driving forces behind the establishment of hospitals in the West, charity and compassion, existed in China and were evident to missionaries when they arrived. The various models of providing welfare services in the West, the use of guilds, the actions of community leaders (in China, the gentry), state and local government, and religious charities all existed in China and had all been involved, at one time or another, in the provision of welfare, including medical, services. This aspect of the missionary hospital was not new. Nor were the methods of financing new: China had financed its welfare activities from subscriptions, donations from individuals, government funds and, in addition, had a long tradition of ensuring ongoing funding by investing in real estate.

And neither was the mission hospital's emphasis on dispensary services alien. Because of the nature of Chinese medicine, medical care had always included dispensary-type services and had not required inpatient accommodation. Jing Shao, in his study, "Hospitalizing Traditional Chinese Medicine" has characterized the practice of Chinese medicine as being largely "'ambulatory,' in that either the patient would walk or be carried to the practitioner, or the practitioner would walk or be carried to the patient." Traditional remedies consisted of herbal prescriptions, which the patient or their family made up and administered at home—hospitalization was unnecessary. For example, when a hospital of Chinese medicine was established at Shasi in Hubei province as late as 1956, the eight beds "essentially provided lodging for patients who had traveled from distant rural areas."[3] Chinese who had had to travel considerable distances to a charity or public dispensary in the nineteenth century would often have found accommodation in one of the inns that abounded in Chinese towns.

So far as patients paying for medical services was concerned, China always provided medicine and medical advice (in a dispensary setting) free of charge. In addition, it had devised other public systems. For example, during the Tang dynasty (618–906 C.E.), "prescriptions together with officially-fixed prices of medicines were engraved on stones erected in public places, and it was decreed that the poor and sick should be able to obtain money from the national treasury to buy them. This publication of official prices was also designed to moderate the cost of medicines sold in private pharmacies."[4] Medical knowledge was also disseminated via such avenues as almanacs and calendars.

A separate nursing profession did not form part of the Chinese system of medical care and, although missionaries undertook training for male nurses, female nurses were not commonly found in hospitals before the 1920s.[5] However, as we have seen, missionaries had accommodated the practice of family and friends caring for the patient in hospital—out of necessity but also, consideration.

It is clear then, that when medical missionaries arrived in the mid to late-nineteenth century the Chinese were not only familiar with forms of institutionalized medical care which had been available in China for hundreds of years, but that the structures, and means for financing charitable works were present in their contemporary society. So, the questions arise; how much did new hospitals established by the Chinese owe their existence and form to the introduced hospital and how much did they owe to indigenous Chinese precursors?

No-one should be surprised to discover that the complex process of establishing the institution of the hospital in China was more than a case of cultural imperialism or of simple transplantation in its entirety into virgin soil. One test of the extent to which the hospital in China was an 'introduced species' is to examine the nature of any institutionalized medical care the Chinese established after the missionaries had been in China for a time.

The first case I will consider is the one with which I opened this book—a *Minzhengbu Yiyuan*,[6] in particular the *Neichengguan yiyuan* 内城官医院, or Inner City Public Hospital, which was established in 1906 in the Manchu, or Tartar, city of Beijing[7]* by the Ministry of Civil Affairs (the *Mingzhengbu*). The German idea that "public health and disease prevention efforts should be directed by the police," which had been adopted in Japan,

*see www.michellerenshaw.com

had gained currency in China since 1902.[8] The Ministry of Civil Affairs, the *Minzhengbu,* was created in 1906 to take responsibility for both the police and "matters relating to public sanitation [which included] the prevention of plague, examination of doctors and inspection of hospitals."[9] In 1906, there was no specific reference to the establishment of hospitals for the poor sick and the ministry "generally encouraged private initiatives to fulfill public functions, including medical relief."[10] The ministry was reorganized in 1913 under a new name, the Ministry of the Interior or *Neiwubu* 内务部, into ten departments. One was the Department of Sanitation and Public Health, the *Weisheng si* 卫生司, under Lin Wenqing 林文庆. It was to supervise the establishment of "workhouses, institutions for the blind, the dumb and the insane" as well as orphanages, and relief for "distressed widows," the poor, and victims of disasters.[11]

As discussed in the introduction to this book, the plan of *the Minzhengbu yiyuan* was unusual. When compared with the plans of mission hospitals discussed in chapters 4 and 5 it becomes even more clear that this hospital took little or nothing from introduced designs. Mullowney provided some information about the workings of this hospital and it seems that the only subsequent discussion is an article by Zhu Xianhua 朱先华 published in the *Zhonghua yishi zazhi* 中华医史杂志 (Chinese Journal of Medical History) in 1985.[12] According to Zhu, in the early days comparatively more people chose Chinese medicine than Western. He attributed this to Western medicine having "only just appeared in my country and was not known or understood by the people." The situation was reversed from the sixth month of 1907 when 6,851 people were treated with Chinese medicine and 7,499 with Western medicine and from then on the preference for Western treatment continued to rise.[13] This trend was confirmed by Mullowney who was told, in 1912, "four-fifths of the patients ask for the Western-trained physician."[14] A group of YMCA students who undertook a survey of hospitals in Beijing in1913 visited this hospital and estimated that of 500 patients, 150 would choose Chinese medicine.[15] A bamboo slip system, like the one the missionaries had appropriated from Chinese practice, was used in this hospital to regulate the order in which patients were attended to. After they were registered they were given slips, red for men and green for women, and special ones for those who had priority for treatment—naval officers, army officers and ordinary soldiers, school students, policemen, and those who were wounded or needed urgent attention.[16]

Unlike outpatients in most mission hospitals, outpatients of the *Minzhengb yiyuan* were not charged a fee. In this respect, the hospital was in line with traditional Chinese practice and did not emulate the foreign example. Inpatients, though, paid a daily fee: first class—$1, second class—50 cents, and third class—15 cents for which they received "meals, medicines, operations, and all medical and surgical attention while in the hospital."[17] The government, via a grant from the *Minzhengbu* of 400 yuan per month, supported the hospital financially as did grateful patients. [18] It does not appear, from the many references to free dispensaries in the contemporary record, that this hospital was an exception in this regard. Isabella Bird, passing through Zhenjiang 镇江 (in Jiangsu) in 1896, for example, reported the existence of "two free dispensaries, with nine doctors in charge. They are open without fees every day, treating about 200 patients, who are not required to pay for their medicines."[19] And, in 1905, before the *Minzhengbu* hospital was opened, N. S. Hopkins reported that "there [were] many free dispensaries opened by the government and the military in [Peking]." Mullowney had been told, however, that the authorities in charge of the *Minzhengbu* hospital were "very seriously contemplating a change [because] they have found, as we have in Western lands, that a great many people abuse the privilege and a great many come for treatment who could easily pay a physician."[20] A similar story had accompanied an illustration of a Chinese hospital in the highly influential magazine from Shanghai, the *Dianshizhai Huabao* 点石斋画报 (1884–1898), in 1885. When it first started, the doctors "chose those who had no money and gave the medicine free of charge." They had become "worried that this might not be fair, and might cause misunderstanding [so] they started to give medicine free of charge to everyone who came." However, between 400 and 500 people came every day to see the doctors, and they were unable to continue the practice. Since the *Ren Ji Shantang* 仁济善堂 had no other way to earn money, they were contemplating limiting free medicine to every other day.[21] (see Plate 24)

In fact, some Chinese dispensaries did charge patients. One such was the Jiukiang 'Red Cross' hospital, run by mission-trained Chinese doctors, supported mainly by subscriptions from merchants and from a "house tax [and] a tax on tea sent to Hupeh." They charged outpatients "eight coppers for the first visit, and four coppers afterwards, but soldiers and police [paid] half rates."[22] Thus, the policies on charging outpatients varied among Chinese hospitals and dispensaries, as they did among mission hospitals, but less so. For the period 1903–1910, I estimate that seventy-four percent of mission hospitals charged a fee for outpatient services whereas it would seem that a much smaller proportion of Chinese dispensaries did so. Because accurate statistical or survey data are not available for Chinese hospitals, it is not possible to make a definitive statement but it would seem highly

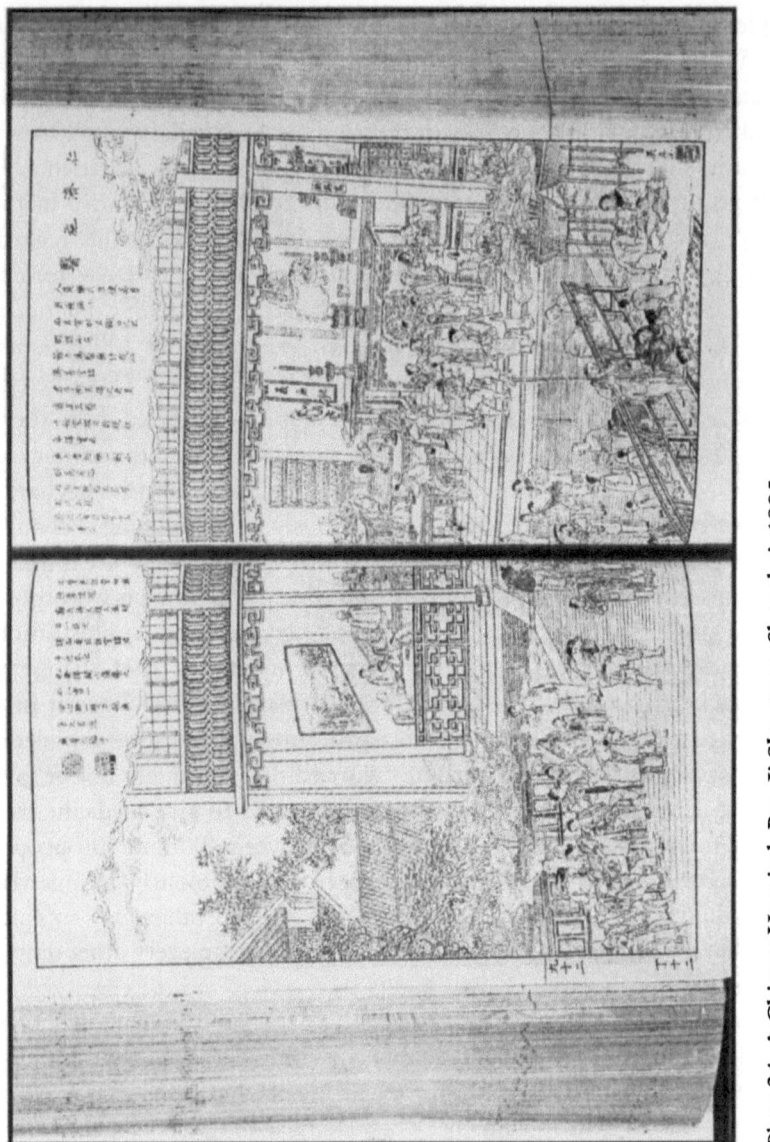

Plate 24. A Chinese Hospital, *Ren Ji Shantang*, Shanghai, 1885
Source: *Dianshizhai Huabao* 2 (1885): 92. Reproduced with the Permission of the Library, School of Oriental and African Studies.

likely that Chinese hospitals relied much less on patients for their financial viability than did mission hospitals.

As for staff, Mullowney had noted that in 1911 the hospital was well catered for with seven Western-trained physicians and three "doctors of the old school." Zhu provides us with more details of the founding doctors. Wu Weiyu 吳為雨 and Xie Kangyou 謝康尤, both graduates in Western medicine from the Beiyang Medical School, had been appointed, in 1906, as chief and deputy medical officer respectively at the Inner City hospital.[23] Tang Jian 唐堅, a doctor with the Public Health Office of the Police Department, took charge of Chinese medicine and was later responsible for setting up a second hospital, the Outer City Hospital, or *Waichengguan yiyuan* 外城官 医院, in the Chinese city.[24] In all, when the hospital was established eight physicians were appointed to treat patients: four for Chinese and four for Western medicine.[25] To F. W. Peabody's eye, "the western men were fairly bright looking men . . . [but] the Chinese doctors were much older and certainly looked much wiser than their western colleagues."[26] Compared with mission hospitals, where up to a third of physicians were women, in these hospitals, as far as we know, they were all men. The hospital also employed many more ancillary staff than a mission hospital could. The *Minzhengbu yiyuan* staff included three pharmacists with eight assistants, six administrative (bookkeeping) staff, and a number responsible for cleaning, running errands, "looking after the fire for tea," and delivering hot water. There was also one chief and six policemen who undertook guard duties.[27]

Just as the mission hospitals had some rules, so did these hospitals. The rules for the *Minzhengbu* hospitals provided that all patients should be given a bath and have their hair washed before being admitted to a ward; inpatients could not leave the hospital at will and could not be discharged without a certificate of cure from a doctor; and visiting friends and relatives had to report to the manager and get permission from the doctor if they wanted to bring a present of food for the patient.[28] It is unlikely that these rules were observed in this hospital any more than they were in a mission hospital.

The picture which emerges from the, admittedly sketchy, first hand accounts is of an institution which was undoubtedly a hospital, but quite distinct from either an American hospital as established by missionaries or a traditional Chinese dispensary.[29]

ALTERNATIVE MODELS

The *Minzhengbu* hospital, however, was not the only form that Chinese hospitals took in the late Qing. In 1902, when the Capital University was established in Beijing, both traditional Chinese and Western Medicine were included in the curriculum with the Chinese put first, "with a view to giving pride of place to Chinese learning with Western study as an essential subsidiary."[30] In 1903, this twin system of medicine was put into practice when a hospital was planned for Jinan, in Shandong, "to be run on native and western lines [in an] old temple."[31] A 1912 survey of medical work in Shandong province briefly described the hospital as having both Chinese and Western departments: the "attendance is very large at the daily dispensaries, amounting at present to forty or fifty thousand a year in the Western department, and half that number on the Chinese side." The hospital side of the institution had not, it was noted, been so largely developed.[32]

John Kerr, a keen observer of the Chinese institutions in Canton, was sure that the emergence of Chinese "native dispensaries and so-called hospitals, which are now quite numerous in South China" was due to the example of foreigners.[33] In an 1899 article, he cited the "Native Dispensary of Canton," or *Aiyutang* 爱育堂, as "a specimen of these institutions." It had been set up in 1871 when Canton already had two missionary hospitals and several dispensaries, the oldest having been there for some thirty-five years. He was interested to explore "how far they are copied from the foreign models and how far native ideas have developed them on new lines." He was clearly not anticipating that any transfer of the Western model would be in its entirety.[34] The administration, finances, and services provided by the *Aiyutang*, according to its annual report for 1887, were not significantly different from those of the dispensaries and benevolent institutions met by missionaries when they arrived in China and were quite unlike the situation in mission hospitals. Management was under the guidance of a board of officials, the *Guangdong shanhou zongju* 广东善后总局, with the work divided into four categories: medical, educational, aid to the poor and "general objects." By far the biggest expenditure—giving aid to the poor—was on the provision of coffins, gravestones, and burial grounds The quality of coffins depended on the status of the poor: the aged poor ($3.62), the "respectable" poor ($2.50), and "friendless paupers" ($1.50). The charity also provided coffins for paupers who died in Kerr's hospital, twenty-six of them in 1887. "General objects" included donations to other charitable causes, for example, 2,000 *taels* ($2,777) to the Viceroy's college and 700 *taels* ($962) to the "Home for the Blind." In previous years "large sums of money had been collected and disbursed for the relief of sufferers from famine and floods, both in this and in the more distant Provinces of the Empire."[35] It would appear that medical aid was restricted to dispensary services. Listed expenditure included 838 *taels* (or $1,163) paid to 4 doctors; 2,975 *taels* (or $3,993) paid for 78,501 prescriptions to be "filled at drug-stores for patients"; and 320 *taels* paid for vaccinations. Chinese practitioners commonly used the 'arm to arm' method of smallpox vaccination and the amount paid by the institution was most likely to have been to mothers of children from whose arm lymph was taken at the rate of 40 *cash* per vaccination according to an 1886 report.[36] The sources of funds for the *Aiyutang* included donations and subscriptions from individuals. However, it also relied on substantial sums from rents—collected from shops and land purchased by, or given to, the institution—and interest on the monies destined to be spent on real estate. As we have seen earlier, reliance on real estate for income was fundamental to Buddhist monasteries and subsequent Chinese benevolent institutions. These last two sources of funds (rents and interest) contributed forty-five percent of the total income for 1887. A further forty-three percent came from the sale of rice (meals), and a mere twelve percent from donations.[37] None was collected from patients. Kerr was impressed with the financial acuity of the managers and interpreted their policy as being, "not to trust to voluntary contributions, but to invest in real estate, so that they will not be dependent on what in a heathen country is well known to be a very uncertain source of support for benevolent purposes."[38]

Another Canton medical welfare institution, the *Fangbiansuo* 方便所, in addition to operating a dispensary, provided accommodation for "friendless paupers who [were] dangerously ill."[39] According to the 1888 report, which gave the name, age and birthplace of each patient along with the outcome of their time in the institution, there had been "243 males and 87 females who recovered and were sent away [and] 469 males and 138 females who died, friendless."[40] The death rate, sixty-five percent, in the *Fangbiansuo* was very different from that in mission hospitals and reflects their different purposes. Mission hospitals sought to minimize the number of patients dying in hospital by either not accepting dying patients in the first place or arranging with family and friends to remove them from hospital prior to death. The high death rate in the *Fangbiansuo* is consistent with its aim of providing a place to die for those who had no family.[41] Kerr came to no definite conclusion about the provenance of these two institutions vis-à-vis Western influence but it would seem that whilst the timing of their establishment may have been influenced by the foreign presence, they owed their form, financing and management to their own Chinese predecessors. Kerr was optimistic about the future of Chinese institutions but would have liked them to have been *more* influenced by the mission example. "The success attained under the control of heathen managers" he said "is an assurance that the same business talent, sanctified by grace and devoted to works of Christian benevolence, will fill this land with institutions for the relief of human suffering in all its forms."[42]

Unlike the *Minzhengbu* hospitals, the institutions Kerr described employed only Chinese traditional medicine as did the "Hospital of Extensive Benevolence (*guangren yiyuan* 广仁医院)" that had been set up in Wuzhou (Guangxi), funded by "native subscription." With its "small, square chambers, without windows, like prison cells," it would appear that the design of the hospital was also closer to the *Minzhengbu* hospital than any foreign example.[43]

A range of circumstances and of motives prompted the establishment of Chinese hospitals. For example, it was an attempt to improve the quality of Chinese traditional medicine that drove the officials and merchants in 1895 at Haikou 海口 on Hainan Island. They considered that the "medical knowledge of the men professing to be native doctors was of the very poorest description" and subscribed money to establish a hospital in a converted government school building. Three doctors were engaged and "medicine and advice [were] given gratis to the poorest applicants." Those who could afford to pay were given prescriptions to be made up at one of the "native drug stores." Aldridge, a Customs Medical Officer, thought that the "chance of obtaining better native treatment has been greatly taken advantage of, and the hospital so far has been a success": 7300 patients had been seen in the three summer months and average monthly attendance since opening had been 1100 patients.[44]

A relatively common strategy emerged where members of the gentry or officials would sponsor a young man, once he had received some training in a mission hospital, to set up his own practice and take in patients. One of the earliest reports of this phenomenon came in 1881 from Hankow, in Hubei. An "old hospital boy [had set up] a hospital for the poor Chinese of the city" using three converted Chinese houses. He was supported by "ten mandarins [who] have given him Tls. 100 each per annum" and he charged a small fee (14 *cash*) for the first visit and another for any medicine.[45] According to Thomas Kirkwood in 1904, it was not the missionary example to which the "talk of starting a hospital in Chungking to be managed wholly by Chinese" was due but to the influence of the local Chinese newspaper and its Japanese editor. The paper was "continually instructing the Chinese, what they have done in Japan. After all the victories of the Japanese against Russia, the Chinese are beginning to think they can follow the example of Japan. And so they mean to begin with a hospital."[46]

In 1910, an institution was founded which does seem to have been directly modeled on a missionary Western-style hospital. This apparently very successful enterprise was established in Cixi 慈溪, a walled city near Ningbo, when two "leading gentlemen," Chen Xiatang 陈夏堂 and Zou Runqing 奏润卿,[47] set up the "Tzeki People's Medical Association" (*Cixi baoli yihui* 慈溪保黎医会).[48] Funded by subscription, they hired Doctor Wu Lianting 吴莲艇, who had been trained by a missionary doctor at Kashing, and, using an adapted ten-room Chinese house, established a "modern western hospital" (*xiandai xiyi yiyuan* 现代西医医院), the *Baoli yiyuan* 保黎医院.[49] The Cixi *Baoli* adopted an interesting approach to patient fees. It seems that the people were initially "somewhat sceptical and slow to avail themselves" of the services but, by "offering free attendance and medicine for two days a week, charging only five cents on the others, and also by judicious use of tickets on the part of the committee, prejudice was removed and people began to flock to the place."[50]

Cody has written, in reference to the adoption of Western education, that those Chinese who wanted to "adopt western learning [built their schools] in what they considered to be the correct western style ... tall, plain houses of wood and plaster with bare roofs of grey tiles."[51] However, it was not until 1912 that any mention can be found of a Chinese-run hospital being housed in anything but Chinese-style buildings. The Cixi Medical Association was reported as having replaced their adapted Chinese house with a "two-storeyed foreign hospital accommodating 27 men and 23 women" in 1912 and, in 1916, they added a "two-storeyed modern building" to their plant.[52] Most of the Chinese who adopted the notion of the hospital as a site for medical treatment do not seem to have felt it necessary to adopt Western architecture along with the package.

Although none of the commentators has provided a comprehensive description of the wards in a Chinese hospital, a picture can be built up from snippets of information contained in their reports from a range of hospitals. The Rockefeller Foundation's representatives, Francis Peabody and R. S. Greene, were suspicious of the "spotless white uniforms" worn by attendants at the Government Hospital at Kaifeng but described the rooms used by the Western-trained doctor responsible for surgery as "clean and neat."[53] A well-financed Government Hospital in Nanking, housed in an "excellent building" with room for 50 patients, only had "about eight patients in a dirty, neglected ward, looking very miserable but lying on excellent iron beds" when Peabody visited in 1914.[54] Dr Kin, (Jin Yamei) the American-trained Chinese doctor in charge of the Peiyang Hospital for Women and Children, did, apparently, "strictly enforce" the rule that "friends of patients are not allowed to stay in the hospital." But she, unlike doctors in other hospitals, had access to a large contingent of women nurses from the training school attached to her hospital and "everything looked very clean" and patients, who were provided with bedding, looked "fairly well cared for."[55] Peabody and Greene were impressed by a hospital in Jiujiang[56] run by two Chinese doctors who had both been trained at the AEM hospital at Anqing. Patients were all bathed on admission and slept on wooden beds; the hospital supplied bedding and clothes "unless their own were clean [and the wards] were about as neat and clean as one can expect in old Chinese buildings."[57] In the Kung Yee hospital at Canton, "maintained by an association of fifty Chinese gentlemen" but under the charge of a foreign physician, Dr Todd, patients were allowed to have only one friend with them at night but "there are more of the family in the room during the day." The wards were "fairly clean considering the good many people in them."[58] Mullowney had been particularly struck by the fact that the *Minzhengbu* hospital was "housed in buildings of Chinese architecture, and enclosed according to Chinese fashion, within high walls."[59] He was impressed by the cleanliness of the hospital: "The most striking thing to one's eye, as one passes from place to place in this half-Eastern, half-Western temple of healing, is the refreshing cleanliness and orderliness of the whole establishment. I have seen very few foreign-managed hospitals in China that are any cleaner, if as clean and hygienically in order, than these hospitals of the *Min Cheng Bu*."[60] He used this observation to reinforce his call for the use of Chinese architecture and for medical missionaries to "learn too, even though it is rather late, that the old Chinese architecture can be used and can be made hygienically clean, and that therefore, it is not perhaps as necessary as some people think, to spend large sums of money in foreign architecture."[61]

Thus, it would seem that the conditions in Chinese hospitals were no more constant, and just as variable, as those encountered in mission hospitals. Just as there was no typical American hospital, nor typical mission hospital, it seems there was no typical Chinese hospital. What emerges is that the Chinese did not adopt a single model; rather, a range of institutions came into being towards the end of the Qing that shared some characteristics of the foreign model with characteristics of earlier indigenous Chinese institutions. If these emergent Chinese institutions indeed resembled the mission hospitals in China it was because the mission hospitals had taken on Chinese characteristics and much in common with Chinese institutions. In other words, the mission hospital was a "sinicized" or "indigenized" hospital. It is also clear that none of the new Chinese hospitals were modeled, absolutely, even on the sinicized mission hospital. Rather, they can be interpreted as examples of syncretism; the Chinese drew on both autochthonous and foreign precursors to create uniquely Chinese institutions.

A friend from Ningxia Autonomous Region, who chooses Chinese or Western medicine at her local hospital depending on the nature of her ailment, explains what has become of that Chinese institution. Wang Zhuqin tells me that in smaller centers, or rural areas, most people still take food in to cook for hospital patients. She says that, although "it is against hospital regulations" they persist because, "if someone is hospitalized and there is nobody from his or her family to take care of him or her, [they] will feel disappointed and at a loss . . . nobody in the world cares about [them]. But if there is a certain person from his or her family cooking or taking care of him or her, he will feel much better. He even gets better sooner. Cooking food for the inpatients is a way of expressing one's love to others. It's also a kind of Chinese tradition."[62]

Appendix

NOTES AND SOURCES FOR FIGURE A: COMPARATIVE CHRONOLOGY

1. Greek *Asclepieia*, or 'healing temples.' See Guenter B. Risse, *Mending Bodies, Saving Souls: A History of Hospitals* (New York: Oxford University Press, 1999), 15–38.

2. Temkin describes the role of "public physician" as dating from the fifth century B.C.E. but there is much debate as to if, or when, they provided a place for patients to recuperate. Miller, for example, acknowledges that physicians performed surgery in their offices, or *iatreia*, but disputes any claim that accommodation was provided in them before the Christian era. Timothy S. Miller, *The Birth of the Hospital in the Byzantine Empire, The Henry E. Sigerist Supplements to the Bulletin of the History of Medicine; New Series, No.10* (Baltimore: Johns Hopkins University Press, 1985), 41–47; Owsei Temkin, *The Double Face of Janus and Other Essays in the History of Medicine* (Baltimore: Johns Hopkins University Press, 1977), 205–6.

3. Based on the *Zhouli*. Lu Gwei-Djen and Joseph Needham, "China and the Origin of Examinations in Medicine," *Proceedings of the Royal Society of Medicine* 56, February (1963): 63–64. See also Ralph C. Croizier, *Traditional Medicine in Modern China: Science, Nationalism, and the Tensions of Cultural Change, Harvard East Asian Series; 34* (Cambridge: Harvard University Press, 1968), 28–29.

4. Based on the *Guanzi*. See, Croizier, *Traditional Medicine*, 29–30; Demieville, *Buddhism and Healing*, 58; K C. Wong and Wu Lien-teh, *History of Chinese Medicine: Being a Chronicle of Medical Happenings in China from Ancient Times to the Present Period*, 2nd. ed. (Shanghai: National Quarantine Service, 1936), 43–44.

5. *Valetudinaria*, or military hospitals, provided for Roman soldiers, gladiators, and by plantation owners, for slaves date from early in the first century C.E. Risse, *Mending Bodies*, 38–59. Thompson and Goldin, who focus on the physical manifestation revealed by excavations, are impressed by the planning and sanitary techniques, as is Scarborough. John Scarborough, "Roman Medicine," in *Aspects of Greek and Roman Life*, ed. Scullard

(London: Thames and Hudson, 1969), 76–79, John D. Thompson and Grace Goldin, *The Hospital: A Social and Architectural History* (New Haven: Yale University Press, 1975), 4–6.

6. From the biography of Han Emperor Hanping 汉平. Ban Gu (32–92), *Han Shu,* (Beijing: Zhonghua shuju, 1975), 353. See Wong and Wu Lien-teh, *History of Chinese Medicine,* 77 and Joseph Needham, *Science and Civilization in China: Biology and Biological Technology,* ed. Nathan Sivin, vol. 6 (Cambridge: Cambridge University Press, 2000), 54.

7. A Royal proclamation of Yongping 永平, in 60 C.E. Wong and Wu Lien-teh, *History of Chinese Medicine,* 138.

8. These small, sometimes short-lived, institutions provided refuge for people who were sick, traveling or elderly. See Granshaw, "The Hospital", 1181; Miller, *Birth of the Hospital,* 21–22; Rosen, "The Hospital: Historical Sociology", 3–4; Temkin, *Double Face of Janus,* 218.

9. *Xenodocheia* or *xenones,* associated with Christian churches from early in the fourth century C.E. Miller cites the *xenon* at Antioch, which was de-scribed in 381 C.E. as being a place where, "every root of evil, the strange forms of disease, and the many causes of depression" could be observed, as being "perhaps a true hospital." Miller, *Birth of the Hospital,* 20–21, George Rosen, "The Hospital: Historical Sociology of a Community Institution," in The Hospital in Modern Society, ed. Eliot Freidson (London: Free Press of Glencoe, 1963), 3–4.

10. According to Wong, the *Liubing guan* 六病馆, or Six Diseases Home, a "charity hospital" was organized by Crown Prince Hui Wen and Prince Jing Ling who were admirers of Buddhism. Prince Jing Ling also established a *"hai"* where he took in the poor and provided them with medicine and clothing. K.C. Wong, "Chinese Hospitals in Ancient Times," *CMJ* 37, no. 1 (1923): 78.

11. The first permanent hospital with a dispensary was established in 491 by Xiao Ziling, "a Buddhist prince of the Southern Qi dynasty." P.Y. Ho and F.P. Lisowski, *A Brief History of Chinese Medicine,* 2nd Edition (Singapore: World Scientific Publishing Co., 1997), 21. See also Needham, *Sc.And Civ.,* Vol. 6, 54.

12. In 510 C.E. "Toba Yu, a prince of Northern Wei" established a "govern-ment hospital" under the auspices of the Ministry of Imperial Sacrifices *(taichangbu).* It was intended for poor or destitute suffering from disabling diseases. Zhen Zhiya, "Zhongguo Gudaide Yiyuan (Ancient Hospitals in China)," *Journal of Beijing College of Traditional Chinese Medicine* 2 (1980): 55; Ho and Lisowski, *Brief History,* 19 and Needham, *Sc. and Civ.,* Vol. 6, 54. Ren Yingqiu describes this establishment as "maybe the earliest type of public hospital." Ren Yingqiu, "Yiyuande," 19.

13. The refuge set up by Xin Gongyi 辛公义. Wong and Wu Lien-teh, *History of Chinese Medicine,* 137.See also Needham, *Sc. and Civ.,* Vol. 6, 54

14. *Nosokomeia,* specifically for the care of the sick developed into late sixth or early seventh-century hospitals like the "Sampson—an institution with a specialized staff of physicians and trained assistants." Miller, *Birth of the Hospital,* 23, 25–27.

15. Christian charitable institutions for orphans, the aged, and foundlings. Ibid. 24–25.
16. There were "400-odd" Hôtels Dieu by the early seventeenth century. Colin Jones, *The Charitable Imperative: Hospitals and Nursing in Ancien Regime and Revolutionary France,* Wellcome Institute Series in the History of Medicine (London; New York: Routledge, 1989), 10.
17. Buddhist temples served as hostels for monks, pilgrims, lay travelers, officials, and students. See Kenneth S. Ch'en, *Buddhism in China: A Historical Survey* (Princeton: Princeton University Press, 1964), 263–64.
18. State-sponsored welfare. Kenneth S. Ch'en, *The Chinese Transformation of Buddhism* (Princeton: Princeton University Press, 1973), 297.
19. *Beitian yuan* or *Beitian fang* (Fields of Compassion). Paul Demieville, *Buddhism and Healing: Demieville's Article "Byo" from Hobogirin,* trans. Mark Tatz (Lanham, Md.: University Press of America, 1985), 58–60; See also Angela Ki Che Leung, "Organized Medicine in Ming-Qing China: State and Private Medical Institutions in the Lower Yangzi Region," *Late Imperial China* 8, no. 1 (1987): 135, Hugh Scogin, "Poor Relief in Northern Sung China," *Oriens Extremus* 25 (1978): 3, and Wong and Wu Lien-teh, *History of Chinese Medicine,* 139.
20. State-sponsored infirmaries established following the proscription of Buddhism in 845 c.e. Scogin, "Poor Relief," 31, Wong and Wu Lien-teh, *History of Chinese Medicine,* 139; and Demieville, *Buddhism and Healing,* 59–60.
21. First Islamic Bimaristan (hospital), at Baghdad at the turn of the ninth century. Michael W. Dols, "The Origins of the Islamic Hospital: Myth and Reality," *Bulletin of the History of Medicine* 61 (1987): 382–84 and Risse, *Mending Bodies,* 125–29.
22. The first Muslim hospital was not widely emulated in the ninth century, and only emerged widely throughout the empire in the tenth century. They were well established in major cities by the twelfth century. Dols, "Origins of the Islamic Hospital," 388.
23. Carlin describes the leper hospitals as "the first and perhaps easiest to distinguish" of the medieval hospitals in England. According to Porter, by early in the thirteenth century some 19,000 leprosaria existed in Europe. As leprosy declined some of these became hospitals for people with other infectious diseases, the insane, or merely indigent. Some were brought into use as quarantine hospitals during the plague of the fourteenth century. Almshouses were by far the most common English medieval welfare institution (67 percent) followed by leper hospitals (31 percent) and refuges for poor pilgrims or travelers (12 percent). Generally, in none of these was medical or nursing care provided. Only ten percent of the medieval institutions provided any form of medical care, those for the "non-leprous sick poor" and, of these, less one fifth were devoted exclusively to the sick. Martha Carlin, "Medieval English Hospitals," in *The Hospital in History,* ed. Lindsay Granshaw and Roy Porter (New York: Routledge, 1989), 23–25.
24. In the official history of the Song, *futian yuan* 幅田院 Blessed Fields (or Good Fortune Home) are already referred to as the "old system" when discussing

the reforms undertaken during the reign of Yingzong 英宗 (1064–1068). Scogin, "Poor Relief," 31.

25. *Huimin yaoju* (惠民药局), or charity pharmacies, which distributed free medicines, particularly during epidemics but at other times for common illnesses, were established at least by the Yuanfeng 元丰 reign (1078–1085) when the publication of state-sponsored books of prescriptions was initiated. Leung, "Organized Medicine," 136–37.

26. *Anle fang* 安乐坊, or peace and happiness ward: set up by "the famous scholar-official" Su Shi (1036–1101) in Hangzhou in 1089." Ibid. 136; Scogin, "Poor Relief," Wong, "Chinese Hospitals in Ancient Times," 139.; Wong and Wu Lien-teh, *History of Chinese Medicine*, 139.

27. *Juyang fa* 居养法, or 'Poorhouse System.' Scogin, "Poor Relief," 32–33.

28. *Anji fang* 安济坊, or 'Peace and Relief Wards or Hospitals.' Ibid: 34–35.

29. St Bartholomew's, London. Porter, *Cambridge Illustrated History*, 212.

30. *Pantocrator Xenon:* Complex Byzantine hospital at Constantinople, Miller's "first modern hospital," founded in 1136. See Miller, *Birth of the Hospital*, 11–29; Rosen, "The Hospital: Historical Sociology," 12–29; Risse, *Mending Bodies*, 125–30.

31. Yüan dynasty military hospitals modeled on *anle fang*. Zhen Zhiya, "Zhongguo gudaide yiyuan": 56.

32. St Maria Nuova established in Florence in 1288. See Henderson, "Hospitals of Florence," 70–71; Granshaw, "The Hospital,"1183–84; Porter, *Greatest Benefit*, 211.

33. Quarantine hospitals: the idea of quarantine, isolation wards, and boards of health were developed in the Italian city states in the fourteenth and fifteenth centuries as a response to the bubonic plague. See Benedict, "Policing the Sick": 62 and Dorothy Porter, "Public Health" in *Companion Encyclopedia of the History of Medicine*, ed. W.F. Bynum and Roy Porter (London: Routledge, 1993), 1232.

34. Yüan emperor Chengzong (r.1295–1308) re-established state hospitals. *Yuan shi*, Song Lian (1310–1381). (Beijing: Zhonghua shuju, 1976) speaks of appointing doctors and setting up the old *huimimyaoju* to distribute medicine to the widowed and poor who are sick. The use of the word "hospital" is K.C. Wong's (unsourced) interpretation. Wong, "Chinese Hospitals in Ancient Times": 80.

35. The monastic hospitals, for example St Thomas, and St. Bartholomew's, were re-established under the auspices of the City of London after a short break following the Reformation and the dissolution of the monasteries. This time they had physicians on the staff so that they could provide specifically for the sick poor. London was an exception to the rest of the country where there were no comparable institutions. Granshaw, "The Hospital," 1184.

36. *Hôpitaux Généraux:* Jones describes the duel role of compassion and control in the establishment of these "catch all institutions," or "hospital-cum-workhouse," by the French state. Jones, *Charitable Imperative*, 39–41.

37. The *Tongshan hui* 同善会, or Society for Sharing Goodness, was the first documented benevolent society. Started in 1590 in Yucheng 虞城, Henan

at the instigation of Ming scholar, Yang Dongming (1548–1624) 杨东明 its charter was to build roads and bridges and distribute alms to the poor and needy. The following year Yang led an elite group to establish a second society, the *Guangren hui* 广仁会, or Society for Spreading Humaneness, in the same city. This time they included medical care for the poor in the charter: effected by the distribution of prescriptions and medicine. Handlin-Smith, "Benevolent Societies": 311; Leung, "Organized Medicine": 145. Rogaski discusses a similar institution, the *Yuli tang,* established in Tianjin in 1687. Rogaski, "From Protecting Life," 82–83.

38. Charitable dispensary set up in a temple by "the late Ming patriot," Qi Biaojia (1602–1645) in Shaoxing in 1636. Ten physicians worked in six-hour rotating shifts. For details of this and similar establishments, see Leung, "Organized Medicine": 145–46.

39. Two medical general hospitals in London: St Bartholomew's and St Thomas's. Granshaw, "The Hospital," 1184.

40. First hospitals in America: Pennsylvania Hospital in 1792, and New York Hospital in 1771. Rosenberg, *The Care of Strangers,* 18–22 and Bordley and Harvey, *Two Centuries of American Medicine,* 57.

41. Free Dispensaries in England and Scotland. 1770, Aldersgate Street Dispensary, London. See Cherry, *Medical Services,* 42; Granshaw, "The Hospital," 1188–89.

42. 1802, London Fever Hospital. Freidson, ed., *The Hospital in Modern Society,* 21.

43. *Puji tang* 普济堂. This general clinic and infirmary was formed from the merging of a dispensary and a charitable institution that provided a medical service. The majority of people were treated as outpatients by "Confucian doctors," but those without families who were seriously ill could be accommodated in "a ward at the rear of the building.' In the mid eighteenth century the Yongzheng 雍正 emperor ordered that these be set up all over the country. Leung, "Organized Medicine": 147–48.

44. Specialized hospitals were 'medicalized' earlier than general hospitals. Granshaw, "The Hospital," 1189–91.

45. Map showing Qing Charitable Institutions with a medical service in the Jiangnan region before 1840. Leung, "Organized Medicine": 148.

46. Peter Parker, the "first medical missionary" arrives and sets up a hospital in Canton, 1834. See "Peter Parker: Bodies or Souls" in Jonathon Spence, To Change China: Western Advisers in China 1620—1960 (London: Penguin Books, 1969), 34–56.

47. Hospitals played a central role in health care by the 1920s. Granshaw, "The Hospital," 1195–56.

Notes

NOTES TO INTRODUCTION

1. Harold Balme, *China and Modern Medicine: A Study in Medical Mission Development* (London: United Council for Missionary Education, 1921), 82–3. At the time Balme was Dean of the School of Medicine and later, President of Shantung Christian University, he had previously been in charge of the American Presbyterian Hospital at Jinan 济南, Shandong.

2. See, for example Ralph C. Croizier, *Traditional Medicine in Modern China: Science, Nationalism, and the Tensions of Cultural Change, Harvard East Asian Series; 34* (Cambridge: Harvard University Press, 1968), 43; Karen Minden, *Bamboo Stone: The Evolution of a Chinese Medical Elite* (Toronto: University of Toronto Press, 1994), 16; and K C. Wong and Wu Lien-teh, *History of Chinese Medicine: Being a Chronicle of Medical Happenings in China from Ancient Times to the Present Period,* 2nd. ed. (Shanghai: National Quarantine Service, 1936), 137.

3. The *Minzhengbu* was created in 1906 to take responsibility for both the police and "matters relating to public sanitation" which included "the prevention of plague, examination of doctors and inspection of hospitals." Montague H.T. Bell and H.G.W. Woodhead, *The China Year Book* (London: George Routledge & Sons, Ltd., 1912), 230. Mullowney had visited at least two other government hospitals in Beijing: the *Waicheng guan yiyuan* 外城官医院, in the Chinese city, and an "Almshouse and Refuge for the Insane," the *fengrenyuan* 疯人院. John J. Mullowney, "Modern Hospitals for Chinese by Chinese," *CMJ* 26, no. 1 (1912): 38.

4. Ronald G. Knapp, Personal Communication, November 2002 See also Ronald G. Knapp, *China's Vernacular Architecture: House Form and Culture* (Honolulu: University of Hawai'i Press, 1989).

5. See John Scarborough, "Roman Medicine," in *Aspects of Greek and Roman Life*, ed. Scullard (London: Thames and Hudson, 1969), 78–79. For a detailed description, plan and explanation see Royal Commission on the Ancient and Historical Monuments of Scotland and (RCAHMS), "Pinnata Castra, Roman Legionary Fortress & Marching Camps, Inchtuthill, Tayside," 2004. <http://www.roman-britain.org/places/pinnata_castra.htm and http://www.roman-britain.org/ glossary_m.htm>(May, 2004).

6. Mullowney, "Modern Hospitals for Chinese by Chinese," 37.

7. Ibid.

8. Ibid.

9. Prince Su he had held the post since July 1907, Montague H.T. Bell and H.G.W. Woodhead, *The China Year Book,* 554. Mullowney, "Modern Hospitals for Chinese by Chinese," 37.

10. Mullowney, "Modern Hospitals for Chinese by Chinese," 39. The *Hou men* 后门, the "back gate" between the Imperial City and Tarter City.

11. Lindsay Patricia Granshaw and Roy Porter, *The Hospital in History, Wellcome Institute Series in the History of Medicine* (London; New York: Routledge, 1989), Guenter B. Risse, *Mending Bodies, Saving Souls: A History of Hospitals* (New York: Oxford University Press, 1999). For an earlier general survey of the history of the hospital see, Eliot Freidson, ed., *The Hospital in Modern Society* (London: Free Press of Glencoe, 1963). A number of general histories and encyclopaedias of medicine deal, *inter alia*, with the history of hospitals, for example W.F. Bynum and Roy Porter, eds., *Companion Encyclopedia of the History of Medicine,* 2 vols., vol. 1 and 2 (London: Routledge, 1993), Steven Cherry, *Medical Services and the Hospitals in Britain* 1860–1939, ed. Michael Sanderson, *New Studies in Economic and Social History* (Cambridge: Cambridge University Press, 1996), Peregrine Horden and Richard Smith, *The Locus of Care: Families, Communities, Institutions, and the Provision of Welfare since Antiquity, Studies in the Social History of Medicine.* (London; New York: Routledge, 1998).

12. Charles E. Rosenberg, *The Care of Strangers: The Rise of America's Hospital System* (New York: Basic Books, 1987), Rosemary Stevens, *In Sickness and in Wealth: American Hospitals in the Twentieth Century* (Baltimore: The Johns Hopkins University Press, 1999).

13. Wong and Wu Lien-teh, *History of Chinese Medicine,* 137. This work, now superseded by contemporary scholarship, provides facts of contemporary events but their extrapolations from ancient texts (see later) are to be treated with caution.

14. Croizier, *Traditional Medicine,* 43.

15. Minden, *Bamboo Stone,* 16.

16. Chapter IV "The Evolution of the Hospital," Balme, *China and Modern Medicine,* 82–106; Wong and Wu Lien-teh, *History of Chinese Medicine.*

17. See for example, *Zhongguo Yixue Shi* (*History of Chinese Medicine*), (Shanghai: Beijing zhongyi xueyuan (Beijing College of Chinese Medicine): Shanghai kexue zhishu chubanshe, 1982), a text book designed for use throughout the whole country. It includes a chronological list of the establishment of medical schools and their hospitals. Similar chronologies are provided in Yu Shenchu, *Zhongguo Yixue Jian Shi* (*a Brief History of Chinese Medicine*) (Fuzhou: Fujian kexue jishu chubanshe, 1983) and *Zhongguo Yixue Baikequanshu,* (Shanghai: Shanghai kexue jishu chubanshe, 1987). Within recent Chinese scholarship a small number of hospitals, which started out under missionary auspices, have been the subject of articles. See Zhu Deming, "Zhejiang Guangji Yiyuan Yu Shengliyiyao Zhuankexuexiao

Shilue (a Brief History of the Zhejiang Central Hospital and Provincial School of Medicine," *Zhonghua yizshi zazhi* 25, no. 1 (1995) and Chen Fenglin, Liu Shiying, and Liang Jun, "Beijing Daoji Yiyuan Kaolue (the Dow Hospital in Beijing)," *Zhonghua yizshi zazhi* 28, no. 3 (1998).

18. For example see Norman Goodall, *A History of the London Missionary Society, 1895–1945* (Oxford: Oxford University Press, 1954), Kenneth Scott Latourette, *A History of Christian Missions in China* (New York: Russell & Russell, 1929), Gustav Warnek, *Outline of a History of Protestant Missions from the Reformation to the Present Time* (Edinburgh and London: Oliphant Anderson & Ferrier, 1901); Irwin T. Hyatt, "Protestant Missions in China, 1877–1890: The Institutionalisation of Good Works," in *American Missionaries in China: Papers from Harvard Seminars,* ed. Liu Kwang-Ching (Cambridge, Mass.: East Asian Research Center, Harvard University, 1966) and Sidney A. Forsythe, *An American Missionary Community in China, 1895–1905* (Cambridge, Mass.: East Asian Research Center, Harvard University, 1971).

19. Known as the Shantung Road Hospital after the erection of a new building in 1861. Wong and Wu Lien-teh, *History of Chinese Medicine,* 379.

20. In particular see Chapter 7, "A Charitable Enterprise: The Chinese Hospital" in Kerrie L. MacPherson, *The Wilderness of Marshes: The Origin of Public Health in Shanghai, 1843–1893,* ed. Wang Gungwu, East Asian Historical Monographs (Hong Kong: Oxford University Press, 1987), 143–71.

21. William Warder Cadbury and Mary Hoxie Jones, *At the Point of a Lancet: One Hundred Years of the Canton Hospital, 1835–1935* (Shanghai: Kelly and Walsh Ltd., 1935); Sara Waitstill Tucker, "The Canton Hospital and Medicine in 19th Century China, 1835–1900." (PhD, Indiana University, 1983); Edward Gulick, *Peter Parker and the Opening of China* (Cambridge, Mass.: Harvard University Press, 1973); Connie Anne Shemo, "An Army of Women: The Medical Ministries of Kang Cheng and Shi Meiyu, 1873–1937 (China)" (PhD, State University of New York at Binghamton, 2002); and Yuet-wah Cheung, *Missionary Medicine in China: A Study of Two Canadian Protestant Missions in China before 1937* (Lanham, Md.: University Press of America, 1988).

22. Caroline Beth Reeves, "The Power of Mercy: The Chinese Red Cross, 1900–1937" (PhD, Harvard University, 1998) and Carol Benedict, "Policing the Sick: Plague and the Origins of State Medicine in Late Imperial China," *Late Imperial China (Ch'ing-Shih Wen-t'i)* 14, no. 2 (1993).

23. Ho Tak Ming, *Doctors in the East: Where West Meets East* (Subang Jaya, Malaysia: Pelanduk Publications, 2001).

24. Ruth Rogaski, "From Protecting Life to Defending the Nation: The Emergence of Public Health in Tianjin, 1859–1953" (PhD, Yale University, 1996), 62. John Kenneth Mackenzie, a Scottish doctor and "devout Christian" was 29 years old when he was transferred from Hankou to establish medical work in Tianjin. He received financial support from the viceroy, Li Hongzhang, who gave him the use of "the recently built Zeng Guofan temple" to set up his initial medical clinic and provided funds to build a new hospital and later, an associated medical school. Rogaski, "From Protecting Life," 114–20. See

also, Mary Isabella Bryson, *John Kenneth Mackenzie: Medical Missionary to China* (London: Hodder and Stoughton, 1891)and Ma Kanwen, "East-West Medical Exchange and Their Mutual Influence," in *Knowledge across Cultures-Universities East and West*, ed. Ruth Hayhoe (Hubei: OISE Press, 1993), 169. Rogaski (Rogaski, "From Protecting Life," 233–36) also describes the failed attempts by the Chinese Chamber of Commerce to establish a Western-style municipal hospital in Tianjin in 1911, in response to fears of the Manchurian plague.

25. Rogaski, "From Protecting Life," 65.

26. Michel Foucault, *The Birth of the Clinic: An Archaeology of Medical Perception*, trans. A.M. Sheridan (London: Routledge, 1973; reprint, 1997).

27. Jonathon Spence, *To Change China: Western Advisers in China 1620–1960* (London: Penguin Books, 1969).

28. Paul A. Cohen, *Discovering History in China: American Historical Writing on the Recent Chinese Past* (New York: Columbia University Press, 1984), 13–14.

29. David Arnold, *Colonizing the Body: State Medicine and Epidemic Diseases in Nineteenth Century India* (Berkeley and Los Angeles, Ca.: University of California Press, 1993), 59.

30. Ibid. 251.

31. Ibid. 253–54.

32. Arthur Jr. Schlesinger, "The Missionary Enterprise and Theories of Imperialism," in *The Missionary Enterprise in China and America*, ed. John K. Fairbank (Cambridge, Mass.: Harvard University Press, 1974), 363.

33. Ibid. 363–64.

34. See James Watson's Introduction to James L. Watson, ed., *Golden Arches East: McDonald's in East Asia* (Stanford, CA: Stanford University Press, 1997), 5 and Sangmee Bak, "McDonald's in Seoul: Food Choices, Identity, and Nationalism," in Golden Arches East: McDonald's in East Asia, ed. James L. Watson (Stanford, CA.: Stanford University Press, 1997), 151.

35. Gael Graham, *Gender, Culture, and Christianity: American Protestant Mission Schools in China, 1880–1930* (New York: Peter Lang Publishing, Inc., 1995), 1.

36. Andrew Porter, "'Cultural Imperialism' and Protestant Missionary Enterprise, 1780–1914," *Journal of Imperial and Commonwealth History* 25, no. 3 (1997): 388.

37. Lian Xi, *The Conversion of Missionaries: Liberalism in American Protestant Missions in China, 1907–1932* (University Park, PA: Pennsylvania State University Press, 1997), 11.

38. See Charles Horner, "China's Christian History," *First Things* 75, no. August/September (1997): 1.

39. Resulted in Clement XI's encyclical *"Ex Illa Die"* issued in 1715. See Dun J. Li, *China in Transition, 1517–1911* (New York: Van Nostrand Reinhold Company, 1969), 22–24.

40. Joanna Waley-Cohen, *The Sextants of Beijing: Global Currents in Chinese History* (New York: W.W. Norton & Company, 1999), 77.

41. In order to distance themselves from Catholics they did not adopt the term *Tianzhu* and the debate turned on whether to use *Shangdi* or *shen* (a generic term for god or spirits). See Paul Rule, "The Chinese Rites Controversy: A Long Lasting Controversy in Sino-Western Cultural History," *Pacific Rim Report, the Center for the Pacific Rim's occasional papers series, no. 23* (2004): 1.

42. See Richard J. Smith, *Fortune-Tellers and Philosophers: Divination in Traditional Chinese Society* (Boulder: Westview Press, 1991), 76.

43. Watson, ed., *Golden Arches East*, 37.

44. Calculated from data compiled using Jos. C Thomson, "Medical Missionaries to the Chinese," *CMMJ* 1, no. 2 (1887); Jos.C. Thomson, "Medical Missionaries to the Chinese," *CMMJ* 4, no. 4 (1890) and "Notices: Arrivals and Departures," *CMMJ* 1–19 (1887–1905).

45. Based on a dataset I constructed from a variety of primary and secondary sources, principally Wong and Wu Lien-teh, *History of Chinese Medicine*, confirmed by reference to individual annual reports and notices in *CMMJ*.

46. Rosenberg, *The Care of Strangers, 5*. Rosen gives a lower number for 1873—149 "hospitals and related institutions" of which one third were for the mentally ill. George Rosen, "The Hospital: Historical Sociology of a Community Institution," in *The Hospital in Modern Society*, ed. Eliot Freidson (London: Free Press of Glencoe, 1963), 25. For 1909 see James Bordley and A. McGehee Harvey, *Two Centuries of American Medicine* (Philadelphia: W.B. Saunders Company, 1976), 60.

47. See Paul A. Cohen, "Foreword," in *An American Missionary Community in China, 1895–1905* (Cambridge, Mass.: East Asian Research Center, Harvard University, 1971).

48. Paul Howard, "Opium Suppression in Qing China: Responses to a Social Problem, 1729–1906 (Qing Dynasty)" (PhD, University of Pennsylvania, 1998), 119.

49. Harold Balme and Milton T. Stauffer, "An Enquiry into the Scientific Efficiency of Mission Hospitals in China" (paper presented at the Annual Conference of the China Medical Missionary Association, Peking, February 20–27, 1920) and Jeffrey W. Cody, "Striking a Harmonious Chord: Foreign Missions and Chinese-Style Buildings, 1911–1949," *Architronic* 5, no.3, 1996. <http://architronic.saed.kent.edu/v5n3/> (December 2002). See also Jeffrey W. Cody, Building in China: *Henry K. Murphy's "Adaptive Architecture,"* 1914–1935 (Hong Kong: The Chinese University Press, 2001).

NOTES TO SECTION I. THE HISTORICAL CONTENT

1. William C. Milne, *Life in China* (London: Routledge, 1857), 47–72. Others who reported or commented on Chinese medical institutions include William Warder Cadbury, John Glasgow Kerr, T. J Preston, Arthur Henderson Smith, and S. Wells Williams.

2. Guenter B. Risse, *Mending Bodies, Saving Souls: A History of Hospitals* (New York: Oxford University Press, 1999), 4.

3. In addition to Risse, histories taking these as their starting point include Lindsay Granshaw, "The Hospital," in *Companion Encyclopedia of the History of Medicine,* ed. W. F.Bynum and Roy Porter (London: Routledge, 1993) and Timothy S. Miller, *The Birth of the Hospital in the Byzantine Empire, The Henry E. Sigerist Supplements to the Bulletin of the History of Medicine; New Series, No.10* (Baltimore: Johns Hopkins University Press, 1985).
4. For the most detailed description of the place of *Asclepieia,* or "healing temples," in the history of hospitals, see Risse, *Mending Bodies,* 15–38.
5. Risse reasons that the Romans were compelled by their feelings of familial responsibility to provide care for their soldiers and slaves who were away from home and their own families. Ibid. 44–6. Others identify a more economic imperative: for example, Thompson notes that slaves and soldiers were valuable assets worth preserving. John D. Thompson and Grace Goldin, *The Hospital: A Social and Architectural History* (New Haven: Yale University Press, 1975), 5. For a more up-to-date assessment of these institutions, see Patricia Baker, "The Roman Military Valetudinaria: Fact or Fiction?," in *The Archeology of Medicine: Proceedings of the Theoretical Archeology Group* (Oxford: 2002).
6. See Risse, *Mending Bodies,* 56–59.
7. Miller, *Birth of the Hospital,* 38–43.
8. Michael W. Dols, "The Origins of the Islamic Hospital: Myth and Reality," *Bulletin of the History of Medicine* 61 (1987): 371.

NOTES TO CHAPTER ONE

1. For example, see generic histories of the Western hospital: Lindsay Granshaw, "The Hospital," in *Companion Encyclopedia of the History of Medicine,* ed. W. F. Bynum and Roy Porter (London: Routledge, 1993), Lindsay Patricia Granshaw and Roy Porter, *The Hospital in History,* Wellcome Institute Series in the History of Medicine (London; New York: Routledge, 1989), Guenter B. Risse, *Mending Bodies, Saving Souls: A History of Hospitals* (New York: Oxford University Press, 1999), George Rosen, "The Hospital: Historical Sociology of a Community Institution," in *The Hospital in Modern Society,* ed. Eliot Freidson (London: Free Press of Glencoe, 1963), Charles E. Rosenberg, *The Care of Strangers: The Rise of America's Hospital System* (New York: Basic Books, 1987). For specific studies, see Martha Carlin, "Medieval English Hospitals," in *The Hospital in History,* ed. Lindsay Granshaw and Roy Porter (New York: Routledge, 1989), Steven Cherry, *Medical Services and the Hospitals in Britain 1860–1939,* ed. Michael Sanderson, *New Studies in Economic and Social History* (Cambridge: Cambridge University Press, 1996), John Henderson, "The Hospitals of Late-Medieval and Renaissance Florence: A Preliminary Survey," in *The Hospital in History,* ed. Lindsay Granshaw and Roy Porter (London: Routledge, 1989), Colin Jones, *The Charitable Imperative: Hospitals and Nursing in Ancien Regime and Revolutionary France, Wellcome Institute Series in the History of Medicine*

(London; New York: Routledge, 1989), Timothy S. Miller, *The Birth of the Hospital,* Owsei Temkin, *The Double Face of Janus and Other Essays in the History of Medicine* (Baltimore: Johns Hopkins University Press, 1977), John D. Thompson and Grace Goldin, *The Hospital: A Social and Architectural History* (New Haven: Yale University Press, 1975) and John Scarborough, "Roman Medicine," in *Aspects of Greek and Roman Life,* ed. Scullard (London: Thames and Hudson, 1969). For the Islamic hospital, see Michael W. Dols, "The Origins of the Islamic Hospital: Myth and Reality," *Bulletin of the History of Medicine* 61 (1987), Toby E. Huff, *The Rise of Early Modern Science: Islam, China, and the West* (Cambridge: Cambridge University Press, 1993) and Lawrence I. Conrad, "Arab-Islamic Medicine," in *Companion Encyclopedia of the History of Medicine,* ed. W. F. Bynum and Roy Porter (London: Routledge, 1993), 715–17.

2. Angela Ki Che Leung, "Organized Medicine in Ming-Qing China: State and Private Medical Institutions in the Lower Yangzi Region," *Late Imperial China* 8, no. 1 (1987), Hugh Scogin, "Poor Relief in Northern Sung China," *Oriens Extremus* 25 (1978).

3. Asaf Goldschmidt, "The Systematization of Public Health Care by Emperor Song Huizong-Benefiting or Policing the Sick" (paper presented at the Tenth International Conference on the History of Science in East Asia, Shanghai, China, 6th October 2002).

4. Song Jiong, "Liang Song Juyang Zhidu De Fazhan-Songdai Guanban Cishan Shiye Chutan (the Development of the Poorhouse System During the Song Dynasty-Initial Discussion of the Song Dynasty Government-Operated Charity Organisation)," *Zhongguoshi yanjiu,* no. 4 (2000).

5. Ren Yingqiu, "Yiyuande Jianli-Bingfang (the Establishment of Hospitals)," *Ming bao yuekan* 57, no. September (1970), Zhen Zhiya, "Zhongguo Gudaide Yiyuan (Ancient Hospitals in China)," *Journal of Beijing College of Traditional Chinese Medicine* 2 (1980).

6. See Figure 1, number 8. There is a wealth of literature devoted to these early Christian institutions dealing with their architecture, modus operandi, clientele, and motivation. I have consulted Carlin, "Medieval English Hospitals," Miri Rubin, "Development and Change in English Hospitals, 1100–1500," in *The Hospital in History,* ed. Lindsay Granshaw and Roy Porter (New York: Routledge, 1989), Eduard Seidler, "Medieval Western Hospitals: Social or Health Care Facilities?," in *History of Hospitals—the Evolution of Health Care Facilities. Proceedings of the 11th International Symposium on the Comparative History of Medicine-East and West,* ed. Yosio Kawakita, Shizu Sakai, and Yasuo Otsuka (Susano-shi, Shizuoka, Japan: Division of Medical History, The Taniguchi Foundation, 1989). See also general histories such as Granshaw, "The Hospital," Risse, *Mending Bodies,* Rosen, "The Hospital: Historical Sociology,".

7. See Figure 1, number 17.

8. See Kenneth S. Ch'en, *Buddhism in China: A Historical Survey* (Princeton: Princeton University Press, 1964), 263–4, for a description of Buddhist temples serving as hostels for monks, pilgrims, lay travelers, officials and students. For a first-hand account of the range of accommodation provided

to travelers in Tang China, including Buddhist "monasteries and cloisters,"
see Ennin and Edwin O. Reischauer, *Diary: The Record of a Pilgrimage to
China in Search of the Law* (New York: Ronald Press Co., 1955), Edwin O.
Reischauer, *Ennin's Travels in T'ang China* (New York: Ronald Press, 1955),
143–52.

9. See Figure 1, number 32.

10. For example, The Foundling Hospital in Florence was commissioned by the
Silk Guild in 1419 and inaugurated on January 25, 1445. Despite its name
it was not really a hospital but a home for abandoned illegitimate children.
See Guido Morozzi and A. Piccini, *Il Restauro Dell'ospedale Di Santa Maria
Degli Innocenti, 1966–1970* (Firenze: Becocci Editore, 1971).

11. Henderson, "Hospitals of Florence," 70–71.

12. "Numbers of inmates varied from around two or three to about thirty, with
an average of ten." Granshaw, "The Hospital," 1184.

13. See Figure 1, number 18.

14. See Figure 1, number 19.

15. See Figure 1, number 30. Founded by Eirene, the wife of John II Comnenos
in 1112 and completed in 1136. Miller, *Birth of the Hospital,* 12–21. See
also Risse, *Mending Bodies,* Chapter 3, 117–65, Rosen, "The Hospital:
Historical Sociology," 4–5; and Temkin, *Double Face of Janus,* 218.

16. See Figure 1, number 22. Rosen, "The Hospital: Historical Sociology," 5–6.

17. See Figure 1, number 21. Huff, *The Rise of Early Modern Science,* 171.

18. Dols, "Origins of the Islamic Hospital," 379.

19. A tutor to the Caliph Harun ar-Rashid. Dols challenges the accepted wisdom
(for example, see Risse, *Mending Bodies,* 125–28) that the "first Muslim
hospital" was founded at Damascus, Syria, in 707 CE under Umayyad
Caliphal-Walid (705–715). Instead he describes that institution as a "shelter
or hospice for lepers." Dols, "Origins of the Islamic Hospital," 378.

20. Dols, "Origins of the Islamic Hospital," 388.

21. For details, see Huff, *The Rise of Early Modern Science,* 171–2.

22. Dols, "Origins of the Islamic Hospital," 387–89. Huff takes a different view:
because the hospitals were religious endowments teaching medicine was "constrained by religious law." Huff, *The Rise of Early Modern Science,* 178.

23. Roy Porter, *The Cambridge Illustrated History of Medicine* (Cambridge:
Cambridge University Press, 1996), 212.

24. See Figure 1, numbers 24–28. I shall resist the temptation to speculate as
to the extent of transfer of medical institutions, as opposed to medical
knowledge, which may have occurred between the Arab world and China
during the times of extensive contact between the two cultures, from the
seventh century. See Jacques Gernet, *A History of Chinese Civilization,*
trans. J.R. Foster (Cambridge: Cambridge University Press, 1985), 287–90.
At least two authors raise the possibility but do not pursue the topic Chen
Haifeng, *Zhongguo Weisheng Baojian Shi* (History of China's Health Care)
(Shanghai: Shanghai kexue jishu chubanshe, 1993) and Ma Kanwen, "East-
West Medical Exchange and Their Mutual Influence," in *Knowledge across
Cultures—Universities East and West,* ed. Ruth Hayhoe (Hubei: OISE Press,
1993).

25. Scogin, "*Poor Relief,*" 35.
26. The modern hospital did not assume the same form in the various countries of Europe: in Germany, for example, research was mainly carried out in the laboratory, whereas, in Britain clinical research was favored and research material, that is, patients, was amply supplied by hospitals.
27. Or "*pauvres malades* (paupers who were sick) in comparison to *malades pauvres* (sick individuals who, incidentally, were poor)." Jones, *Charitable Imperative,* 2.
28. Jones puts forward evidence from seventeenth and eighteenth-century French hospitals to counter the portrayal of the "pre-clinical hospital" as a "death-trap." In his view many historians have relied too heavily on the rhetoric of hospital reformers rather than closely examining "the daily realities of hospital life" in making their claims. See Ibid. 11–12 and chapter II, "Hospital Nursing": 89–208.
29. Li Liangsong, "Luelun Zhongguo Gudai Dui Zhuanran Bingrende Anzhi Ji Zhuanran Bingyuan (a Brief Discussion on Ancient Chinese Infectious Hospital and Setting Down for Patients with Infectious Diseases)," *Zhonghua yizshi zazhi* 27, no. 1 (1997): 33.
30. Sometimes referred to as the *Chou guan* or *Zhou guan li.* Michael Loewe, ed., *Early Chinese Texts: A Bibliographic Guide, Early Chinese Special Monograph Series* (Berkeley: The Society for the Study of Early China and Institute of Asian Studies, University of California, 1993), 24.
31. Ibid.
32. D. C. Lau, *Guanzi Zhuzi Suoyin* (a Concordance to the Guanzi), ed. D. C. Lau and Zhen Fangzheng, ICS Ancient Chinese Texts Concordance Series: Philosophical Works: No. 37 (Hongkong: The Commercial Press, 2001), 127–28. Interpreted by K.C. Wong, "Chinese Hospitals in Ancient Times," CMJ 37, no. 1 (1923): 77.
33. William G. Boltz, "Chou Li," in *Early Chinese Texts: A Bibliographic Guide,* ed. Michael Loewe (Berkeley: The Society for the Study of Early China and Institute of Asian Studies, University of California, 1993), 25–26.
34. Lu and Needham translate the term *jiyi* 疾医, as "State Physicians." Lu Gwei-Djen and Joseph Needham, "China and the Origin of Examinations in Medicine," *Proceedings of the Royal Society of Medicine* 56, February (1963): 63–64. Veith has translated the relevant section of the *Zhou li* and compared it with the Song dynasty "statesman and political and social reformer" Wang An-shih's (王安石 (1021–1086) "New Interpretation of the Government of the Chou Dynasty" (周官新义). She translates *jiyi* as "the doctor of the common diseases." All agree that they were "charged with attending to the diseases of the mass of the people." Ilsa Veith, "Texts and Documents: Government Control and Medicine in Eleventh Century China," *Bulletin of the History of Medicine* 14, no. 2 (1943): 165.
35. For example, see Ralph C. Croizier, *Traditional Medicine in Modern China: Science, Nationalism, and the Tensions of Cultural Change, Harvard East Asian Series; 34* (Cambridge: Harvard University Press, 1968), 28.
36. A pre-Han text attributed to Guan Zhong (d. 645 B.C.E.), but which Rickett describes as having been written by several unknown authors over a long

period of time: between the fourth and first centuries B.C.E. or "Warring States" period. W. Allyn Rickett, "Kuan Tzu," in *Early Chinese Texts: A Bibliographic Guide*, ed. Michael Loewe (Berkeley: The Society for the Study of Early China and Institute of Asian Studies, University of California, 1993), 244–49. Wong, "Chinese Hospitals in Ancient Times," 77, K.C. Wong, "Four Milleniums (Sic) of Chinese Medicine," *The Lancet* (1929): 158.

37. Presumably Wong is distinguishing here between the tenth-century B.C. clinic mentioned earlier and a "hospital." Wong, "Four Milleniums (Sic) of Chinese Medicine," 158.

38. Despite these reservations, he does acknowledge, "the mere existence of such concrete ideas is an interesting reflection of social values." W. Allyn Rickett, *Guanzi: Political, Economic, and Philosophical Essays from Early China: A Study and Translation.*, 2 vols., vol. 2 (Princeton: Princeton University Press, 1998), 227.

39. See Figure 1, number 4. D. C. Lau and Chen Fangzheng, *Zhouli Zhuzi Suoyin* (a Concordance to the Zhouli), Chinese University of Hong Kong Institute of Chinese Studies the ICS Ancient Chinese Texts Concordance Series. Classics: No. 4. (Hong Kong: The Commercial Press, 1993), 127–28.

40. Rickett, *Guanzi*, 227–29. Demieville, in his essay on the role of Buddhism in healing, cites the same section but describes the Guanzi as a "work of purely utopian character . . . largely apocryphal and this passage (about the hospitals) may be a late addition under the buddhist (sic) influence." Paul Demieville, *Buddhism and Healing: Demieville's Article "Byo" from Hobogirin*, trans. Mark Tatz (Lanham, Md.: University Press of America, 1985), 58.

41. T.J. Preston, "The Chinese Benevolent Institutions in Theory and Practice," *Chinese Recorder and Missionary Journal* 28 (1907): 245–48.

42. Elsewhere the text addresses a responsibility to "inquire after the sick," which involves an official visiting sick persons, over ninety years old, daily; over eighty, every other day and so on. See Rickett, "Kuan Tzu (in Loewe)," 230.

43. See Figure 1, number 6. *Han Shu*, (Zhonghua shuju chuban, 1975), 353. This interpretation is taken from Joseph Needham, *Science and Civilization in China: Biology and Biological Technology*, ed. Nathan Sivin, vol. 6 (Cambridge: Cambridge University Press, 2000), 54, who points out that "it seems, this was only a provisional measure, not the foundation of an institution." Wong interprets the section as "Emperor Han Ping, issued a proclamation to the effect that "all infected persons should be sent to empty outhouses where treatment will be provided." Wong, "Chinese Hospitals in Ancient Times," 77. Li describes the reference as the first recorded account of a specialized institution set up to take in acutely sick people for treatment. Li Liangsong, "Ancient Chinese Infectious Hospital," 33.

44. Wong, "Chinese Hospitals in Ancient Times," 78. Because Wong fails to give the precise source, or the Chinese original, of this quotation it is difficult to assess the reliability of his interpretation.

45. See Figure 1, numbers 1 and 5.

46. Granshaw, "The Hospital," 1181.

47. By Basil the Great. Nurses and attendants provided medical care. Temkin, *Double Face of Janus,* 218.
48. See Figure 1, numbers 8 and 9.
49. Henderson, "Hospitals of Florence," 63.
50. See Figure 1, numbers 14 and 15. Miller, *Birth of the Hospital,* 22–23, Risse, *Mending Bodies,* 122, Rosen, "The Hospital: Historical Sociology," 4.
51. Miller, *Birth of the Hospital,* 22–5, Rosen, "The Hospital: Historical Sociology," 4. For detailed treatment of the early Christian institutions see Risse, *Mending Bodies,* particularly chapter 2; Miller, *Birth of the Hospital,* chapter 2; and Rosen, "The Hospital: Historical Sociology," 4–5.
52. Miller, *Birth of the Hospital,* 25.
53. See Figure 1, number 14.
54. See Figure 1, number 16.
55. See also Carole Reeves, *Egyptian Medicine* (Princes Risborough: Shire Publications, 1992), 22–25.
56. See Risse, *Mending Bodies,* 44–47.
57. See Figure 1, number 11.
58. See Figure 1, number 12. Needham, *Sc. and Civ.,* Vol. 6, 54.
59. Or perhaps he set up the refuge on his own volition. See Figure 1, number 13.
60. Wei Zheng (580–643), "Sui Shu," (Beijing: Zhonghua shuju, 1973), 1681. See also Needham, *Sc. and Civ.,* Vol. 6, 54.
61. Imperial patronage was given an initial impetus by Empress Wu, who took over in 683 C.E. and, in 691, decreed that Buddhism take priority over Taoism. She was forced to abdicate in 705 but, after a short period of decline, with the accession of Xuan Zong, in 712, Buddhism was returned to its previously privileged position, albeit with certain state controls. Ch'en, *Buddhism in China,* 220–24.
62. Ibid. 295.
63. See Figure 1, number 19. The Tang government co-operated with, subsidized and helped administer the monasteries. See Scogin, "Poor Relief," 30.
64. Kenneth S. Ch'en, *The Chinese Transformation of Buddhism* (Princeton: Princeton University Press, 1973), 295–96.
65. Ibid. 297. According to Demieville, a "lay commissariat" created, between 701 and 705, by the Empress Wu had administered these "hospitals." Demieville, *Buddhism and Healing,* 59–60. Needham, on the other hand interprets the memorial to mean "ever since Chang-an had been the capital (i.e. since the beginning of the Western Wei in 534). Needham, *Sc. and Civ.,* Vol. 6, 54. Scogin has a slightly different interpretation. He reads the memorial as advising the closure of the institutions, which he describes as being operated already by Buddhists in co-operation with the state, because of corrupt practices and the fact that "small acts of charity" were not an alternative to "good government." Scogin, "Poor Relief," 30.
66. Ch'en, *Chinese Transformation,* 300, Scogin, "Poor Relief," 31.
67. Ch'en discusses the various political and economic forces that led to the restriction, from around 841, and the eventual proscription of Buddhism. Ch'en, *Buddhism in China,* 226–33. See also Gernet, *Chinese Civilization,* 294–96.

68. Scogin, "Poor Relief," 31.
69. Needham, *Sc.And Civ.,* Vol. 6, 54.
70. See Figure 1, number 20. Scogin, "Poor Relief," 31.
71. See Demieville, *Buddhism and Healing,* 58–60; Leung, "Organized Medicine," 135; Scogin, "Poor Relief," 31; K C. Wong and Wu Lien-teh, *History of Chinese Medicine: Being a Chronicle of Medical Happenings in China from Ancient Times to the Present Period,* 2nd. ed. (Shanghai: National Quarantine Service, 1936), 139.
72. France led the way in using the hospital as the preferred site for the teaching of medicine but it was not until the 1790s that clinical practice was formally incorporated into French medical education. Jones, *Charitable Imperative,* 16–17. For the most persuasive case for hospital teaching, put by a contemporary practitioner, see Phillippe Pinel, *The Clinical Training of Doctors: An Essay of 1793. Edited and Translated, with an Introductory Essay by Dora B. Weiner, trans. Dora B. Weiner, The Henry Sigerist Supplement to the Bulletin of the History of Medicine; New Series, No. 3* (Baltimore: The Johns Hopkins University Press, c.1980). Employing the hospital, and its patients, as a site for research was not to emerge America until the late nineteenth century. Rosenberg, *The Care of Strangers,* 151–53.
73. Seidler, "Medieval Western Hospitals," 8.
74. "The recipients of [medieval] charity were held to represent Christ himself, and indeed the whole movement of charitable giving was predicated upon the equation between Christ and the pauper." Jones, *Charitable Imperative,* 1.
75. See Figure 1, number 36. Ibid. 5. Jones does, however, warn against "overestimating the judicial and repressive dimensions" of these institutions. Jones, *Charitable Imperative,* 8.
76. See Figure 1, number 24. Goldschmidt translates the term as "Blessed Field Houses." Goldschmidt, "Systematization of Public Heath," 2.
77. The reign of Yingzong (英宗), during which Wang An-shi was most influential. For a summary of Ying Zong's life and work, see Veith, *"Texts and Documents,"* 159–61.
78. Scogin, "Poor Relief," 31.
79. See Figure 1, number 27. Scogin appears to be basing this statement on the existence of a 1098 imperial edict issued by Zhezong (C.E. 1086–1100) that describes a "government charity system designed to provide shelter and health care for the poor and indigent." According to Goldschmidt, the edict was not implemented until Huizong's reign (1100–1129). Goldschmidt, "Systematization of Public Heath," 5–6.
80. For interpretations of the text, see Ibid. 8 and Scogin, "Poor Relief," 33.
81. Translation according to Leung, "Organized Medicine," 136. Goldschmidt uses the term "Peace and Happiness Hospital." Goldschmidt, "Systematization of Public Heath," 7.
82. See Figure 1, number 26. For a detailed account of Su Shih's public-health work in Hangzhou, where "he put through . . . a clean water system and a hospital, dredged the salt canals, reconstructed West lake, successfully stabilized the price of grain . . . and worked for famine relief," see Lin Yutang,

The Gay Genius: The Life and Times of Su Tungpo (London: William Heinemann Ltd., 1948), chapter 22 "Engineering and Famine Relief": 263–76.

83. Based on "surviving records" see Goldschmidt, "Systematization of Public Heath," 7 Also Leung, "Organized Medicine," 136 Scogin, "Poor Relief," 32.

84. Wong and Wu Lien-teh, *History of Chinese Medicine,* 139, Wong, "Chinese Hospitals in Ancient Times," 80.

85. See Figure 1, number 28. Literally, "Rest and Relief Office," Goldschmidt, "Systematization of Public Heath," 5.

86. In response to a memorial from "Wu Juhou (1037–1113), the governor of the capital prefecture." For a translation of the relevant section of the memorial, see Ibid. 7–8.

87. Scogin, "Poor Relief," 34–35. Scogin is basing his 'description' on the recommendations specified in Wu's memorial rather than of an actual institution. Goldschmidt, however, provides sources for the record of the establishment of "hospitals" at Hebei (in 1902) and Hangzhou (1904). Goldschmidt, "Systematization of Public Heath," 8.

88. Collected Administrative Documents from the Song, compiled by various authors between the years 978–1243 and edited by Xu Song (fl. 1781–1848).

89. Leung, "Organized Medicine," 136. See also Goldschmidt, "Systematization of Public Heath," 9.

90. Excavations in 1985, 1993 and 1994 of "an ancient graveyard ... at Xiangyang in Shanxi province" unearthed 849 tombs "with records of burial dating to the years 1105–1116." Goldschmidt, "Systematization of Public Heath," 1, 10.

91. See Figure 1, number 25. According to the *Fujian Shengzhi–Weisheng Zhi* (*Gazetteer of Fujian–Public Health*), (Zhonghua shuju, 1995), 251, this generic name was not adopted in Fujian until the Ming dynasty. In the early Song they were called *maiyaoju* 卖药局 which was later changed to *hejiju* 和济局. Somewhat surprisingly, Goldschmidt does not include these agencies as part of his "public health system."

92. Leung, "Organized Medicine," 135.

93. On the basis of an entry for 1284 in the *Xin Yuanshi,* Zhen Zhiya attests the existence of special hospitals for military men in the late Yuan. Zhen Zhiya, "Zhongguo Gudaide Yiyuan," 56.

94. See Leung, "Organized Medicine," 139–42 for a summary of the role of the Ming State in the provision of medical relief. Gong Chun has described the provision of medical aid to the military during the Ming. See Gong Chun, "Mingdai Junyi Zuzhide Tedian (Characteristics of the Military Medical Organisation in the Ming Dynasty)," *Zhonghua yizshi zazhi* 17, no. 1 (1987).

95. See Figure 1, numbers 37 and 38. For an analysis of this phenomenon see Joanna F. Handlin-Smith, "Benevolent Societies: The Reshaping of Charity During the Late Ming and Early Ch'ing," *The Journal of Asian Studies* 46, no. 2 (1987). See also Leung, "Organized Medicine," 139–40.

96. See Figure 1, numbers 43 and 45.

97. See Leung, "Organized Medicine," 163, for a comprehensive list of welfare institutions established before 1840 in the Jiangnan Region that provided medical care.

NOTES TO CHAPTER TWO

1. "Description of the City of Canton," *Chinese Repository* 2, no. 10 (1833): 263.
2. Ibid.
3. "Charitable Institutions," *Chinese Repository* 2, no. 8 (1833): 195.
4. William C. Milne, "Notices of Seven Months' Residence in the City of Ningbo, Continued," *Chinese Repository* 16, no. 1 (1847): 26–27.
5. Ibid. 30.
6. For an explanation of what constituted the gentry in Qing China, see T'ung-Tsu Ch'u, *Local Government in China under the Qing* (Cambridge, Mass.: Council on East Asian Studies, Harvard University Press, 1988), 169–73.
7. Wang Mien, who wrote the preface to the 1842 report, described himself as "the promoted prefect of Suchau, assistant superintendent of the granaries, acting prefect of the independent prefecture of Taichang, formerly the acting prefect of Shanghai." Wang Mien, "Preface to the Report of the Foundling Hospital at Shanghai," *Chinese Repository* 14, no. 4 (1845): 180.
8. Angela Ki Che Leung, "Relief Institutions for Children in Nineteenth-Century China," in *Chinese Views of Childhood,* ed. Anne Behnke Kinney (Honolulu: University of Hawaii Press, 1995)
9. Ibid. 263.
10. Wang Tsinchin, "Report of the Foundling Hospital at Shanghai," *Chinese Repository* 14, no. 4 (1845): 180–93.
11. Ibid. 182. The 1842 Report contained financial and statistical information covering each year from 1839 to 1842 inclusive.
12. "Regulations, Etc., of Hall of United Benevolence for the Relief of Widows, the Support of the Aged, Providing of Coffins, Burial-Grounds, Etc.," *Chinese Repository* 20, no. 8 (1846): 402.
13. Shin-ping-yuen, "Report of the Public Dispensary Attached to the Poo-Yuen-Tang at Shanghai, for the 25th Year of Taoukwang, (1845)," *Chinese Repository* 17, no. April (1848): 193.
14. William Lockhart, "Report of the Medical Missionary Society's Hospital at Shanghai. From 1st May, 1844, to 30th June, 1845," *Chinese Repository* 15, no. 6 (1846): 289.
15. Shin-ping-yuen, "Report of the Public Dispensary Attached to the Poo-Yuen-Tang at Shanghai, for the 25th Year of Taoukwang, (1845)," 199.
16. Ibid. 197–98.
17. Lockhart, "Medical Missionary Hospital—Shanghai, 1845," 289.
18. He described guilds as "more properly insurance companies, which give aid to their members if in distress" and "companies" as being "got up for special occasions, such as for the relief of poverty by famine, flood or war, and dispensaries for the poor in times of pestilence." John Glasgow Kerr,

"The Native Benevolent Institutions of Canton, Part 1," *China Review* 2 (1873): 89.

19. Ibid. 89, 91.
20. John Glasgow Kerr, "Benevolent Institutions of Canton," *China Review* 3 (1874–75): 112–13. For the history of this institution see Elizabeth Sinn, *Power and Charity: The Early History of the Tung Wah Hospital Hong Kong,* ed. Wang Gungwu, 1989 *East Asian Historical Monographs* (Hong Kong: Oxford University Press, 1989).
21. Kerr, "Benevolent Institutions of Canton," 112–14.
22. Ibid. 112–15.
23. S. Wells Williams, *The Middle Kingdom: A Survey of the Geography, Literature, Social Life, Arts and History of the Chinese Empire and its Inhabitants,* 2 vols. (New York: Paragon Book Reprint Corp., 1895; reprint, 1966), 266.
24. John Glasgow Kerr, "The Bubonic Plague," *CMMJ* 8, no. 4 (1894): 180.
25. John Glasgow Kerr, "Is It an Advance?," *CMMJ* 3, no. 2 (1889): 66–67.
26. Williams, *The Middle Kingdom:* 263–64, 66.
27. For an overview of Chinese charitable and welfare activities, see chapter XV, "Benevolence," in Arthur Henderson Smith, *Chinese Characteristics* (Shanghai: North China Herald and S.C. & C. Gazette, 1890), 68–73.
28. T. J. Preston, "The Chinese Benevolent Institutions in Theory and Practice," *Chinese Recorder and Missionary Journal* 28 (1907): 249–53.
29. Colin Jones, The Charitable Imperative: (London; New York: Routledge, 1989), 32.

NOTES TO SECTION II. THE PHYSICAL HOSPITAL

1. The miasma from sick people were seen as particularly morbid and dangerous as they were the body's way of ridding itself of disease by elimination noxious matter so that it may regain health. Charles E. Rosenberg, The Care of Strangers, 125.
2. Based on a photograph reproduced in *The Lancaster General Hospital: Thirteenth Annual Report,* (Lancaster: Press of the New Era Printing Company, 1906), foll. 40. See also Marcus Whiffen, *American Architecture since 1780: A Guide to the Styles* (Cambridge, Mass.: M.I.T. Press, 1969), 159–60 and Adrian Forty, "The Modern Hospital in England and France: The Social and Medical Uses of Architecture," in *Buildings and Society: Essays on the Social Development of the Built Environment,* ed. Anthony D. King (London: Routledge & Keegan Paul, 1980), 69–72.
3. A.E. Hertzler, *The Horse and Buggy Doctor* (New York and London: Harper & Bros., 1938) quoted in James Bordley and A. McGehee Harvey, *Two Centuries of American Medicine* (Philadelphia: W.B. Saunders Company, 1976), 279. On Hertzler, see also Thomas Neville Bonner, *The Kansas Doctor: A Century of Pioneering* (Lawrence: University of Kansas Press, 1959), 1, 252–54.
4. Rosenberg 118–19.

5. Bonner, *The Kansas Doctor: A Century of Pioneering*, 91.

6. The most significant of these being the Johns Hopkins Hospital built in Baltimore between 1876 and 1885. The design process for Johns Hopkins is discussed in detail in John D. Thompson and Grace Goldin, *The Hospital: A Social and Architectural History*, 175–87.

7. Hugh Small, *Florence Nightingale, Avenging Angel* (London: Constable, 1999), 91–92.

8. Rosenberg, *The Care of Strangers*, 124.

9. According to Traux, a word coined by James Young Simpson: gangrene was the rotting away of flesh while the person was alive; erysipelas-started as a skin infection and spread to the membranes of the heart, lung, and brain. Accompanied by high fevers and rigors, or shivering fits, it was frequently fatal and extremely contagious. Most hospitals had erysipelas wards. Because it seemed to occur more frequently at particular times of the year some hospitals did not perform operations during certain seasons. Rhoda Traux, *Joseph Lister: Father of Modern Surgery* (London: George G. Harrap & Co. Ltd, 1947) 34–35, 116.

10. Simpson's plan to erect small iron huts had "won some powerful support-ers, who were clamouring that infected hospitals should be destroyed, but Lister had never liked the idea" Ibid. 89. On Lister and antiseptic surgery, see Guenter B. Risse, *Mending Bodies*, 373–78 and Peter Stanley, *For Fear of Pain: British Surgery, 1790–1850* (New York: Rodopi, 2003), 131–58.

11. "On the Effects of the Antiseptic System of Treatment upon the Salubrity of a Hospital." Quoted in Traux, *Joseph Lister: Father of Modern Surgery*, 144–45.

12. Pasteur, in an address to a meeting of the International Medical Congress in London in 1881 expressed his satisfaction with the acceptance of the germ theory by the medical profession in England. In particular, he recalled "the lively feeling of satisfaction I experienced when your great surgeon Lister declared that that my publication in 1857 on milk fermentation had inspired him with his first ideas on his valuable surgical method. Louis Pasteur, "The Germ Theory," *Lancet* (1881): 271.

13. Milburn, "A Comparative Study of Modern English, Continental and American Hospital Construction," *JRIBA* 8, no. 3 (1913) Quoted in Jeremy Taylor, *The Architect and the Pavilion Hospital: Dialogue and Design Creativity in England 1850–1914* (London: Leicester University Press, 1997), 50.

14. James Y. Simpson, *Anaesthesia, Hospitalism, Hermaphroditism, and a Proposal to Stamp out Smallpox and Other Contagious Diseases*, ed. W.G. Simpson (New York: D. Appleton, 1872) and, on Erichson, see Risse, *Mending Bodies*, 367.

NOTES TO CHAPTER THREE

1. Except for Hong Kong ceded to Britain in 1842 under the terms of the Treaty of Nanjing.

2. Anthony D. King, *Colonial Urban Development: Culture, Social Power and Environment.* (London: Routledge & Kegan Paul, 1976), 17.

3. Rhoads Murphey, *The Outsiders: The Western Experience in India and China* (Ann Arbor: The University of Michigan Press, 1977), 103.

4. See Jurgen Osterhammel, "Semi-Colonialism and Informal Empire in Twentieth-Century China: Towards a Framework for Analysis," in *Imperialism and After: Continuities and Discontinuities,* ed. Wolfgang J. Mommsen and Jurgen Osterhammel (London: Allen and Unwin, 1986).

5. Murphey, *The Outsiders,* 21–22.

6. Su Gin-Djih, *Chinese Architecture: Past and Contemporary* (Hong Kong: The Sin Poh Amalgamated (H.K.) Ltd., 1964), 127.

7. King, *Colonial Urban Development,* 17.

8. The exception was Hong Kong. When it became a crown colony Britain assumed control over all aspects of life, including the health of the Chinese population.

9. Murphey, *The Outsiders,* 21–22.

10. Cited in Pat Barr, *To China with Love* (London: Secker & Warburg, 1972), 84.

11. Headquartered in Boston, Massachusetts, the ABCFM entered China in 1830 when Rev. E. C. Bridgman (the first American missionary to China) arrived in Canton. Samuel Couling, *The Encyclopaedia Sinica* (Shanghai: Literature House, Ltd., 1917; reprint, 1964), 15–17. For an analysis of the backgrounds and opinions of missionaries with the ABCFM in the period immediately following the focus of this study, see Janet Elaine Heininger, "The American Board in China: The Missionaries' Experiences and Attitudes, 1911–1952" (PhD, University of Wisconsin-Madison, 1981).

12. E.G. Ruoff, ed., *Death Throes of a Dynasty: Letters and Diaries of Charles and Bessie Ewing, Missionaries to China* (Kent, Ohio: The Kent State University Press, 1990), 170.

13. Ibid.

14. "Walks About Canton-Extracts from a Private Journal," *Chinese Repository* 4, no. May (1835): 45.

15. John Glasgow Kerr, "History of Medical Missionary Society's Hospital, Canton," *CMMJ* 10, no. 1, 3 (1896): 55.

16. H.T. Whitney, "Medical Missionary Work in Foochow," *CMMJ* 3, no. 3 (1889): 85–86.

17. Karen K. Marcus, "Twentieth Century Chinese Architecture: Examples and Their Significance in a Modern Tradition" (Master of Science in Architecture Studies, Massachusetts Institute of Technology, 1988), 141.

18. Su Gin-Djih, *Chinese Architecture: Past and Contemporary,* 129.

19. Headquartered in New York, the American Presbyterian Mission (North), the "largest denominational mission in China, started work in Macau in 1843 and in Canton in 1847. Couling, *The Encyclopaedia Sinica,* 18–22. Photograph used on the front cover of pamphlet, *Hospitals in China, Medical Mission Series* (Philadelphia, Pa.: The Woman's Foreign Missionary Society of the Presbyterian Church, 1912).

20. With headquarters in Boston, Massachusetts the ABFMS started work at Hongkong in 1842 and Canton in 1844. Couling, *The Encyclopaedia Sinica*, 13–15. Photograph reproduced in J.S. Grant, "Hua Mei Hospital (Viewed from the River), Ningbo: Built in Stages from 1902," in *Wha Mei Hospital Report for 1913* (Ningpo: American Baptist Foreign Missionary Society, 1914).

21. The Methodist Episcopal Mission (South) had its headquarters in Nashville, Tennessee and entered China in 1842. See Couling, *The Encyclopaedia Sinica*, 364–65.

22. *Soochow Hospital, 1883–1933: Fiftieth Anniversary*, (Board of Missions of Methodist Episcopal Church, South, 1933).

23. Qualifications M.D., D.D. He left Suzhou in 1885 on account of his family's health. In 1898 he became General Secretary of the Board of Missions and was elected Bishop in 1910. He died in Yokahama in 1921 and his ashes were returned to Shanghai. Ibid.

24. Harold N. Jr. Cooledge, *Samuel Sloane: Architect of Philadelphia, 1815–1884* (Philadelphia: University of Pennsylvania, 1986), 78. The *Lancet* published a major series of articles, in 1881, which extensively surveyed the contemporary knowledge, represented the culmination of this debate. See Frederic J. Mouat, "On Hospitals: Their Management, Construction, and Arrangements in Relation to the Successful Treatment of Disease," *Lancet* (1881).

25. Cooledge, *Samuel Sloane*, 76–77.

26. Paul A. Cohen, *Discovering History in China: American Historical Writing on the Recent Chinese Past* (New York: Columbia University Press, 1984), 44. For a contemporary summary of the rights of foreigners, especially missionaries, under the various treaties see Gilbert Reid, "Chinese Law on the Ownership of Church Property in the Interior of China: Section I—the General Right Established," *Chinese Recorder and Missionary Journal* 20, no. 9, 10 (1889): 420–26.

27. J. Howie, "First Impressions and Experiences in Chang-Poo," *CMMJ* 4, no. 1 (1890): 2.

28. Reproduced in Chinese with a translation in R.J. Davidson, "Letter to the Editor," *Chinese Recorder and Missionary Journal* 20, no. 4 (1889): 184–85.

29. H.T. Whitney, "History of Medical Work in Shaowu," *CMMJ* 2, no. 3 (1888): 121.

30. Edward H. Hume, *Doctors East Doctors West: An American Physician's Life in China* (New York: W.W. Norton and Co., 1946), 41.

31. Edward H. Hume, "Opening of the Yale Mission Hospital, Changsha, Hunan," *CMMJ* 22, no. May, No. 3 (1908): 184.

32. See photograph in Lian Xi, *The Conversion of Missionaries: Liberalism in American Protestant Missions in China, 1907–1932* (University Park, PA: Pennsylvania State University Press, 1997), 34. See photograph of West Archway Street in Hume, *Doctors East Doctors West*, 1946, between 96 and 97.

33. Elliott I. Osgood, "Tisdale Hospital, Chuchow," *CMJ* 25, no. 6 (1911): 413.

34. See Gilbert Reid, "Chinese Law on the Ownership of Church Property in the Interior of China: Section II—Special Limitations to the General Right," *Chinese Recorder and Missionary Journal* 20, no. 9,10 (1889) especially page 455 where Reid explains that in the Chinese code and various Treaties when the word "sell" was used it was often accompanied by the words to 'lease' or 'mortgage' so he advised missionaries to "adopt an expression which gives no offence," for example "perpetual lease."

35. He could house fifty patients in this building which was later incorporated into a larger complex built with funds sourced from philanthropists, Mr and Mrs James Tisdale of Kentucky. Osgood, "Tisdale Hospital, Chuchow," 414–15.

36. W.E. Macklin, "Hwaiyuan Hospital Opening: Letter to the Editor," *CMMJ* 24, no. 5 (1910): 374.

37. Claude M. Lee, *Leaves from the Notebook of a Missionary Doctor* (Shanghai: American Church Mission, 1932), 11. The American Church Mission (full name Domestic and Foreign Missionary Society of the Protestant Episcopal Church in the USA), another Anglican organization, had its headquarters in New York and had entered China in 1835 but the first "tentative" medical work was not started until 1845. Couling, *The Encyclopaedia Sinica*, 144–46.

38. A.M. Jefferys, "Formal Opening of St. Andrew's Dispensary, Wusieh, Kiangsu," *CMMJ* 22, no. 3 (1908): 185.

39. Lee, *Leaves from the Notebook*, 13.

40. Ibid. 19–20.

NOTES TO CHAPTER FOUR

1. H.N. Kinnear, *A Year of Waiting: The Thirty-First Annual Report of Ponasang Missionary Hospital for the Year Ending December 1902* (Foochow: American Board of Commissioners for Foreign Missions (A.B.C.F.M.), 1902), 18.

2. G.F. De Vol, "Resolution Endorsed By Kuling Medical Conference: Hospital Plans" *CMMJ* 17, no. 4 (1903).

3. "The Medical Conference of 1907" *CMMJ* 20, no. 1 (1906): 41. See also Samuel Cochran, "Letter to the Editors: Hospital Plans," *CMMJ* 20, no. 3 (1906), Lucy E. Harris, "T'ung-Chuan-Fu, Szechuan," *CMMJ* 18, no. 3 (1904), W. Hamilton Jefferys and James L. Maxwell, *The Diseases of China* (Philadelphia: P. Blakiston's Son & Co., 1910), Richard Wolfendale, "An Ideal Medical Missionary Hospital," *CMMJ* 17, no. 1 (1903).

4. The most influential and comprehensive papers published during this period included: James Butchart, "Hospital Construction: Paper Read at the Medical Missionary Association, 1901," *CMMJ* 15, no. 2 (1901), Kenneth J. Mackenzie, "The Construction of Hospitals," *CMMJ* 1, no. 2 (1887); Edmund Lee Woodward, "Mission Hospital and Dispensary Construction in China: Paper Read at Medical Missionary Conference at Shanghai, 1907," *CMJ* 21, no. 5 (1907). The collected wisdom was summarized by Jefferys and Maxwell, *Diseases of China*, 1910, 661–97.

5. The London Missionary Society was interdenominational but the majority of missionaries belonged to the Congregational Church of Great Britain. See Samuel Couling, *The Encyclopaedia Sinica* (Shanghai: Literature House, Ltd., 1917; reprint, 1964), 313–15. It was established in, Bristol, by a group led by Baptist minister, John Ryland, at the urging of his friend, William Carey (an indigo planter in Bengal), in 1794. See Tom Hiney, *On the Missionary Trail: A Journey through Polynesia, Asia, and Africa with the London Missionary Society* (New York: Grove Press, 2000), 4–7.

6. Mackenzie, "The Construction of Hospitals," 78. Annmarie Adams' work on the role of doctors as architects in the West is pertinent here. See Annmarie Adams, *Architecture in the Family Way: Doctors, Houses, and Women 1870–1900* (Montreal: McGill-Queens University Press, 1996), particularly Chapter 2, Doctors as Architects: 36–72.

7. Robert E. Speer, "Lu Taifu," Charles Lewis M.D. *A Pioneer Surgeon in China* (New York: The Board of Foreign Missions Presbyterian Church in the USA, c.1930), 47.

8. Ibid. 65.

9. Emma Betow, "Margaret Eliza Nast Memorial Hospital," *CMMJ* 20, no. 4 (1906): 156. Emma Betow was the physician in charge. K C. Wong and Wu Lien-teh, *History of Chinese Medicine:* 586. Details of the structure and work of the MEM (with headquarters in New York and in China from 1847) are to be found in Couling, *The Encyclopaedia Sinica,* 362–64.

10. According to Couling, members of this society "wished to be known as 'Disciples of Christ' or, more simply 'Christians.'" Headquartered in Cincinnati, Ohio, it was a relatively late entrant to China and its first missionary was a (Canadian) physician, W. E. Macklin, who started the medical work at Nanjing 南京. Couling, *The Encyclopaedia Sinica,* 187.

11. Butchart, "Hospital Construction," 97.

12. Harold Balme, F.R.C.S., D.P.H., was in charge of the Union Medical College at Jinan in Shandong which was run under the auspices of the APM and the (English) Baptist Missionary Society (BMS).

13. Harold Balme and Milton T. Stauffer, "An Enquiry into the Scientific Efficiency of Mission Hospitals in China" (paper presented at the Annual Conference of the China Medical Missionary Association, Peking, February 20–27, 1920).

14. William Lennox conducted a less ambitious "self-survey" twelve years later. William G. Lennox, "A Self Survey by Mission Hospitals in China," *CMJ* 46 (1932).

15. Liang Ssu-ch'eng, *A Pictorial History of Chinese Architecture: A Study of the Development of its Structural System and the Evolution of its Types.* (Cambridge, Massachusetts: M.I.T. Press, 1984); Su Gin-Djih, *Chinese Architecture: Past and Contemporary.* Andrew Boyd's book has a similar emphasis. Andrew Boyd, *Chinese Architecture and Town Planning: 1500 B.C.–A.D. 1911* (London: Alec Tiranti, 1962).

16. Of the Department of Architecture at the Hong Kong Chinese University.

17. Jeffrey W. Cody, "Striking a Harmonious Chord: Foreign Missions and Chinese-Style Buildings, 1911–1949," *Architronic* 5, no.3, 1996. <http://architronic.saed.kent.edu/v5n3/> (2002).

18. The so-called May 4th Movement grew out of disillusionment with the West after World War I and culminated with student demonstrations in Beijing on May 4, 1919. It involved attacking Confucianism; initiating a vernacular style of writing, and promoting science.

19. For a detailed examination of one of the most prominent of these adaptive architects, Henry K. Murphy, see Jeffrey W. Cody, *Building in China: Henry K. Murphy's "Adaptive Architecture," 1914–1935* (Hong Kong: The Chinese University Press, 2001).

20. A.P. Peck, "Concerning Williams' Hospital, P'ang Chuang Station, in Shantung, of the North China Mission A.B.C.F.M.," *CMMJ* 1, no. 1 (1887): 66.

21. Mackenzie, "The Construction of Hospitals," 77.

22. Mary Isabella Bryson, *John Kenneth Mackenzie: Medical Missionary to China* (London: Hodder and Stoughton, 1891), 379–80.

23. Mackenzie, "The Construction of Hospitals," 78

24. Dugald Christie, *Thirty Years in the Manchu Capital, 1883–1913. Being the Recollections of Duguld Christie CMG, FRCS, FRCP Edin., Edited by his Wife* (London: Constable and Company, 1915), 23.

25. Speer, *"Lu Taifu," Charles Lewis*, 33.

26. Quoted in James Bordley and A. McGehee Harvey, *Two Centuries of American Medicine*, 280.

27. Harold Balme, *China and Modern Medicine*, 88–89.

28. H.D. Porter, "The Medical Arm of the Missionary Society," *CMMJ* 9, no. 4 (1895): 267.

29. This commonly held belief was expressed by S. Wells Williams: secular culture, in comparison with Christianity "never presents to the mind those sanctions for upholding and reverencing the truth which are alone found in the word of God." Christianity, in his view, is the foundation of the civilizations of the most advanced countries. Cited by Forsythe at Sidney A. Forsythe, *An American Missionary Community in China, 1895–1905*, 20–21, fn 54, 99.

30. Jefferys and Maxwell, *Diseases of China*, 1910, 670.

31. Ronald G. Knapp, *China's Old Dwellings* (Honolulu: University of Hawai'i Press, 2000), 141–43.

32. Edmund Lee Woodward, "St. James' Hospital, Ngankin, China," *CMMJ* 17, no. 1 (1903).

33. Woodward, "Hospital and Dispensary Construction, 1907," 253.

34. Ibid. p. 257. His rejection of Chinese building styles and materials did not extend to the plan of his hospital, which did allow for the complete separation of the sexes.

35. "The Opening of the Pingyin Hospital," *CMMJ* 23, no. 6 (1909): 408. The Church of England Mission, North China (C of EM (NC)) was often referred to as the Society for the Propagation of the Gospel in Foreign Parts (SPG). The society had its headquarters in London and although they had entered China in 1863 did not start work until twelve years later in 1875. Couling, *The Encyclopaedia Sinica*, 117–8.

36. Even in the most Western of hospital complexes the Chinese-style entrance gate often served to acknowledge their location in China and their Chinese patients. See photographs at www.michellerenshaw.com

37. Stephen C. Lewis, "Opening of the American Presbyterian Hospital at Chenchow, Hunan," *CMMJ* 22, no. 4 (1908)
38. Knapp, *Old Dwellings*, 223–24.
39. Cody, "Striking a Harmonious Chord.," Gael Graham, *Gender, Culture, and Christianity: American Protestant Mission Schools in China, 1880–1930* (New York: Peter Lang Publishing, Inc., 1995), 85.
40. Butchart, "Hospital Construction," 99.
41. Professor of Church History, Oberlin College, Ohio, later to become secretary of the China division of American Board of Commissioners for Foreign Missions.
42. In North China—following the destruction by Boxers.
43. E.G. Ruoff, ed., *Death Throes of a Dynasty,* 128.
44. Ibid.
45. C.M. Lacey Sites, "The New Methodist Hospital at Yen-Ping, Fuh-Kien," *CMMJ* 20, no. 4 (1906): 211. See also J. E. Skinner, "The Alden Speare Memorial Hospital, Yen-Ping, China," *CMMJ* 18, no. 4 (1904).
46. Ling Oi Ki, *The Changing Role of the British Protestant Missionaries in China, 1945–1952* (London: Associated University Press, 1999), 193.
47. Although widespread, these non-load-bearing walls were not universal throughout China and "solid, load-bearing walls have a long history . . . and are far more common . . . than is generally acknowledged in studies of Chinese buildings." They are more commonly found in North China where they are used for the back and sidewalls to provide a barrier to the "predictably steady and cold northwest winds." Knapp, *Old Dwellings,* 170.
48. The *jian* 间, or the "span between two lateral columns or pillars that constitutes a bay" is not a fixed length: in the south it typically varies between 3.6 and 3.9 metres and in the north, 3.3 and 3.6 metres.
49. Butchart, "Hospital Construction," 99. The walls of the St James Hospital at Anqing were "of the usual Chinese style—hollow—up to the level of the top floor being filled with rubble, clay, clay and mortar, making it a heavy wall." "St James' Hospital, Ngankin, China," *CMMJ* 18, no. 3 (1904): 133.
50. Claude M. Lee, *Leaves from the Notebook,* 1932), 20.
51. Peck, "Concerning Williams' Hospital, 1887," 66.
52. Mackenzie, "The Construction of Hospitals," 78.
53. Ibid.
54. For a detailed description of the methods of ventilation utilizing "roof-top transoms" which take "advantage of differential pressure within the building [and the] careful alignment of open doors" in Chinese building, see Knapp, *Old Dwellings,* 240–43.
55. Mackenzie, "The Construction of Hospitals," 78.
56. Ibid. His hospital is described in Bryson, *John Kenneth Mackenzie: Medical Missionary to China,* 380.
57. "Missionary News," *Chinese Recorder and Missionary Journal* 22, no. 7 (1891): 339. The British Treaty of 1858 established that 1 Chinese foot = 14.1 inches. Julean Arnold, *China: Commercial and Industrial Handbook, Trade Promotion Series–No. 38* (Washington: Department of Commerce, USA, 1926), 792.

58. J.H. McCartney, "First (1892) Annual Report: Chungking Hospital, Methodist Episcopal Church, South," *CMMJ* 7, no. 4 (1893): 275.

59. Anne Fearn, who served as a doctor at this hospital for 14 years from 1893, described the buildings as "close to the canal, spacious affairs, architectural hybrids of the East and the West." Anne Walter Fearn, *My Days of Strength: A Woman Doctor's Forty Years in China* (London: Robert Hale Ltd., 1940), 41. MEM (S), which was headquartered in Nashville, Tennessee, had entered China in 1848 and medical work was their first initiative: first in Shanghai but later moved to Suzhou. Couling, *The Encyclopaedia Sinica*, 364–65.

60. Mildred M. Phillips, "The Hospital for Women at Soochow," *CMMJ* 3, no. 1 (1889).

61. Butchart, "Hospital Construction," 98.

62. Balme and Stauffer, "Enquiry: Scientific Efficiency, 1920," 9.

63. Peck, "Concerning Williams' Hospital, 1887," 66–67.

64. Butchart, "Hospital Construction," 99–100; Mackenzie, "The Construction of Hospitals," 78.

65. Edmund Lee Woodward, "The Practice of Asepsis in Mission Hospitals in China," *CMMJ* 18, no. 1 (1904): 256.

66. Speer, *"Lu Taifu," Charles Lewis*, 70.

67. For example, Elliott I. Osgood, "Tisdale Hospital, Chuchow," *CMJ* 25, no. 6 (1911): 415; W.E. Macklin, "Hwaiyuan Hospital Opening: Letter to the Editor," *CMMJ* 24, no. 5 (1910): 374.

68. Phillips, "The Hospital for Women at Soochow," Varnish made from the sap of *Rhus vernicifera* with the peculiarity that it only hardens in a moist atmosphere. Couling, *The Encyclopaedia Sinica*, 587.

69. Butchart, "Hospital Construction," 100.

70. For his solution see Jefferys and Maxwell, *Diseases of China*, 677–80.

71. Butchart, "Hospital Construction," 102.

72. "The Opening of the Pingyin Hospital," 409.

73. Guenter B. Risse, *Mending Bodies*, 367.

74. The disposal of sewerage from hospitals was particularly problematic as Nathaniel Bercovitz (with the APM on Hainan Island) pointed out. In the absence of a method of rendering human waste from sick people safe to use, he proposed a system of disposal into a septic tank that "does away with the use of faeces as fertilizer." Nathaniel Bercovitz, "Studies in Sanitation in China: 1 the Disposal of Sewage in Institutions," *CMMJ* 31, no. 5 (1918).

75. Boyd, Chinese Architecture and Town Planning: 1500 B.C.–A.D. 1911, 83.

76. In the new Chongqing hospital, built by Dr Hall in 1902 the separate buildings were replaced by a single, four storeyed, "grey brick with white stone trimming" building in the shape of a cross. Those functions, which had been housed separately from the ward buildings: kitchen, wash house, dining room, store rooms, bathroom, and laundry were located in the basement and a strong room, morgue and gymnasium had been added. J. H. McCartney, 12th (1902) *Annual Report of Chungking General Hospital of the Methodist Episcopal Church* (Shanghai: American Presbyterian Mission Press, 1903), 1–2.

77. Butchart, "Hospital Construction," 98.

78. Osgood, "Tisdale Hospital, Chuchow," 415, Speer, *"Lu Taifu," Charles Lewis*, 48 and McCartney, *The 12th (1902) Annual Report*, 2.
79. Balme and Stauffer, "Enquiry: Scientific Efficiency, 1920," 4.
80. "Opening of the New Union Medical College Hospital, Tsinanfu," *CMJ* 30, no. 1 (1916): 49.
81. The CPM was based in St. Louis, Missouri but united with the APM (N) in 1906 and the plant, staff and converts were transferred. Couling, *The Encyclopaedia Sinica*, 137. O.T. Logan, "Westminster Sunday School Hospital, Changteh, Hunan," *CMJ* 30, no. 5 (1916): 353.

NOTES TO CHAPTER FIVE

1. Jeffrey W. Cody, "Striking a Harmonious Chord."
2. The name was taken from the literary name for Hunan province, *Hsiang* and *Ya* from *Yali* (the transliteration of Yale). It was used from the time Hume established his first hospital in 1908 and was chosen to symbolize the co-operation envisaged between "the citizens of Hunan and the Yale University Mission." Edward H. Hume, *Doctors East Doctors West*, 177–78.
3. For a summary of the history of this institution, see William Reeves, "Sino-American Cooperation in Medicine: The Origins of Hsiang-Ya (1902–1914)," in *American Missionaries in China: Papers from Harvard Seminars*, ed. Liu Kwang-Ching (Cambridge, Mass.: East Asian Research Center, Harvard University, 1966) and F. C. Yen, "An Example of Co-Operation with the Chinese in Medical Education: Paper Read at Biennial Conference of the CMMA, Shanghai, February, 1915," *CMMJ* 31, no. 3 (1917).
4. Cody, "Striking a Harmonious Chord."
5. Jeffrey W. Cody, Building in China, 37. Lian Xi, *The Conversion of Missionaries*, 35–36.
6. Cody, "Striking a Harmonious Chord."
7. Hume, *Doctors East Doctors West*, 175. Edward Stephen Harkness (1874–1940, an American philanthropist was born in Cleveland, Ohio. He inherited a fortune from his father, a partner of John D. Rockefeller, Sr. His extensive philanthropies, many of them anonymous, were extended especially to colleges, hospitals, and museums. *The Columbia Encyclopedia, Sixth ed.* (New York: Columbia University Press, 2002).
8. Hume, Doctors East Doctors West, 1946, 176.
9. Edward H. Hume, *Hsiangya Hospital, Changsha, (Hunan)* (New York: W.W. Norton and Co., 1946).
10. This criticism is less harsh than that Gwendolyn Wright found among French colonial architects in Indochina, for whom "the worst architectural sin . . . was any intrusion of Indochinese architectural motifs . . . The result of such a merging of cultures, in architectural as in racial terms, was branded with the epithet *"metis."* Gwendolyn Wright, *Politics of Design in French Colonial Urbanism* (Chicago: University of Chicago Press, 1991), 179.
11. Su Gin-Djih, *Chinese Architecture*, 130. The curve of the traditional Chinese roof is not a mere decorative device. Buildings in China were commonly

wooden structures and the overhanging eaves served to protect the walls from rain. The eaves were swept upwards to permit light to enter the interior, despite the overhang. The gap between the top of the wall and the roof also allowed cross-ventilation of the building. In addition, the concave curve of the roof meant that the Chinese semi-cylindrical tiles could be fitted together "snugly for watertightness." Liang Ssu-ch'eng, *A Pictorial History of Chinese Architecture*, 12.

12. Cody, "Striking a Harmonious Chord."
13. Shattuck was Hussey's professor and the president of the Chicago Art Institute. Hussey had undertaken commissions for the YMCA while he was still a student at the Chicago School of Architecture at the Art Institute after winning several design competitions. Harry Hussey, *My Pleasure and Palaces: An Informal Memoir of Forty Years in Modern China*, 1st ed. (New York: Doubleday and Company, 1968), 46–50. The YMCA wished to avoid problems encountered by other organizations which had drawings prepared by architectural firms in America but were not familiar with Chinese landscape, conditions, skills or materials. Cody, "Striking a Harmonious Chord."
14. The first ACM Wuchang hospital for men, started in rented premises in 1874, was replaced by a purpose-built hospital (St. Peter's) in 1894. A hospital for women was opened in 1883. "General Hospital American Church Mission, Wuchang, Hupeh," *CMMJ* 33, no. 1 (1919): 72.
15. In particular, by the Special Committee on Business and Administrative Efficiency. The CCC was established in 1913, under the presidency of Dr. John R. Mott, to help carry out, inter alia, the recommendations of the Missionary Conference held in Shanghai, to "promote co-operation and co-ordination among the Christian forces of China [and] serve as a clearing house for information." Samuel Couling, *The Encyclopaedia Sinica*, 97–98. E.C. Lobenstine, "Letter to the Editor: Relief for Missionary Builders," *Chinese Recorder and Missionary Journal* 46, no. 9 (1915): 578–79 and "A Missionary Architectural Firm," *Chinese Recorder and Missionary Journal* 46, no. 11 (1915).
16. Led by "His Excellency Chou Hsueh-hsi, Minister of Finance under President Yuan Shik-Hai" and Wu Lien-teh. For the others members, a description of the lead up to building and costs, see Wu Lien-teh, *Plague Fighter: the Autobiography of a Modern Chinese Physician* (Cambridge [Eng.]: W. Heffer, 1959), 460–46. See also Wu Lien-teh, "The Central Hospital of Peking," *CMMJ* 31, no. 4 (1917): 352–54.
17. "Peking Union Medical College," *CMJ* 35, no. 4 (1921): 485. See W.W. Peter, "The Conference and Dedication at Peking," *CMJ* 35, no. 5 (1921) for a description of the formalities and the conference called to mark the occasion. Part of the complex had been opened since September 1919. "Peking Union Medical College," 457.
18. Ronald G. Knapp, *China's Old Dwellings*, 62.
19. Curator, Collection of Eastern Art, Ashmolean Museum, Oxford. Peter C. Swann, *Chinese Monumental Art* (London: Thames and Hudson, 1963), 232.

20. Francesca Bray, "Chinese Health Beliefs," in *Religion, Health and Suffering,* ed. John R. Hinnells and Roy Porter (London and New York: Kegan Paul International, 1999), 200.

21. Andrew Boyd, *Chinese Architecture and Town Planning: 1500 B.C.–A.D. 1911* (London: Alec Tiranti, 1962), 45 and Knapp, *Old Dwellings,* 22.

22. Wu Lien-teh, "The Central Hospital of Peking," 461.

23. Logan H. Roots, *Our Plan for the Church General Hospital, Wuchang: A Statement of the Most Urgent Needs in the District of Hankow, Leaflet 211* (New York: The Board of Missions, c. 1916)

24. See "General Hospital American Church Mission, Wuchang, Hupeh," and Roots, *Our Plan.*

25. Hussey, *My Pleasure and Palaces,* 230–32.

26. Robert E. Speer, *"Lu Taifu," Charles Lewis,* 48.

27. Roger S. Greene, "Letter to Rt Rev. H. L. Roots, Bishop of Hankow," (April 29, 1915).

28. Logan H. Roots, "Letter to Roger S. Greene," (June 25, 1915).

29. Guenter B. Risse, *Mending Bodies,* 469.

30. Milburn, "A Comparative Study of Modern English, Continental and American Hospital Construction," 271.

31. Wu Lien-teh, *Plague Fighter,* 463. I have found no other reference to this objection and in traditional courtyard houses some buildings faced east and west.

32. "Opening of the New Union Medical College Hospital, Tsinanfu," *CMJ* 30, no. 1 (1916): 72.

33. See the specified minimum requirements for a small hospital set out in a design competition held by the publishers of the journal, *The Modern Hospital* in 1923. *Architectural Designs for a Small Hospital,* (Chicago: The Modern Hospital Publishing Co., 1923), 104.

34. Roots, *Our Plan,* 10.

35. Wu Lien-teh, *Plague Fighter,* 462–63.

36. Nearly three feet above the street level. Ibid. 463.

37. A clinic, located in the "southern and more crowded section of Peking, where paying and non-paying patients were seen" fed the hospital. Ibid. 465.

38. Interestingly, there are no chimneys shown on the drawing, which raises the question of whether they were simply omitted from the drawing, from the building altogether, or were somehow hidden to lend a Chinese look to the roofline.

39. Mary Latimer James, "Mary Latimer James, M.D.," *Medical Woman's Journal,* October (1945): 55–56. James, a graduate of Bryn Mawr (1904) and the Women's Medical College of Pennsylvania (1907) was appointed to the hospital in 1914 and stayed for 25 years.

40. Wu Lien-teh, *Plague Fighter,* 460–62.

41. Roots, *Our Plan,* 4.

42. Hussey, *My Pleasure and Palaces,* 216.

43. Ibid. 224. The PUMC was the result of a union of North China Education Union (comprising the ABCFM, LMS, and APM in Beijing) using the medical schools of the AMEM, Peking University and LMS. A new College had

been opened in 1906. See Ernest J. Peill, "The New Union Medical College in Peking," *CMMJ* 20, no. 1 (1906): 122–24.
44. See Hussey, *My Pleasure and Palaces*, 224–25.
45. Ibid. 209–11.
46. Mr. Charles A. Coolidge of Shipley, Putnam and Coolidge of Boston, consulting architect to the Rockefeller Foundation, PUMC.
47. Hussey, *My Pleasure and Palaces*, 210.
48. Ibid. 237. Swann describes the Forbidden City as being "dominated by the red buildings whose tints are often toned down by sun and rain to brownish reds or greys and the whole crowned by yellow glazed tiles which glitter in the sunlight." Swann, *Chinese Monumental Art*, 240.
49. Hussey, My Pleasure and Palaces, 216.
50. Ibid. 229.
51. George N. Kates, *The Years That Were Fat: The Last of Old China* (Cambridge, Mass.: The M.I.T. Press, 1952; reprint, 1976), 76.
52. Hussey, *My Pleasure and Palaces*, 220, 30.
53. Ibid. 234.
54. Shattuck and Hussey Architects, "Letter to Robert H. Kirk (Rockefeller Foundation)," (Rockefeller Archive Centre, New York.: August 9, 1918).
55. Hussey, *My Pleasure and Palaces*, 234–35. Not everyone working on the building would agree that the story of the bricks was so simple. The "timekeeper" at Shattuck and Hussey was concerned that they had been overcharged by the supplier. See J. W. Smith, "Letter to Weaver (Rockefeller Foundation) Concerning Financial and Contractural Issues," (Rockefeller Archive Centre, New York.: April 27, 1918).
56. Hussey, *My Pleasure and Palaces*, 237–38. Hussey, in his autobiography, does not mention that the supply of these tiles was to become another source of conflict between himself and the Rockefeller Foundation. Hussey's "honesty" was questioned in relation to the letting of the tile contract. He was eventually replaced by the China Medical Board because of a number of indiscretions and problems with staff and other contractors. See Edwin R. Embree, "Letter to R.S. Greene (Rockefeller Foundation) on Behalf of the Building Committee of the Peking Union Medical College," (Rockefeller Archive Centre, New York.: April 3, 1918). In addition, concern was expressed as to the quality of the tiles supplied: tests had shown that they "did not ring clear, and [were] extremely porous, absorbing under test a large quantity of water." Shattuck and Hussey Architects, "Letter to Robert H. Kirk (Rockefeller Foundation)," (Rockefeller Archive Centre, New York.: August 13, 1918).
57. Hussey, *My Pleasure and Palaces*, 229.
58. "Entrance to the Anatomy Building," *CMJ* 35, no. 4 (1921): 416.
59. Peter, "The Conference and Dedication at Peking,"
60. See color photograph at Photograph Collection, William H. Welch, "View of the Peking Union Medical College, Circa 1921.," 2000. <http://medical archives.jhmi.edu/welch/travelph.htm> (December 2003).
61. John A. Snell, *Report of the Soochow Hospital, Soochow, China* (Shanghai: The Oriental Press, 1919), 5.

62. It is not obvious from either the drawing or photographs whether or not the whole was enclosed in a compound.
63. See Liang Ssu-ch'eng, *A Pictorial History of Chinese Architecture*, 21.
64. See Knapp, *Old Dwellings*, 22–24.
65. O.T. Logan, "Five Years' Experience in Aseptic Surgery in an Inland Hospital," *CMJ* 30, no. 1 (1916): 21.
66. "Opening of the New Union Medical College Hospital, Tsinanfu," 52–53.

NOTES TO SECTION III. FINANCING THE HOSPITAL ENTERPRISE

1. Rosemary Stevens, *In Sickness and in Wealth*, 20.
2. The Federal government provided a few hospitals, for example, for merchant sailors, the army, and "blacks freed from slavery after the Civil War." Ibid. 29. The census was conducted by the U.S. Department of Commerce and Labor, Bureau of the Census. The report was entitled Benevolent Institutions (Washington D.C.: Government Printing Office. 1905). See Stevens, *In Sickness and in Wealth*, 23–24.
3. I have adopted the term secular to avoid the confusion inherent in Steven's use of "private-non-ecclesiastical," for what are variously called voluntary, charitable, or community hospitals.
4. Stevens, *In Sickness and in Wealth*, 24.
5. Ibid. 20. According to Rosenberg this type of hospital only became widespread during the last decade of the nineteenth century and the first decade of the twentieth century. Charles E. Rosenberg, *The Care of Strangers*, 402 n2.
6. In addition to the secondary sources, I draw on the following primary sources for patterns of income and expenditure in a representative range of contemporary American hospitals. *Auburn City Hospital: Thirty-First Annual Report of the Board of Managers* (Year Ended September 30, 1910), (Auburn, N.Y.: Knapp, Peck & Thomson, Printers, 1910), *First Annual Report of the Elliot City Hospital, Keene, N.H. For the Year Ending, December 1, 1893*, (Keene: City of Keene, New Hampshire, 1894), *The Lancaster General Hospital, Report of the Babies' Wards Post-Graduate Hospital*, (New York: n.p., 1917), *Sisters of Mercy, Annual Report of St John's Hospital and Training School for Nurses: October 1913–September 1914* (St Louis, Missouri: 1915), *Sixth Annual Report of the Highland Hospital, Fall River, Mass.*, (Fall River, Massachusetts: 1915).
7. Calculated from plans reproduced in *Lancaster Hospital, 1906*, foll. 56.
8. Ibid. 47–50.
9. For the most thorough examination of the history of the financial and administrative aspects of the American hospital system in the early twentieth century see Stevens, *In Sickness and in Wealth*, esp. chapter 2. See also Rosenberg, *The Care of Strangers*, esp. chapter 10 and Guenter B. Risse, *Mending Bodies*, esp. Chapter 9.
10. Rosenberg, *The Care of Strangers*, 244–45. Sandra Opdycke details the methods employed by New York hospitals to "pay the bills." See Sandra

Opdycke, *No One Was Turned Away: The Role of Public Hospitals in New York City since 1900* (Oxford: Oxford University Press, 1999), 55–58.

11. Stevens, *In Sickness and in Wealth*, 24.
12. Ibid. 25.
13. *Auburn City Hospital*, 1910, 12.
14. In the beginning people who endowed these beds could, if they wished, designate a particular, or class of, beneficiary. However, this practice gradually disappeared coinciding with the emergence of the policy of admitting patients based on medical grounds rather than on recommendation of a hospital benefactor.
15. *Report of the Babies' Wards Post-Graduate Hospital*, 31–39.
16. "Miscellany," *CMMJ* 11, no. 3&4 (1897): 263 and Rosenberg, *The Care of Strangers*, 316.
17. For example, according to the summary of the statistical returns from 126 hospitals in China for 1910 there were a little over 50,000 hospital in-patients compared to nearly or a total of 850,000 out-patients—220,000 new, and at least 630,000 returning. "[Medical Mission] Statistics for the Year, 1910," *CMJ* 25, no. 5 (1911).

NOTES TO CHAPTER SIX

1. See Joanna Waley-Cohen, *The Sextants of Beijing: Global Currents in Chinese History* (New York: W.W. Norton & Company, 1999), 64–70 and Jacques Gernet, *China and the Christian Impact: A Conflict of Cultures* (Cambridge: Cambridge University Press, 1985), 15–16.
2. "Why Medical Missionaries Are in China?," *CMMJ* 14, no. 4 (1900): 279.
3. John Glasgow Kerr, "Self-Support in Mission Hospitals," *CMMJ* 9, no. 3 (1895): 136.
4. A.P. Peck, "The Development of the Medical Department of a Mission Station," *CMMJ* 16, no. 1 (1902): 14.
5. The participants in the debate on fees were overwhelmingly American. Of the sixteen who played the most prominent roles in print whose nationality I have been able to determine, ten were American, two Canadian, three British, and one Chinese trained in America. Of the twelve Americans and Canadians, only three took a stand against charging fees whereas two of the three British did. This section is based largely on the arguments put forward in significant articles published in the *CMMJ*, supplemented with material from the annual reports of a number of hospitals.
6. The hospital had been established just beyond the West Gate of Shanghai's Chinese city in 1885. Kenneth Scott Latourette, *A History of Christian Missions in China* (New York: Russell & Russell, 1929), 456.
7. Elizabeth Reifsnyder, "Methods of Dispensary Work," *CMMJ* 1, no. 2 (1887): 67–68.
8. See for example, the summary of a symposium held in 1910. C.W. Service, "A Symposium on Methods of Raising Money Amongst the Chinese for

Medical Work: Read at the West China Missionary Conference, 1908," *CMJ* 24, no. 1 (1910).

9. For example, see Rosemary Stevens, *In Sickness and in Wealth*, 42 for a description of the turn-of-the-century American hospitals' reluctance to accept "free" patients on the basis that to do so would pauperize them, that is create an underclass, or lead to "charity abuse."

10. Horace A. Randle, "How to Encourage the Chinese to Subscribe toward the Support of Medical Missionary Work among Them: Paper Read at the Shantung Medical Missionary Conference, 1898," *CMMJ* 13, no. 1&2 (1899): 16.

11. Kerr, "Self-Support, 1895," 136.

12. The only missionary society to have its headquarters in China (Shanghai) but with offices in Great Britain, USA, Australia and New Zealand, the CIM was started in England. It was interdenominational and employed missionaries of any nationality. See Samuel Couling, *The Encyclopaedia Sinica*, 98–100.

13. A.W. Douthwaite, "The C.I.M. Hospital and Dispensary at Chefoo.," *CMMJ* 8, no. 2 (1894): 137.

14. S. R Hodge, "The Church's Duty in Relation to Medical Missions, and the Principles Upon Which Such Missions Should Be Conducted.," *CMMJ* 5, no. 3 (1891): 141.

15. A medical missionary with the Canadian Methodist Mission at Chengdu in Sichuan, Kilborn wrote an exhaustive article on the issue of "self-support" in mission hospitals published at the height of the debate in 1901. Omar L. Kilborn, "Self-Support in Mission Hospitals," *CMMJ* 15, no. 2 (1901).

16. Ibid. 94.

17. "Miscellany," *CMMJ* 11, no. 3&4 (1897): 262–65.

18. Randle, "How to Encourage the Chinese, 1899," 14. Evidence that he was at odds with his fellow medical missionaries in his views is provided in a news item to the effect that Randle, formerly with the CIM and the American Southern Baptists, was "constrained by the change in his theological views" to sever connection with the Mission—to do independent work. "News," *CMMJ* 14, no. 1 (1900): 71.

19. Wesleyan Methodist Missionary Society (WMMS) had its headquarters in London and had been in China since 1852. After his time at Foshan, Roderick Macdonald was appointed to open medical work in Wuchow in 1898, but was murdered by pirates in 1906. Couling, *The Encyclopaedia Sinica*, 598.

20. Roderick MacDonald, "Wesleyan Missionary Hospital, Fatshan, China, 1893," *CMMJ* 8, no. 2 (1894): 134. Another who put this view strongly was George Cox of the CIM who wrote that the pay system "lifted them [Chinese] from the moral beggary of which we see so much." Geo. A Cox, "Out-Patient Department of Medical Work," *CMMJ* 16, no. 2 (1902): 129.

21. George A Stuart, "The Wuhu General Hospital: 1891–1893," *CMMJ* 8, no. 2 (1894): 128.

22. Kilborn, "Self-Support, 1901," 96.

23. H.T. Whitney, "To What Extent Is Charity Incumbent Upon Medical Missionaries?," *CMMJ* 8, no. 4 (1894): 185.
24. Stuart, "The Wuhu General Hospital: 1891–1893," 128–29.
25. Stevens, *In Sickness and in Wealth*, 19.
26. Ibid. 25.
27. Theoretically, 1,000 (copper) cash, the currency used by the common people, was equivalent to one tael. In the beginning, the Yaoling Hospital in Shandong charged "all worm-patients and men with venereal disease." Later, when they opened a new hospital they instituted a fee regime for all outpatients, viz. "50 Shantung cash a visit; worm-patients and malarial cases paying fifty cash extra, and venereal patients 500 cash." "Report of the Lao-Ling Medical Mission, 1905," *CMMJ* 20, no. 6 (1906): 270. Huntley "always charged for venereal diseases: two hundred cash per week or a compound fee of one thousand cash." George A. Huntley, "Our out-Patient Work," *CMMJ* 16, no. 2 (1902): 113.
28. Kilborn, "Self-Support, 1901," 93. Cox observed that all his Chinese syphilitic patients, who paid a deposit ($2 Mex.) before being prescribed for, "pay readily and it has a good moral effect on them." Cox, "Out-Patient Department, 1902," 129.
29. W. Hamilton Jefferys and James L. Maxwell, *The Diseases of China*, 576.
30. This did not necessarily apply to those patients who employed the popular contemporary method of committing suicide: eating opium. Ida Kahn, for instance, reported that she never charged "anything for the suicide cases which come to our dispensary, because such emergencies must be treated too spontaneously for determining charges." Ida Kahn, "Self-Supporting Medical Missionary Work," *CMMJ* 19, no. 6 (1905): 224.
31. Kilborn, "Self-Support, 1901," 94. A Lyall reported that he charged most opium-smokers $1 on admission as they came in large numbers and "were very unsatisfactory patients." A. Lyall, "Swatow Medical Mission," *CMMJ* 4, no. 1 (1890): 28.
32. *The Lancaster General Hospital*, 53, 27–41.
33. J.H. McCartney, "Medical Work," *CMMJ* 13, no. 3 (1899): 98.
34. Philip B. Cousland, "Medical Training of Native Preachers," *CMMJ* 16, no. 1 (1902): 69.
35. McCartney, "Medical Work," 98.
36. Luella M. Masters, "The "Pay Doctor" in China," *CMMJ* 16, no. 1 (1902): 3.
37. This is not to imply that the "females" were practitioners of "official" medicine as Leung elaborates: "even though in China 'official' medicine was particularly difficult to define, all agreed women did not belong." Angela Ki Che Leung, "Organized Medicine" 153–54.
38. Ibid. 146.
39. H.T. Whitney, "The Self-Supporting System in Medical Work," *CMMJ* 8, no. 2 (1894): 94.
40. Masters, "The "Pay Doctor" in China," 2.
41. The Wesleyan Missionary Conference had decided, in 1881, that all hospital expenses should be met from patient fees and subscriptions. MacDonald,

"Wesleyan Missionary Hospital, Fatshan, China, 1893," 134. For a description of Chinese methods of paying doctors: a fee wrapped in red paper; contract for a cure in a specified time; and paying to be kept in good health, see Jos. C Thomson, "Native Practice and Practitioners: Paper Read at Medical Missionary Association Conference, Shanghai May 1890," *CMMJ* 4, no. 3 (1890): 33.

42. Chas. Wenyon, "Wesleyan Missionary Hospital, Fatshan, South China: Report 1890," *CMMJ* 5, no. 2 (1891): 123.
43. McCartney, "Medical Work," 99.
44. Ibid.
45. Kahn, "Self-Supporting Medical Missionary Work," 223–24.
46. Hodge, "The Church's Duty, 1891," 141.
47. B.C. Atterbury, "Gratuitous Treatment," *CMMJ* 8, no. 2 (1894): 121.
48. William Warder Cadbury and Mary Hoxie Jones, *At the Point of a Lancet: One Hundred Years of the Canton Hospital, 1835–1935* (Shanghai: Kelly and Walsh Ltd., 1935), 188.
49. Mary W. Niles, "Native Midwifery in Canton," *CMMJ* 4, no. 2 (1890): 52.
50. MacDonald, "Wesleyan Missionary Hospital, Fatshan, China, 1893," 135.
51. Atterbury, "Gratuitous Treatment, 1894," 122.
52. Kahn, "Self-Supporting Medical Missionary Work," 225.
53. Huntley, "Our out-Patient Work," 113.

NOTES TO CHAPTER SEVEN

1. See J.H. McCartney, "First (1892) Annual Report: Chungking Hospital, Methodist Episcopal Church, South," *CMMJ* 7, no. 4 (1893).
2. J.H. McCartney, *Chungking Men's Hospital (1912), (Gouldy Memorial)* (Shanghai: Methodist Publishing House, 1912), 2.
3. J.H. McCartney, *Second (1893) Annual Report: Chungking Hospital of the Methodist Episcopal Church* (Chongqing: Methodist Episcopal Church, 1893), 10.
4. The accounts include amounts of 672.70 and 262.50 *taels* under revenue attributed to "medicines from the Missionary Society and Women's Foreign Mission Society" respectively so we must assume that they donated medicines in kind rather than grants of money. These amounts represented almost twenty percent of the total current expenditure-calculated by taking total listed expenses less "patient's board" (which was fully covered by direct charges); "expenses under special gifts" (which are assumed to be for capital items), but including an amount of 859.98 *taels,* which was applied against the salary of the physician).Thus, the claim of "not one cent" was accurate but somewhat misleading. J.H. McCartney, *Annual Report (1898) of the West China Medical Mission, Methodist Episcopal Church* (Shanghai: American Presbyterian Mission Press, 1899), 16.
5. McCartney, *Second (1893) Annual Report,* 3. "Chair money" referred to the cost of hiring a chair to transport him from the hospital to the home he was visiting.

6. The various forms of currency are discussed later in this chapter. Until 1908, when he conformed to the norm and reported in Mexican dollars, McCartney reported using the local Chongqing *tael*. The exchange rate between cash and the Chongqing *tael* varied between 1200 *cash* in 1897 and 1240 in 1905. See J. H. McCartney, *Sixth (1897) Annual Report of the General Hospital of the Methodist Episcopal Church, Chungking, China:* (Shanghai: American Presbyterian Mission Press, 1898), J.H. McCartney, *15th Annual Report (1905) of the Chungking General Hospital for Men of the Methodist Episcopal Church* (Shanghai: Methodist Publishing House, 1905). In most reports, he gave sufficient information for the exchange rate to be ascertained and it was relatively stable at $1.00 Mexican being equivalent to 0.70 *taels*.

7. McCartney, *Second (1893) Annual Report*, 10.

8. McCartney, *Annual Report (1898)*, 2.

9. Ibid. 6–7.

10. I have not been able to include the money spent by Chinese in the Drug Store because, although references were sometimes made to the turnover, it was not included in the financial statements as a discrete item. As will be seen, the turnover was substantial and so the Chinese contribution to the hospital was more significant than would appear from figure 2.

11. J. H. McCartney, *Annual Report (1901) of the General Hospital, Methodist Episcopal Church, Chungking, China* (Chongqing: The West China Missionary News Office, 1901), 7.

12. McCartney, Annual Report (1898), 9.

13. J. H. McCartney, *12th (1902) Annual Report of Chungking General Hospital of the Methodist Episcopal Church* (Shanghai: American Presbyterian Mission Press, 1903), 6.

14. *Gouldy Memorial Hospital, Methodist Episcopal Church, Chungking, West China, 1908,* (n.p., 1908), 16–17.

15. McCartney, *Chungking Men's Hospital (1912)*, 35.

16. McCartney, *Annual Report (1901)*, 3.

17. *Gouldy Memorial Hospital, 1908*, 8–9.

18. McCartney, *The 15th Annual Report (1905)*, 2.

19. McCartney, *Chungking Men's Hospital (1912)*, 18.

20. See Robert Bickers, *Britain in China: Community, Culture and Colonialism 1900–1949*, ed. John M. MacKenzie, *Studies in Imperialism* (Manchester: Manchester University Press, 1999).

21. "The Commercial Value of the Missionary," *North China Herald and S.C. & C. Gazette,* July 10 1901, 55.

22. Arthur J. Brown, "The Motive of the Missionary Enterprise" *Chinese Recorder 25*, no. 9 (1904): 445.

23. Isabella Bird, *The Yangtze Valley and Beyond: An Account of Journeys in China, Chiefly in the Province of Sze Chuan and among the Man-Tze of the Somo Territory, 1899* (London: Virago Press Ltd; reprint, 1985), 45.

24. Thomas Gillison, "Charging for Drugs," *CMMJ* 16, no. 1 (1902): 20–1. Geo. A Cox, "Out-Patient Department of Medical Work," *CMMJ* 16, no. 2 (1902), E.M. Merrins, "Foreign Patent Medicines in China—Editorial,"

CMMJ 31, no. 4 (1917), "Mistakes of Some Missionaries," *North China Herald and S.C. & C. Gazette,* 24 July 1901; Arthur Jr. Schlesinger, "The Missionary Enterprise and Theories of Imperialism," in *The Missionary Enterprise in China and America,* ed. John K. Fairbank (Cambridge, Mass.: Harvard University Press, 1974).

25. McCartney, *The 12th (1902) Annual Report,* 6.
26. McCartney, *Annual Report (1901),* 4.
27. *Gouldy Memorial Hospital,* 7.
28. Henry Fowler, "Hiao-Kan Medical Mission: Annual Report," in *China India & Local Reports: 1905* (London: London Mission Society, 1905).
29. E.G. Ruoff, ed., *Death Throes of a Dynasty,* 154.
30. Ibid. 160, 62.
31. Current expenses did not include salaries for professional staff employed by the missionary society. I have also excluded any contributions made towards these salaries by the hospital. To calculate the average percentage I have omitted the foreign donations made in 1902 because the total foreign donation, $6,900 Mex., was allocated to a special building fund and it has not been possible to isolate the sum of subscriptions used for hospital running costs.
32. John G. McEllhenney, "200 Years of United Methodism: An Illustrated History," 1984. Available from <http://www.cros.net/wdrown/archives.htm>
33. Estimated from seven of the years for which Chinese subscriptions applied to current expenses can be determined. In 1901 and 1902 donations were included in the special building fund account.
34. Equivalent to $200 Mex. and $140 Mex. respectively. ·
35. J.H. McCartney, *Report (1911) of the Chungking Men's Hospital, Gouldy Memorial* (Shanghai: Methodist Publishing House, 1912), 1, 7.
36. Due to a large, one-off, donation of 1,000 *taels* from the gentry of Jiangbei partly in compensation for the loss of property and life, and to establish the new dispensary mentioned previously.
37. Sometimes McCartney listed donations from Chinese separately from his American supporters but in the main, I have had to rely on the names on the lists in his annual reports to identify the national source of the funds. Arthur Peill, at Cangzhou 滄州 in Hebei, had found that printing his annual reports in Chinese and distributing them among officials and gentry had resulted in "considerable enlightenment and in an increasing number of donations for our work" Arthur D Peill, "Hospital Reports: Roberts' Memorial Hospital, T'sang-Chow," *CMMJ* 20, no. 1 (1906): 45.
38. The large foreign contributions raised in 1901 and 1902 coincided with a drive for funds for building of a new hospital.
39. McCartney, *Chungking Men's Hospital (1912),* 9.
40. Included patient fees plus board but not purchases from the drug store or donations. Extracted from financial data included in Annual Reports, Chungking Hospital, 1897–1912.
41. Calculated using information from Treasurer's Report *The Lancaster General Hospital,* 5–6. Thus, the Lancaster Hospital's patient-fee income, in 1906, fell within the range of that for charity hospitals in America in 1904.

42. Extracted from financial data included in Annual Reports, Chungking Hospital, 1897–1912.
43. McCartney, *Second (1893) Annual Report,* 4–5.
44. Extracted from financial data included in Annual Reports of the Chunking Hospital, 1893–1912.
45. "Medical [Mission] Statistics for 1903," *CMMJ* 19, no. 1 (1905). Before 1903, lists of medical missionaries with, variously, their missionary society, "station," qualifications, dates of arrival and/or departure were published in the journal. See Jos. C Thomson, "Medical Missionaries to the Chinese," *CMMJ* 1, no. 2 (1887); Robert Case Beebe, "The Medical Missionary Association of China: List of Members," *CMMJ* 11, no. 2 (1897); Jos.C. Thomson, "Medical Missionaries to the Chinese," *CMMJ* 4, no. 4 (1890); and "List of Members of the China Medical Missionary Association," *CMMJ* 15, no. 2 (1901).
46. "Among the places which have not sent in reports are Chefoo, Chungking, Amoy, Peking, Tientsin, Chentu, cities where some of the larger hospitals in China are located . . . other cities . . . have failed to include some . . . such as Shanghai and Foochow." *"Medical [Mission] Statistics for 1903,"* 27.
47. "Fees and charges" in this context was a loose term covering any payment at all which could include payments for board, for some medicines or for dispensary visits.
48. "Medical [Mission] Statistics for 1904," *CMMJ* 19, no. 4 (1905); "Medical [Mission] Statistics for 1906," *CMJ* 21, no. 3 (1907); and "Medical Mission Statistics, 1905," *CMMJ* 20, no. 6 (1906).
49. The 1907 report provided only statistical information about patients and surgical operations and was not completely up-to-date, information having been compiled from that collected in 1907, supplemented with 1905 and 1906 data. "Medical Mission Statistics, 1907," *CMJ* 22, no. 3 (1908) and "[Medical Mission] Statistics for the Year, 1910," *CMJ* 25, no. 5 (1911).
50. John L. Carey, "The First National Association," in *The U.S. Accounting Profession in the 1890s and Early 1900s,* ed. Stephen A. Zeff (New York: Garland Publishing, Inc., 1988), 389.
51. Ibid. 397–98.
52. Mary E. Murphy, "Founding Fathers of the American Accounting Profession," in *The U.S. Accounting Profession in the 1890s and Early 1900s,* ed. Stephen A. Zeff (New York: Garland Publishing, Inc., 1988), 386.
53. Gary Giroux, "Great Events in Business and Accounting History." <http://acct.tamu.edu/giroux/timeline.html> (2002).
54. Montague H.T. Bell and H.G.W. Woodhead, *The China Year Book* (London: George Routledge & Sons, Ltd., 1912), 273–77.
55. "The Statistics Again," *CMJ* 21, no. 6 (1907). There was a third category of hospital where patients were responsible for their own food. The arrangements concerning food are discussed in the next chapter.
56. "Missionaries and Accuracy," *CMJ* 29, no. 3 (1915).
57. A German missionary society that worked in Guangdong province.
58. It is difficult to make a definite statement about the application of fees because of obvious inadequacies in the design of the questionnaire. I have

assumed that a response provided under the heading "charges for dispensary patients" of 10 *cash* means that the charge was made for each visit unless otherwise indicated. Twenty-three, out of twenty-seven that gave details of fees, charged for dispensary visits in 1904. Sixty-eight, out of seventy-four that gave details of fees, charged in 1906.

59. "Soochow Hospital, Methodist Episcopal Church, South," *CMMJ* 18, no. 2 (1904): 56. The fees had increased to $1 and 10 cents respectively when a representative of the Rockefeller Foundation visited in 1915 to assess their application for funding. *"Soochow Hospital. Southern Methodist Mission,"* (c.1915).

60. Omar L. Kilborn, "Self-Support in Mission Hospitals," *CMMJ* 15, no. 2 (1901): 93.

61. Francis F. Tucker, "Letter to the Editor: Record Forms," *CMMJ* 18, no. 2 (1904): 94.

62. Five and fifteen times his normal dispensary registration fee respectively. Kilborn, "Self-Support, 1901," 93.

63. Estimated to be equivalent to 350 *cash*. Cox, "Out-Patient Department, 1902," 129.

64. H.W. Boone, "How Can the Medical Work Be Made More Helpful to the Cause of the Church in China?," *CMMJ* 8, no. 1 (1894): 16.

65. The figures that follow are calculated by combining the results of the 1904, 1905 and 1906 surveys. Twenty-seven of the ninety hospitals provided information on two occasions and twenty-six, on all three. Of the remaining thirty-seven, ten responded only in 1904, one in 1905 and twenty-six in 1906 only. Not all who responded gave information about dispensary fees. We could assume that the five that did not answer the specific question charged no fee, but I have excluded them from the analysis.

66. Extracted from Medical Mission Statistical Surveys for 1904, 1905 and 1906 published in *CMMJ*.

67. Based on an analysis of "duration of mission" and fee charging policy. The founding year of eighty-six of the ninety-six hospitals were determined using a variety of sources including Kenneth Scott Latourette, *A History of Christian Missions in China,* K C. Wong and Wu Lien-teh, *History of Chinese Medicine* and "[Medical Mission] Statistics for the Year, 1910."

68. The interdenominational Missionary Societies included: the London Missionary Society, The China Inland Mission, the American Board of Commissioners for Foreign Missions and the Yale Foreign Missionary Society which together accounted for twenty-one of the ninety-two hospitals. Only one did not charge a fee.

69. British Methodists included the English Methodists (New Connection) hospital at Yaoling in Shandong and the Wesleyan Methodist Church Men's hospital at Hankou in Hubei.

70. Included both the American Presbyterian Mission, headquartered in New York, which was the largest denominational mission in China and the American Presbyterian Mission (South), which had its headquarters in Nashville Tennessee. Samuel Couling, *The Encyclopaedia Sinica,* 18–23.

71. I have combined the results for seven English Presbyterian, two United Free Church of Scotland, two Irish Presbyterian, and one Church of Scotland Mission hospitals.

72. See Charles E. Rosenberg, *The Care of Strangers,* 316–22 for an examination of the place of the outpatient department in America. Granshaw discusses the setting up of dispensaries by private practitioners in Britain in the eighteenth century in Lindsay Granshaw, "The Hospital," 1188–89.

73. See Rosemary Stevens, *In Sickness and in Wealth,* 48–9 and 373 fn. 87.

74. Robert Case Beebe, "Hospitals and Dispensaries," *CMMJ* 15, no. 1 (1901): 7.

75. An exception was the Pennsylvania Hospital where outpatients were given a prescription to be "compounded at a drug store." The 1908 annual report attributes the relatively low level of medical versus surgical cases seen during the year to the cost of medicine being beyond the means of many potential patients who went to other dispensaries in the city that supplied medicine free or at a nominal cost. *Report of the Board of Managers of the Pennsylvania Hospital Comprising the Report of the Department for the Sick and Wounded and the Departments for the Insane, West Philadelphia,* (Philadelphia: J.B. Lippincott Company, 1908), 8–9.

76. W. Hamilton Jefferys and James L. Maxwell, *The Diseases of China,* 592.

77. Jeffreys notes that this is the most commonly administered treatment for round worms, Ascaris lumbricoides, but warns against indiscriminate use. Ibid. 169

78. "Medical [Mission] Statistics for 1906." Some specifically mention that they only charge for patients with venereal diseases.

79. He answered "$4 per month board," "150–2000 cash a month," and " 80–2000 cash per day" to the question "Inpatient Fees?" in the 1904, 1905 and 1906 surveys respectively. "Medical [Mission] Statistics for 1904"; "Medical [Mission] Statistics for 1906"; "Medical Mission Statistics, 1905."

80. *Architectural Designs for a Small Hospital,* 104.

81. Calculated from floor plans reproduced in *Lancaster Hospital, 1906,* foll. 56.

82. *Sixth Annual Report of the Highland Hospital, Fall River, Mass.,* (Fall River, Massachusetts: 1915).

83. James Butchart, "Hospital Construction: Paper Read at the Medical Missionary Association, 1901," *CMMJ* 15, no. 2 (1901): 98.

84. "The Opening of the Pingyin Hospital," *CMMJ* 23, no. 6 (1909): 408.

85. "The American Baptist Mission Hospital: Shaohsing, Chekiang," *North China Herald and S.C. & C. Gazette,* March 25 1910. The architects for the Alden Speare Memorial Hospital, run by Methodist Episcopalians at Yen-ping in Fujian, anticipated the possibility that smaller rooms could become desirable and designed wards that they could be easily "divided at any time." J.E. Skinner, "The Alden Speare Memorial Hospital, Yen-Ping, China," *CMMJ* 18, no. 4 (1904): 163.

86. Richard Wolfendale, "An Ideal Medical Missionary Hospital," *CMMJ* 17, no. 1 (1903): 21.

NOTES TO SECTION IV. THE PATIENT'S EXPERIENCE

1. See Roy Porter, *The Cambridge Illustrated History of Medicine*, 140, Roy Porter, *The Greatest Benefit to Mankind: A Medical History of Humanity from Antiquity to the Present* (London: Harper Collins, 1997), 606. The Canton hospital reported in 1900 that they had acquired an X-ray machine for $750 'through the liberality of some Chinese friends.' 'Hospital Reports: Summary,' *CMMJ* 14, no. 3 (1900): 204.
2. Rosemary Stevens, *In Sickness and in Wealth*, 18.
3. An X-ray machine, given by late 'Tao tai of Ningpo,' needed 'accumulators' [batteries] that had to be taken to Shanghai regularly to be charged as they had no dynamo to make power. A.F. Cole, *Twentieth Annual Report: C.M.S. Hospital, Ningpo* (Ningpo: C.M.S. Medical Mission, 1906), 10. Balme's survey found, as late as 1919, that of the 188, who answered the question, 115 (61 percent,) hospitals still relied on kerosene oil for lighting and two used acetylene. Harold Balme and Milton T. Stauffer, 'An Enquiry into the Scientific Efficiency of Mission Hospitals in China' (paper presented at the Annual Conference of the China Medical Missionary Association, Peking, February 20–27 1920), 19–20.

NOTES TO CHAPTER EIGHT

1. Omar L. Kilborn, *Heal the Sick: An Appeal for Medical Missions in China* (Toronto: Missionary Society of the Methodist Church, 1910), 189.
2. Many hospitals also ran "district" dispensaries in surrounding villages and some held clinics in centers further away on a less regular basis. Both acted as avenues for admittance to hospital, as did physicians' visits to patients' homes.
3. For a description of the forces involved in the demise of the public dispensary, see Charles E. Rosenberg, *The Care of Strangers*, 316–22.
4. See Paul Starr, *The Social Transformation of American Medicine* (New York: Basic Books, Inc., 1982), 181–84.
5. Most mission societies required all their workers to undergo a minimum of one years' language study, and many required two. See Appendix II, "Information Regarding Medical Missionary Service in China," Note 7 in Harold Balme, *China and Modern Medicine: A Study in Medical Mission Development* (London: United Council for Missionary Education, 1921), 212–14. Alfred Hogg thought that "[t]o attack a local dialect with eight tones, and no colloquial dictionary to assist one, is about enough for the first year's work." Charles Johnson, at Yizhoufu, spent his mornings in language study and, while prevented from work due to the Boxers, "read some medical books in Chinese so as not to forget." Alfred Hogg, "Letter to the Editor: Wenchow Hospital," *CMMJ* 13, no. 1&2 (1899) and Charles F. Johnson, "Hospital Reports: Medical Work at I-Chow-Fu," *CMMJ* 19, no. 5 (1905): 209.
6. George A. Huntley, "Our out-Patient Work," *CMMJ* 16, no. 2 (1902): 113. Other missionaries did not report this practice and Huntley might have

been referring to the ritual burning of paper with characters. The Chinese so revered the written word that people were employed by benevolent institutions to collect such paper. See William C. Milne, "Notices of Seven Months' Residence in the City of Ningbo, from December 7th, 1842, to July 7th, 1843," *Chinese Repository* 13, no. 1,2,3,7 (1844): 30.

7. An exception was Omar Kilborn at Chengdu who reported that the women, who constituted 20–30 percent of his patients, were all seen before the first man. Kilborn, *Heal the Sick,* 1910, 189.

8. George Hadden, "The Registration of Out-Patients," *CMMJ* 31, no. 1 (1917): 27–28.

9. D. Duncan Main, "An Out-Patient Day at the Hangchow Hospital, 12th February, 1889," *CMMJ* 3, no. 4 (1889): 113.

10. An inveterate traveler, Isabella Lucy Bird, (1831–1904), married Dr John Bishop in 1881 but he died five years later and she "set off on her travels" to Tibet, Persia, Kurdistan, Korea and, in 1896, the interior of China. Isabella Bird, *The Yangtze Valley and Beyond*

11. W. Hamilton Jefferys and James L. Maxwell, *The Diseases of China,* 667. He did mention that Shanghai was the only city where such segregation of the sexes in the waiting room was unnecessary. Presumably, by 1910, the Chinese who lived within the foreign concessions were sufficiently used to the ways of Western missionaries.

12. "The Opening of St James' Hospital, Anking," *CMJ* 22, no. 1 (1908): 117.

13. "St James' Hospital, Ngankin, China," *CMMJ* 18, no. 3 (1904): 134.

14. A. M. Jefferys, "Formal Opening of St. Andrew's Dispensary, Wusieh, Kiangsu," *CMMJ* 22, no. 3 (1908): 185.

15. "Opening of the New Union Medical College Hospital, Tsinanfu," *CMJ* 30, no. 1 (1916): 50

16. T. W. Ayers, "Warren Memorial Hospital, Hwang-Hein, Shantung," *CMMJ* 20, no. 1 (1906): 49.

17. "The Medical Missionary and the Anti-Foreign Riots in China," *CMMJ* 7, no. 2 (1893): 110.

18. "Mistakes of Some Missionaries," *North China Herald and S.C. & C. Gazette,* 24 July 1901, 171–72.

19. A.F. Cole, *Twentieth Annual Report: C.M.S. Hospital, Ningpo,* 8.

20. From the beginning, medical missionaries tried to find young, preferably "Christian" Chinese men, to train as assistants. Some formalized the training and conducted classes in the rudiments of western medicine, anatomy and science. These formed the basis of the small medical schools which proliferated before the arrival of the Rockefeller Foundation into China, in 1914, after which larger, "Union" medical schools were established on a more substantial basis.

21. Cole, *Twentieth Annual Report: C.M.S. Hospital, Ningpo,* 2.

22. He did have a special room for surgical dressing, a private room for "special examinations" and a dark room for eye patients. Kilborn, *Heal the Sick,* 1910, 188.

23. Elizabeth Reifsnyder, "Methods of Dispensary Work," *CMMJ* 1, no. 2 (1887): 68

24. Jos. C Thomson, "Native Practice and Practitioners: Paper Read at Medical Missionary Association Conference, Shanghai May 1890," *CMMJ* 4, no. 3 (1890): 197. For a description of a typical consultation with a Chinese doctor, see S. M. Hillier and J. A Jewell, *Health Care and Traditional Medicine in China, 1800–1982*, 4–5.
25. Reifsnyder, "Methods of Dispensary Work," 69.
26. Edward H. Hume, *Doctors East Doctors West*, 56.
27. Geo. A Cox, "Out-Patient Department of Medical Work," *CMMJ* 16, no. 2 (1902): 129.
28. In order to answer the question, he visited most hospitals in Shandong, Tianjin, and Peking as well as holding discussion with a "a dozen or more medical men sojourning at their summer retreat." Charles K. Roys, "Some Dispensary Methods," *CMMJ* 21, no. 3 (1907): 110.
29. Ibid. 110–12.
30. "Medical [Mission] Statistics for 1906," *CMJ* 21, no. 3 (1907).
31. Rosemary Stevens, *In Sickness and in Wealth*, 33.
32. *The Lancaster General Hospital*, 53.
33. *Auburn City Hospital*, 27.
34. *Sisters of Mercy, Annual Report of St John's Hospital*, 20.
35. *Report of the Board of Managers of the Pennsylvania Hospital*, 64–83.
36. Jefferys and Maxwell, *Diseases of China*, 1910, 573–74.
37. "A New Hospital in Central China, the Hospital of the American Baptist Mission at Hanyang Formally Opened," *CMJ* 21, no. 1 (1907): 123.
38. "Tsing-Kiang-Pu (Qingjiangbu) Hospital," *CMMJ* 19, no. 1 (1905): 33.
39. Frances F. Cattell, "Work in and About Soochow," *CMMJ* 16, no. 2 (1902): 103.
40. Claude M. Lee, *Leaves from the Notebook*, 21.
41. A.F. Cole, *Twenty-Fourth Annual Report: C.M.S. Hospital, Ningpo*, 1. Even as late as 1920, 9.5% of hospitals replying to a survey question had no facility at all to bath patients; only 40 percent bathed patients on admission; and less than 20 percent of hospitals had baths with running water. Harold Balme and Milton T. Stauffer, "An Enquiry into the Scientific Efficiency of Mission Hospitals in China," 21–22.
42. J.H. McCartney, "First (1892) Annual Report: Chungking Hospital, Methodist Episcopal Church, South," *CMMJ* 7, no. 4 (1893): 275.
43. D. Duncan Main, "Short Sketch of Work in the Hangchow Medical Mission," *CMMJ* 23, no. 1 (1909): 11.
44. James Butchart, "Hospital Construction," 101.
45. Harold Balme, "Efficient Mission Hospitals: The Irreducible Minimum," *CMJ* 33, no. 6 (1919): 572.
46. Rosenberg, *The Care of Strangers*, 292.
47. Main, "Short Sketch of Work in the Hangchow Medical Mission," 11.
48. *Twenty-Sixth Annual Report: CMS Hospital, Ningbo*, (Ningpo: C.M.S. Medical Mission, 1912), 11.
49. Jefferys advised his fellow medical missionaries to ask for a deposit (his was two dollars) before a patient could be admitted to the wards or find someone to act as guarantor. Jefferys and Maxwell, *Diseases of China*, 1910, 7.

50. Dugald Christie, *Thirty Years in the Manchu Capital,* 61.
51. *Twenty-Sixth Annual Report: CMS Hospital, Ningbo,* 2.
52. "Hospital Reports," *CMMJ* 13, no. 1&2 (1899): 61
53. William Wilson, "Hospital Reports: Sui-Ting-Fu, Wan Hsien, via Ichang," *CMMJ* 19, no. 2 (1905): 122.
54. "Hospital Reports: Summary," *CMMJ* 14, no. 3 (1900).
55. "Correspondence from Chinkiang," *CMMJ* 2, no. 1 (1888): 75.
56. "Hospital Reports: Church of Scotland, Ichang," *CMMJ* 20, no. 2 (1906): 99.
57. Lillie E.V. Saville, "Hospital Reports: London Mission Women's Hospital, Peking, Annual Report, 1905," *CMMJ* 20, no. 4 (1906): 188.
58. A.W. Douthwaite, "China Inland Mission Hospital and Dispensary, Chefoo: 1887 Report.," *CMMJ* 1, no. 2 (1887): 83.
59. H.L. Canright, "Chen-Tu Report," in *Annual Report (1898) of the West China Medical Mission, Methodist Episcopal Church* (Shanghai: American Presbyterian Mission Press, 1898), 19.
60. Ayers, "Warren Memorial Hospital, Hwang-Hein, Shantung," 49.
61. Refers to outpatients. "Notes and Items: St Luke's Hospital, Shanghai," *CMMJ* 2, no. 3 (1888): 120.
62. Rosenberg, *The Care of Strangers,* 298.
63. Average occupancy of the Pennsylvania Hospital for the Insane during 1908 was 457.
64. Average occupancy during 1910 was 42.
65. In the Elliot City Hospital the ratio of men to women was 2.3 to 1 and it was 1.7 to 1 in the Pennsylvania Hospital. *First Annual Report of the Elliot City Hospital, Keene, N.H. For the Year Ending, December 1, 1893,* (Keene: City of Keene, New Hampshire, 1894) and *Report of the Pennsylvania Hospital, 1908,* In the Pennsylvania Hospital for the Insane there were three women to every two men. More dramatically, women outnumbered men in the private hospital (Highland Hospital) by two to one.
66. Women and children were generally accommodated together.
67. "[Medical Mission] Statistics for the Year, 1910," *CMJ* 25, no. 5 (1911). A number of the fifty-five hospitals which reported having beds for both men and women had them in separate hospital buildings or compounds. If a hospital reported beds under one heading only it has been assumed that this was a single sex hospital. The statistics compiled by Balme in 1920, from information provided by almost twice as many hospitals (195 hospitals), showed that a larger majority, 126 (65%), catered for both men and women, there were relatively few, 33 (17%), hospitals exclusively for men and marginally more, 36 (18%) catering solely for women. Balme and Stauffer, "Enquiry: Scientific Efficiency, 1920," 8.
68. "[Medical Mission] Statistics for the Year, 1910."
69. Actually 1: 2.78. The corresponding ratios of female to male inpatients for 1904, 1905, and 1907 were 1: 3.75; 1: 5.35; and 1: 2.71. Source: Constructed from data included in Medical Mission Statistics, 1904–1910. A note to the 1910 statistics explains that a few hospitals failed to divide patients into male and female. In those cases all were counted as male. The way that the

data are presented makes it impossible to remove these hospitals from the set. Thus, the resultant ratios may be skewed slightly in favor of the number of male patients.

70. Church of England Mission in North China, "somewhat incorrectly called the S.P.G. Mission" Samuel Couling, *The Encyclopaedia Sinica*, 27, 117.

71. A. Marston, "Peking S.P.G. Hospital," *CMMJ* 14, no. 3 (1900): 206.

72. Margaret H. Polk, "Women's Medical Work," *CMMJ* 15, no. 2 (1901): 114.

73. The David Gregg Hospital for Women (1903); the Hackett Medical College for Women; The Turner School for Nurses, with the Perkins Memorial Building containing maternity and children's wards at Canton.

74. *Hospitals in China, Medical Mission Series* (Philadelphia, Pa.: The Woman's Foreign Missionary Society of the Presbyterian Church, 1912), 5.

75. Mary Brown, "The Training of Native Women as Physicians," *CMMJ* 12, no. 4 (1898): 179.

76. H.T. Whitney, "Medical Missionary Work in Foochow, II," *CMMJ* 3, no. 4 (1889): 86.

77. Kate Woodhull, "The Field Women of Foochow," *CMMJ* 16, no. 1 (1902): 44–45.

78. "Hospital Reports: Church of Scotland, Ichang," 97.

79. Jefferys and Maxwell, *Diseases of China*, 1910, 670–71.

80. Mildred M. Phillips, "The Hospital for Women at Soochow," *CMMJ* 3, no. 1 (1889): 30. See also discussion in Jefferys and Maxwell, *Diseases of China*, 1910, 683–84.

81. The preferred term for themselves: "not that one objects to washlady, saleslady, etc., but woman is a grand word, and let us use the grandest word we can find." Francis F. Tucker and Emma Boose Tucker, "Letter to the Editor," *CMJ* 22, no. 1 (1908).

82. Jos. C Thomson, "Medical Missionaries to the Chinese," *CMMJ* 1, no. 2 (1887): 56.

83. More than "twenty-five of her sex ... have since followed her." B.C. Atterbury, "Medical Missionary Work in Pekin," *CMMJ* 1, no. 3 (1887): 113.

84. See for example Mary Roth Walsh, "Feminist Showplace," in *Women and Health in America: Historical Readings,* ed. Judith Walzer Leavitt (Madison, Wisconsin: University of Wisconsin Press, 1984).

85. Anne Houston-Patterson, "Fifty Three Years a Doctor," *Medical Woman's Journal,* no. August (1944): 31.

86. Cora Bagley Marrett, "On the Evolution of Women's Medical Societies," in *Women and Health in America: Historical Readings,* ed. Judith Walzer Leavitt (Madison, Wisconsin: University of Wisconsin Press, 1984), 431.

87. Starr, *Social Transformation,* 117. Many of the remainder closed following the Flexner Report, Medical Education in the United States and Canada (1910) which recommended the consolidation of medical schools, their association with universities, the upgrading of facilities and the employment of full-time teachers rather than practicing physicians. Roy Porter, *The Greatest Benefit to Mankind,* 358.

88. Starr, *Social Transformation,* 124.
89. Houston-Patterson, "Fifty Three Years," 31.
90. "The second national census to identify physicians by sex." Marrett, "On the Evolution of Women's Medical Societies," 429–30.
91. Although the percentage was considerably higher in some major cities:18.2 percent in Boston, 19.3 percent in Minneapolis and 13.8 percent in San Francisco. Starr, *Social Transformation,* 117.
92. For example, of the sixty women medical women in Boston in 1892 three quarters of them were homeopaths. Marrett, "On the Evolution of Women's Medical Societies," 430.
93. At the time homeopathy still vied with allopathy, or "regular," medicine and was associated with some prestigious institutions. When all female physicians were included, the percentage was slightly higher and ranged from five to nine per cent. Ibid.
94. Paul A. Varg, *Missionaries, Chinese and Diplomats: The American Protestant Missionary Movement in China, 1890–1952* (Princeton, New Jersey: Princeton University Press, 1958), vii–viii.
95. Ruth J. Abram, *"Send Us a Lady Physician": Women Doctors in America, 1835–1920* (New York: W.W. Norton & Company, 1985), 182.
96. See Sara Waitstill Tucker, "Opportunities for Women: The Development of Professional Women's Medicine at Canton, China, 1879–1901," *Women's Studies International Forum* 13, no. 4 (1990) for an overview of the advantages afforded American women who treated and trained Chinese women in Canton.
97. See E.G. Ruoff, ed., *Death Throes of a Dynasty,* 2.
98. The Hospital was in North Jiangsu. Houston-Patterson, "Fifty Three Years," 31.
99. There was "said to have been twenty-two women physicians in China by 1890." Kenneth Scott Latourette, *A History of Christian Missions in China,* 457. A count of female members of the China Medical Missionary Society, published in 1890, reveals twenty-seven current members. Jos.C. Thomson, "Medical Missionaries to the Chinese," *CMMJ* 4, no. 4 (1890): 231–35.
100. For example, see E.H. Edwards, "Work among Women," *CMMJ* 1, no. 3 (1887).
101. Mary J. Davidson, "Medical Work Amongst Women by Women: Paper Read at the West China Conference, 1899," *CMMJ* 13, no. 3 (1899): 77–78.
102. Ibid. 83.
103. Figure constructed from a count of new arrivals (that is, I have removed returning missionaries) in *CMMJ* (1865–1912) supplemented and checked against data included in Marshall Broomhall, ed., *The Chinese Empire: A General Survey and Missionary Survey* (London: Morgan & Scott, 1907) and K C. Wong and Wu Lien-teh, *History of Chinese Medicine.*
104. Based on my research, in 1890, the percentage of physicians who were women was 21.4 percent. The corresponding percentages in 1897, 1901, 1906 and 1910 were 22.3, 27.1, 33.5 and 31.5. According to the China Mission Handbook, Shanghai, 1896, which gave "for the first time a bird's-eye view, as comprehensive as it is trustworthy, of evangelical mission work

in China" the ratio of female to male physicians was higher than membership of the Association would indicate: of the 183 medical missionaries, 59 or 32% were women and was almost the same in 1898. Gustav Warnek, *Outline of a History of Protestant Missions from the Reformation to the Present Time* (Edinburgh and London: Oliphant Anderson & Ferrier, 1901), 295, 97. The CMMA failed to conform to its constitution and publish an alphabetical list of members annually, so I rely on figures gleaned from the statistical returns for 1906, 1907 and 1910, which do not include all hospitals. In these returns, the number of women is more likely to be understated than the number of men because, in the case of a hospital with both men and women's departments, often it was only the man who was named as physician. For example, McCartney is the only physician recorded in connection with the Chunking Hospital where Dr Agnes Edmonds was in charge of the women's hospital from 1903. I have attempted to remedy such omissions by checking details from annual reports of individual hospitals, annual reports of the major missionary associations, newspaper articles and various accounts in the *CMMJ* and *CMJ*. The figures for 1906 and 1910 were derived from those hospitals that responded to the surveys (in 1910 returns were received from 126 hospitals, representing 175 of the 415 medical missionaries in China). Broomhall, who provides a summary of statistics collected from all missionary societies reveals a total of 298 medical missionaries of whom 75 (25%) were women in 1906. Broomhall, ed., *The Chinese Empire*, 36–39.

105. *Seventeenth Annual Report of the Directors of the Maine General Hospital*, (Portland: Stephen Berry, 1887).
106. *Lancaster Hospital, 1906.*
107. *Report of the Pennsylvania Hospital, 1908.*
108. *Auburn City Hospital, 1910.*
109. *Sixth Annual Report of the Highland Hospital, Fall River, Mass.*
110. *Annual Report of the Medical Director of Bloomingdale Hospital, White Plains-New York*, (White Plains, NY: 1925).
111. *Report of the Babies' Wards Post-Graduate Hospital.*
112. Extracted from table in Broomhall, ed., *The Chinese Empire*, 36–9 whom, as noted above, underestimated the number of women physicians.
113. Sophia Jex-Blake, "Letter to the Editor, Medical Women," *Lancet*, no. 8 November (1873).
114. Starr, *Social Transformation*, 117.
115. McCartney, in 1893, described Chongqing as "one of the best fields that could be afforded to a lady physician in China." J. H. McCartney, *Second (1893) Annual Report*, 2.
116. Abram, *"Send Us a Lady Physician"*, 172.
117. Susan B. Tallmon, *Glimpses of Lintsingchow Hospital: Being an Attempt to Show Briefly What Has Been Done, What We Are Trying to Do, and a Hint of What May Be Done* (Lintsingchow: A.B.C.F.M., 1910), 3.
118. Ibid. 23. It was more common in mixed sex hospitals for the number of men to far exceed that of women whether the physician was a man or a woman.

119. *Centers of Compassion: Our Hospitals in China,* (Boston, Mass.: Woman's Foreign Missionary Society, Methodist Episcopal Church, c. 1913), 13.

120. Before the hospital opened, both women spent one year in China "studying the language, observing the ways of the people and medical missionary methods." J.W. Davis, "The Opening of the Tooker Memorial Hospital, Soochow," *CMMJ* 14, no. 1 (1900): 58.

121. Reifsnyder, "Methods of Dispensary Work," 69.

122. The same held true for all women missionaries. In 1906, when there were 1,101 married and 471 single men, there were 971 "single ladies" and 75 "lady physicians," that is 1,037 single women. Data extrapolated from Broomhall, ed., *The Chinese Empire,* 36–39.

123. Figures derived from a count of arrivals noted above. There was insufficient information to determine the marital status of 51 of the men. It was the policy of most missionary societies to send out married men, to provide stability and a helpmeet for the man and as an example to the Chinese of the "Christian family." See also Jane Hunter, *The Gospel of Gentility: American Women Missionaries in Turn-of-the-Century China* (New Haven and London: Yale University Press, 1984), 11. Statistics for all missionaries (including physicians) are available for 1906 that imply a higher rate of marriage among men: 1,572 men, 1,101 wives, that is 70 percent married, 30 percent single or unaccompanied by wives.

124. J. Preston Maxwell, "Hospital Reports: Eng-Chhun Hospital," *CMMJ* 20, no. 3 (1906): 144.

125. Polk, "Women's Medical Work," 116.

126. Brown, "The Training of Native Women as Physicians," 179–80.

127. Dominique Hoizey and Marie-Joseph, *A History of Chinese Medicine,* trans. Paul Bailey (Vancouver: UBC Press, 1993), 151.

128. Dana L. Robert, *American Women in Mission: A Social History of their Thought and Practice,* ed. Wilbert R. Shenk, *The Modern Mission Era, 1792–1992: An Appraisal* (Macon, Georgia: Mercer University Press, 1997), 183.

129. Ibid. 185.

130. "Drs. Ida Kahn and Mary Stone," *CMMJ* 10, no. 4 (1896). An early account of the work of Mary Stone is to be found in Edward Carter Perkins, *A Glimpse of the Heart of China* (New York, Chicago: Fleming H. Revell Company, 1911) and these two remarkable women are the subjects of a recent study, Connie Anne Shemo, "An Army of Women: The Medical Ministries of Kang Cheng and Shi Meiyu, 1873–1937 (China)" (PhD diss., State University of New York at Binghamton, 2002).

131. Polk, "Women's Medical Work," 112–13.

132. Tallmon, *Lintsingchow Hospital,* 14.

133. See Walsh, "Feminist Showplace."

134. Regina Markell Morantz and Sue Zschoche, "Professionalism, Feminism, and Gender Roles: A Comparative Study of Nineteenth-Century Medical Therapeutics," in *Women and Health in America: Historical Readings,* ed. Judith Walzer Leavitt (Madison, Wisconsin: University of Wisconsin Press, 1984), 412–15. Their study involved a comparison (based on clinical records) of the New England Hospital (founded in Boston in 1862), one of the

first "hospitals for women and children staffed by women physicians," with the Boston Lying-In Hospital, one of the teaching facilities of the Harvard Medical School (staffed by men).

135. See Sidney A. Forsythe, *An American Missionary Community in China, 1895–1905,* 17.

136. J.H. McCartney, "Medical Work," *CMMJ* 13, no. 3 (1899): 99.

137. Robert Case Beebe, "Hospitals and Dispensaries," *CMMJ* 15, no. 1 (1901): 12–13.

138. "The Emmanuel Movement," *CMJ* 23, no. 2 (1909): 112.

139. The story of the triumph of the medical over the religious in the notion of a "medical missionary" is told in Theron Kue-Hing Young, "The William Osler Medal Essay: A Conflict of Professions: The Medical Missionary in China, 1835–1890," *Bulletin of the History of Medicine* 47, no. 3 (1973).

140. The following is based on data extracted from "[Medical Mission] Statistics for the Year, 1910," between 338–39.

141. The results are skewed in favor of the larger hospital, which had the resources and interest in responding to the survey. In any event, only 99 of the approximately 400 hospitals in China at the time supplied information.

142. The modal (most frequently occurring) size of a women's hospital was 10–19 beds and the median size had between 20 and 29 beds.

143. The modal size of a men's hospital was 30–39 beds and the median size, between 50 and 59 beds.

NOTES TO CHAPTER NINE

1. John Glasgow Kerr, "The Native Benevolent Institutions of Canton, Part 1," 157.

2. S. R Hodge, "The Church's Duty in Relation to Medical Missions, and the Principles Upon Which Such Missions Should Be Conducted.," *CMMJ* 5, no. 3 (1891): 141.

3. R.G.K., "Editorial: Cleanliness," *CMMJ* 15, no. 2 (1901): 156.

4. Arthur Stanley, "Chinese Hygiene," *CMMJ* 17, no. 1 (1903).

5. W. Hamilton Jefferys, "Editorial: Chinese Hygiene, by Dr. Arthur Stanley, M.D. Health Officer of Shanghai," *CMMJ* 17, no. 4 (1903): 166.

6. Cecil J. Davenport, "Hospital Reports," *CMMJ* 18, no. 3 (1904): 156.

7. Douglas M. Gibson, "The Old-Time Hospital and Assistants," *CMJ* 33, no. 5 (1919).

8. Isabella Bird, *The Yangtze Valley and Beyond,* 42–45.

9. Ibid. 466.

10. *Sisters of Mercy, Annual Report of St John's Hospital,* 14–15.

11. L.G. Thacker, "How Best to Obtain and Conserve Results in the Evangelistic Work among Hospital Patients," *CMJ* 26, no. 6 (1912): 341.

12. A. Marston, "Peking S.P.G. Hospital," *CMMJ* 14, no. 3 (1900): 206.

13. Alfred Hogg of Wenchow Hospital reported, in 1898, that their bedsteads from England were iron, with wooden bottoms and straw mattresses. Alfred Hogg, "Letter to the Editor: Wenchow Hospital," *CMMJ* 13, no. 1&2 (1899)

14. *Twenty-Sixth Annual Report: CMS Hospital, Ningbo*, 5.

15. W. H. Park and J. A. Snell, *Medical Work: Soochow Hospital Report,* (Suzhou: Board of Missions of the Methodist Episcopal Church, South, The China Conference, 1914), 1.

16. Robert E. Speer, *"Lu Taifu," Charles Lewis*, 34.

17. H.D. Porter, "The Medical Arm of the Missionary Society," *CMMJ* 9, no. 4 (1895): 267. Twenty years later, Miss Hope Bell was to observe, "It is a mistake to think that Chinese patients prefer little hard pillows: they much prefer softer and larger ones." E. Hope Bell, "Nursing Requirements in Our Mission Hospitals," *CMJ* 29, no. 3 (1915): 176.

18. Richard Wolfendale, "An Ideal Medical Missionary Hospital," *CMMJ* 17, no. 1 (1903): 9.

19. Luella M. Masters, "The "Pay Doctor" in China," *CMMJ* 16, no. 1 (1902): 3.

20. J.W. Davis, "The Opening of the Tooker Memorial Hospital, Soochow," Not all advocated routinely burning the straw mattress, Mabel Poulter, who, by 1916, had Lawson Tait iron beds, advised sunning the straw mattresses, and washing mats with Jeyes fluid. She only burned them if they were soiled. Mabel C. Poulter, "Obstetrical Experiences in a Chinese City," *CMJ* 30, no. 2 (1916): 78.

21. Harold Balme, "Efficient Mission Hospitals" 572.

22. A.W. Douthwaite, "China Inland Mission Hospital and Dispensary, Chefoo: 1887 Report.," *CMMJ* 1, no. 2 (1887): 83

23. A.P. Peck, "Concerning Williams' Hospital" 66

24. A.P. Peck, "The Development of the Medical Department of a Mission Station," *CMMJ* 16, no. 1 (1902): 14.

25. Sewell McFarlane, S, "Opening of the Chi-Chou Mission New Hospital," *CMMJ* 8, no. 4 (1894): 220.

26. A. F. Cole, *Twenty-Fourth Annual Report: C.M.S. Hospital, Ningpo*, 4.

27. Henry Fowler, "Hiau-Kan L.M.S. Hospital," *CMMJ* 16, no. 3 (1902): 151.

28. Josephine M. Bixby, "Kieh-Yang Hospital Report," *CMMJ* 19, no. 6 (1905): 262.

29. "Rules for Companions to Patients" Sisters of Mercy, St. John's Hospital, 21. The companion was not allowed unfettered access to the patient; they needed the physician's permission. See also "Rules for Private Patients" *Auburn City Hospital: Thirty-First Annual Report*, 29.

30. For details, see John Z. Bowers, *When the Twain Meet: The Rise of Western Medicine in Japan* (Baltimore: Johns Hopkins University Press, 1980), 68.

31. Cited in "Discussion on Women's Medical Work by Polk," *CMMJ* 15, no. 4 (1901): 299.

32. In 1912 Arthur Tatchell, of the Hodge Memorial Hospital at Hankow, bemoaned the lack of nurses in most hospitals and called for the training of male nurses. He noted that "the time has not arrived when men patients can be nursed by women nurses" although he had successfully employed maybe the first English matron in a men's hospital to train male nurses ten years earlier. W. Arthur Tatchell, "The Training of Male Nurses," *CMJ* 26, no. 5 (1912): 271.

33. Margaret H. Polk, "Women's Medical Work," 114.
34. A. F. Cole, *Twenty-Third Annual Report: C.M.S. Hospital, Ningpo* (Ningpo: C.M.S. Medical Mission, 1909), 15. See also Harold Balme and Milton T. Stauffer, "An Enquiry into the Scientific Efficiency of Mission Hospitals in China" 15–16. and W. Hamilton Jefferys and James L. Maxwell, *The Diseases of China*, 7.
35. Lillie E.V. Saville, "Hospital Reports: London Mission Women's Hospital, Peking, Annual Report, 1905," *CMMJ* 20, no. 4 (1906): 188.
36. Bixby, "Kieh-Yang (1905)," 262.
37. Peck, "The Development of the Medical Department of a Mission Station," 14.
38. Kingston De Gruche, *Doctor Apricot of "Heaven Below": The Story of the Hangchow Medical Mission (C.M.S.)*, Third ed. (London & Edinburgh: Marshall Brothers, Ltd., 1910), 140.
39. In Balme's survey in 1920, 70% of kitchens were situated in "out-houses"; 94% used "native stoves"; and only 33% were screened from flies and mosquitoes. Balme and Stauffer, "Enquiry: Scientific Efficiency, 1920," 17–18.
40. Mary Latimer James, "What Is—and What Should Be," in *Our Plan for the Church General Hospital, Wuchang: A Statement of the Most Urgent Needs in the District of Hankow, Leaflet 211* (New York: The Board of Missions, c. 1916), 6.
41. Bixby, "Kieh-Yang (1905)," 263.
42. *Auburn City Hospital, 1910*, 29.
43. *The Lancaster General Hospital*, 54.
44. Bixby, "Kieh-Yang (1905)," 236.
45. John A. Snell, *Report of the Soochow Hospital, Soochow, China* (Shanghai: The Oriental Press, 1919), 2.
46. Balme, "Irreducible Minimum, 1919," 272–73.
47. Three, who have written general histories of the hospital, Guenter B. Risse, *Mending Bodies*, Charles E. Rosenberg, *The Care of Strangers*, Rosemary Stevens, *In Sickness and in Wealth*, while they mention it in the text, do not include a reference to diet or nutrition in their indexes.
48. *Auburn City Hospital, 1910*, 37.
49. Ibid. 22.
50. William Augustus Guy and John Harley, eds., *Hooper's Physician's Vade Mecum: A Manual of the Principles and Practice of Physic*, Tenth ed., vol. 1 (New York: William Wood & Company, 1884). The original by Hooper, first published in 1823, by 1884 was in its tenth edition, revised by Guy and Harley.
51. See Ibid. 217–22.
52. Henry M. Lyman et al., *The Practical Home Physician and Encyclopedia of Medicine* (London: World Publishing Co., c.1900), 1073–75.
53. Extracted from LMS Hospital Report for 1897–98 by the Editor of *CMMJ*. "Hospital Reports," *CMMJ* 13, no. 1&2 (1899): 56–57.
54. Fred H. Judd, "Dieting Patients: Letter to the Editor," *CMMJ* 20, no. 6 (1906).

55. Fred H. Judd, "Enhancing the Value of the Medical Conference: Letter to the Editor:," *CMJ* 25, no. 6 (1911).

56. See, Erwin H. Ackerknecht, *Therapeutics: From the Primitives to the 20th Century with an Appendix: History of Dietetics* (New York: Hafner Press, 1973), 171–86.

57. In 1861, delegates from the Women's Central Association of Relief from New York proposed that the Secretary of War establish a Commission, which, inter alia, would "enquire into the subjects of diet, cooking, cooks . . . crude, unvaried, or ill-cooked food." The United States Sanitary Commission was the result but the emphasis was on soldiers in the field rather than hospitals per se. The resulting Regulations for the Medical Department of Military Forces included rudimentary instructions relating to the preparation of food and to diet: for example "the diet of the patients will be divided into full, half, and low . . . to each ten patients, for example, on low diet, a certain quantity of tea, sugar, &c. To each ten on half diet, a certain quantity of rice, milk, &c." R.W. Gibbes, "Regulations for the Medical Department of the Military Forces of South Carolina," 1861. available from <URL: http://docsouth.unc.edu/gibbes/gibbes.html> (2002). McCool dates attention to the diet of wounded soldiers to the Spanish-American War when "'dietists' provided nutrition support for the wounded" and claims that "it was not until World War I that the American Red Cross established the first qualifications for dieticians assigned to Army-based hospitals." Audrey. C. McCool, "The Heritage of Army Dietetics" *Journal of American Dietetic Association* 97, no. 10 (1997), 1080.

58. For discussion of Chinese Traditional Medicine and its relation to foods, see E.N. Anderson, "Fishing People's Medicine: Variations on Chinese Themes" (paper presented at the Association of Asian Studies, Pacific Coast Branch, Bellingham, WA, 2002), Francesca Bray, "Chinese Health Beliefs," in *Religion, Health and Suffering,* ed. John R. Hinnells and Roy Porter (London and New York: Kegan Paul International, 1999), Paul U. Unschuld, "The Chinese Reception of Indian Medicine in the First Millenium A.D.," *Bulletin of the History of Medicine* 53 (1979); and Manfred Porkert and Dr. Christian Ullmann, *Chinese Medicine,* trans. Mark Howson (New York: Henry Holt and Company, 1982), and Paul U. Unschuld, *Medicine in China* (Berkeley: University of California Press, 1985).

59. See Porkert and Ullmann, *Chinese Medicine,* 203.

60. E.N. Anderson, Personal Communication, June 7, 2002.

61. Cynthia J Brokaw, "Commercial Publishing in Late Imperial China: The Zou and Ma Family Businesses of Sibao, Fujian," *Late Imperial China* 17, no. 1 (1996): 49–50.

62. Wei Shang, "Writing, Reading, and Constructing the Everyday World: Studies of Late Ming and Early Qing Reading Materials," 1997. <http://www.aasianst.org/absts/1997abst/China/c153.htm> (October 2002).

63. Jefferys and Maxwell, *Diseases of China,* 1910, 656 fn.

64. J.H. McCartney, *Second (1893) Annual Report,* 2.

65. Calculated using reported expenditure on various classes of food included in Gouldy Memorial Hospital, Methodist Episcopal Church, Chungking, West China, 1908, (n.p., 1908), 16–17.

66. Jonathon Spence, "Ch'ing," in *Food in Chinese Culture: Anthropological and Historical Perspectives*, ed. K.C.Chang and Eugene N. Anderson (New Haven: Yale University Press, 1977), 268–70.

67. Mary Stone, "Hospital Dietary in China," *CMJ* 26, no. 5 (1912): 299.

68. Ibid. 300–1. Neal presented results of a survey and analysis of the Chinese diet in terms of the calorific value to help physicians design adequate, balanced diets for patients in hospital. James Boyd Neal, "Diet Lists for Use in the Hospital of the Union Medical College, Tsinan, Shantung," *CMJ* 30, no. 1 (1916). After the article by Stone, this appears to be the first serious attempt to deal with the issue of diet by medical missionaries in China.

69. Anderson, "Fishing People's Medicine," 5.

70. Ibid. 4–5.

71. Stanley, "Chinese Hygiene," 58.

72. Anne Walter Fearn, *My Days of Strength*, 64–65.

73. Anderson, "Fishing People's Medicine," 10.

74. See Rosenberg, *The Care of Strangers*, Chapter 12, 286–309.

75. Ibid. 298.

76. *Lancaster Hospital*, 1906, 53.

77. Ibid. 53–54.

78. See *Auburn City Hospital, 1910*, 29, 46.

79. Rosenberg, *The Care of Strangers*, 298.

80. McCartney, *Second (1893) Annual Report*, 2.

81. Richard J. Smith, *Fortune-Tellers and Philosophers: Divination in Traditional Chinese Society* (Boulder: Westview Press, 1991), 18, 39–40.

82. Ibid. 74–75.

83. Ibid. 82.

84. A. P. Parker, "Chinese Almanac," *The Chinese Recorder* 19, no. 2 (1888): 61.

85. Smith, *Fortune-Tellers and Philosophers*, 87.

86. I have not been able to locate a copy of McCartney's calendars and he does not make it clear whether they were Christian or Chinese. It is most likely that it followed the example of the simple calendar, produced by the American Presbyterian Press at Shanghai, which included both Chinese and Western months and days. "English and Chinese Calendar: 1893," (Shanghai: American Presbyterian Mission Press, 1893).

87. Gouldy Memorial Hospital, Methodist Episcopal Church, Chungking, West China, 1908, 7."

88. E.M. Merrins, "Foreign Patent Medicines in China-Editorial," *CMMJ* 31, no. 4 (1917): 317.

89. "North China Mission American Board: Resolution," *Chinese Recorder* 22, no. 7 (1891): 342

90. Originally published in the Edinburgh M.M. Society's Quarterly Paper. P. Anderson, "Foreign Nurses for Chinese Hospitals," *CMMJ* 10, no. 1 (1896).

91. Jefferys and Maxwell, *Diseases of China*, 1910, 7.

92. Thacker, "How Best to Obtain, 1912," 341.

93. Jefferys and Maxwell, *Diseases of China*, 1910, 8.

94. Rosenberg, *The Care of Strangers*, 289.

95. Zhao Hongjun, "Jindai Zhongxiyi Lunzheng Shi (History of the Modern Controversies over Chinese vs. Western Medicine) Introduction and Summary by Nathan Sivin," *Chinese Science* 10 (1991): 22.

96. According to Thomson, the use of moxa "dates to periods long preceding the dawn of actual history, and which seems peculiarly Chinese" and was "prepared by making a small cone of the flowers of amaranthus, or of the downy fibres of the bruised stem of a species of artemisia, and is used by setting this cone on fire on the part affected." Jos. C Thomson, "Surgery in China: Section I—the History and Present Position of Chinese Native Surgery," *CMMJ* 6, no. 4 (1892): 226. Joseph Needham wrote that "the acupuncture technique, was from ancient times onward thought most valuable in acute diseases, while moxa was considered more appropriate in chronic ones, and even for prophylactic purposes too." Joseph Needham, *Science in Traditional China: A Comparative Perspective* (Cambridge, Massachusetts: Harvard University Press, 1981), 85. See also discussion: Christopher Cullen et al., "Discussion: Relative Lack of Dissection in China," *EASCI Discussion List* (2000).

97. Omar L. Kilborn, *Heal the Sick,* 197.

98. As Rosenberg pointed out, in relation to antebellum hospitals in America, many "surgical" patients were admitted but few operations undertaken. Treatment more often consisted of "diet and rest, the regular changing of dressings, and the healing powers of nature." Rosenberg, *The Care of Strangers,* 28.

99. J. S. Grant, *"Wha Mei Hospital Report for 1915,"* (Ningbo: American Baptist Foreign Missionary Society, 1916), J. S. Grant, *Wha Mei Hospital Report for 1916 in Connection with the American Baptist Foreign Missionary Society, Ningpo, China* (Shanghai: Presbyterian Mission Press, 1917).

100. Park and Snell, "Medical Work: Soochow Hospital Report," 3.

101. "Hospital Reports: St. Luke's Hospital for Chinese, Shanghai," *CMMJ* 18, no. 1 (1904): 38.

102. John A. Anderson, "Medical Work at T'ai Chow-Fu," *CMMJ* 19, no. 5 (1905): 212.

103. Cole, *Twenty-Third Annual Report: C.M.S. Hospital, Ningpo,* 15.

104. Eliza Wells, "London Missionary Society, Report for 1904, Hongkong," (Hongkong: LMS, 1904).

105. Robert Case Beebe, "Hospital Reports: Philander Smith Memorial Hospital, Nanking," *CMMJ* 1, no. 3 (1887): 178.

106. Francis F. Tucker and Emma Boose Tucker, "Williams' Hospital of the American Board," *CMMJ* 19, no. 6 (1905): 258–59.

107. "Hospital Reports: Fifty-Ninth Annual Report of the Chinese Hospital (Shantung Road) Shanghai, 1905," *CMMJ* 20, no. 5 (1906): 231–32.

108. Calculated from a count of cases recorded. *Auburn City Hospital, 1910,* 26. It is appropriate to use the Auburn City Hospital for comparison as its statistics compare favorably with the 19 days, which was the "average length of stay in non-sectarian institutions," in 1904. Risse, *Mending Bodies,* 471. The equivalent statistics for the Lancaster Hospital reveal a similar story: in 1905–1906, when there were two surgical cases for every medical case, the

average length of stay was 17.95 days. Calculated from data contained in *Lancaster Hospital, 1906,* 42. In St. Johns, several years later in 1913–1914, the medical to surgical ratio was still in the same range (1:2.1) and the average length of stay was shorter again at 17.0 days. *Sisters of Mercy, St. John's Hospital,* 39.

109. *Auburn City Hospital, 1910,* 26.

110. Extracted from Chungking Hospital Reports 1901–1911.

111. "Hospital Reports: London Mission Men's Hospital at Hankow," *CMMJ* 18, no. 3 (1904): 149.

112. John A. Snell, *Report of the Soochow Hospital, Soochow, China* (Shanghai: The Oriental Press, 1917), 7–8.

113. Opened in 1898, for history see C. C. Seldon, "Work among the Chinese Insane and Some of Its Results," *CMMJ* 19, no. 1 (1905).

114. Opened in 1899. For history see John E. Kuhne, "The Leper Asylum at Tungkun," *CMMJ* 21, no. 1 (1907) and G Olpp, "The Rhenish Mission Hospital, Tungkun," *CMMJ* 23, no. 3 (1909).

115. Main's men's hospital (1884) grew out of an Opium Refuge (1881) to which was added a women's hospital (1894). In addition to the "Convalescent and Fresh-air Homes," he established small leper asylums (1889), a Maternity Hospital (1906). D. Duncan Main, "Short Sketch of Work in the Hangchow Medical Mission," *CMMJ* 23, no. 1 (1909). For a more complete history, see De Gruche, *Doctor Apricot.*

116. Jefferys and Maxwell, *Diseases of China,* 1910, 523.

117. He reported "almost daily [being] forced to turn away needy cases; many of them suffering constant agony." Samuel Cochran, "Fifth Report of the Hwai-Yuen Hospital, September 1, 1905–April 30th, 1906," *CMMJ* 21, no. 2 (1907): 98.

118. Jefferys and Maxwell, *Diseases of China,* 1910, 523.

119. For an overview of the rise of specialization in Western hospitals, see Rosenberg, *The Care of Strangers,* 169–75.

120. See chapter III, Unofficial Physicians—The Traditional Physicians in Late Imperial Chinese Society, of Chang Che-Chia, "The Therapeutic Tug of War: The Imperial Physician-Patient Relationship in the Era of Empress Dowager Cixi (1874–1908) (Ching-Qing)" (PhD, University of Pennsylvania, 1998), 55–83.

121. Ibid. 76.

122. H. Barton, *Twenty-Ninth Annual Report: C.M.S. Hospital, Ningpo* (Ningpo: C.M.S. Medical Mission, 1915), 9.

123. Cole, *Twenty-Third Annual Report: C.M.S. Hospital, Ningpo,* 5.

124. Bill Purves describes how his workers organized buying trips for the factory he managed in the late 1980s in western Guangdong. Bill Purves, *Barefoot in the Boardroom: Venture and Misadventure in the People's Republic of China* (Sydney: Allen & Unwin, 1991), 136–37.

125. "Methodist New Connection Mission, Laoling," *Chinese Recorder* 1892.

126. A. Lyall, "Swatow Medical Mission," *CMMJ* 4, no. 1 (1890): 27.

127. Cecil J. Davenport, "L.M.S. Hospital, Wuchang," *CMMJ* 19, no. 6 (1905): 265.

128. William Wilson, "Hospital Reports: Sui-Ting-Fu, Wan Hsien, via Ichang," *CMMJ* 19, no. 2 (1905): 122.

129. Francis F. Tucker, Emma Boose Tucker, and Myra L. Sawyer, *A Chinese Revolution in Physical Well-Being at Pangkiachwang Shantung, China, 1911–1912* (Williams Hospital of the American Board, 1912), 8–9.

130. Samuel Cochran, "Hospital Reports: Hwai-Yuen Hospital, An-Hui," *CMMJ* 19, no. 2 (1905): 121.

131. Speer, *"Lu Taifu," Charles Lewis,* 84.

132. Arthur D Peill, "Roberts' Memorial Hospital, T'sang-Chou," *CMMJ* 18, no. 2 (1904): 99.

133. John A. Snell, "The City Hospital: Paper Read at the Annual Conference of the China Medical Missionary Association, Peking, 1920.," *CMMJ:* Hospital Supplement (1921): 43–44.

134. "L.M.H., Hiau-Kan Annual Report," *CMMJ* 17, no. 3 (1903): 125.

135. Henry Fowler, "L.M.S. Hiau Kan Medical Mission Report for 1902," in *China India Local Reports, 1913* (London: London Mission Society, 1913), 7.

136. "L.M.H., Hiau-Kan Annual Report," 125.

137. A.F. Cole, *Twentieth Annual Report: C.M.S. Hospital, Ningpo* (Ningpo: C.M.S. Medical Mission, 1906), 4.

138. Cole, *Twenty-Third Annual Report: C.M.S. Hospital, Ningpo,* 14.

139. See, James L. Watson, "The Structure of Chinese Funerary Rites: Elementary Forms, Ritual Sequence, and the Primacy of Performance," in *Death Ritual in Late Imperial and Modern China,* ed. James L. Watson and Evelyn S. Rawski (Berkeley: University of California Press, 1988), 8, James L. Watson, "Funeral Specialists in Cantonese Society: Pollution, Performance, and Social Hierarchy," in *Death Ritual in Late Imperial and Modern China,* 122–23.

140. Susan Naquin, "Funerals in North China: Uniformity and Variation," in *Death Ritual in Late Imperial and Modern China,* ed. James L. Watson and Evelyn S. Rawski, 38.

141. Ministry of the Interior, "Regulations for Dissection in China: Issued by Ministry of the Interior, Nov. 22nd, 1913. Government Gazette 563. Supplementary Regulations Issued April 22, 1914. Order No. 85 of the Board of the Interior," *CMMJ* 30, no. 2 (1916): 126–30.

142. James Butchart, "Hospital Construction" 101–2.

143. J.H. McCartney, *Annual Report (1901) of the General Hospital, Methodist Episcopal Church, Chungking, China* (Chongqing: The West China Missionary News Office, 1901), 2.

144. "Disposal of Patients Dying in Hospital," *CMMJ* 14, no. 3 (1900): 197.

145. Ibid. 198.

146. C.W. Somerville, *Report of the London Mission Men's Hospital, Wuchang* (Shanghai: American Presbyterian Press, 1905), 7.

147. Risse, *Mending Bodies,* 104–5.

148. Rosenberg, *The Care of Strangers,* 292–93.

149. For example see George Hadden, "The Registration of out-Patients," *CMMJ* 31, no. 1 (1917), George Hadden, "A Standard Clinical Chart," *CMMJ* 32, no. 6 (1918), Carl A. Hedblom, "Hospital Efficiency in China," *CMJ* 30, no.

4 (1916), L.F. Heimburger, "The Value of Hospital Records," *CMMJ* 35, no. 3 (1921).

150. For the situation regarding the lack of laundry facilities in Chinese hospitals, see F.E. Dilley, "The Hospital Laundry," *CMMJ* 32, no. 5 (1918).

NOTES TO CONCLUSION

1. Eleanor Chestnut, "Medical Work in Lien-Chow, Kwangtung," *CMMJ* 14, no. 2 (1900): 123.
2. The twelfth-century Byzantine hospital, the Pantocrator and tenth-century Muslim Bimaristans, excepted.
3. Jing Shao, "'Hospitalizing' Traditional Chinese Medicine: Identity, Knowledge and Reification" (PhD, University of Chicago, 1999), 118–19.
4. Arab and Persian merchants, who traveled widely in China in the ninth century, witnessed and reported on all these measures." Angela Ki Che Leung, "Organized Medicine in Ming-Qing China" 135.
5. The question of women nursing men was still a topic of discussion in 1919. See Edith J. Haward, "Is China Ready for Women Nurses in Men's Hospitals?," *CMMJ* 33, no. 2 (1919).
6. Except for a cursory mention in general histories of Chinese medicine and studies focusing on particular aspects of the history of Western medicine in China, the *Minzhengbu* hospitals have received little attention. For example, Dominique Hoizey and Marie-Joseph, *A History of Chinese Medicine,* implies that the Chinese established hospitals in some twelve cities but no mention is made of who was responsible for them. Wu Lien-teh lists the hospitals with which he was associated after the 1911 bubonic plague provided the impetus for their establishment in Wu Lien-teh, *Plague Fighter,* 448–69 but does not mention the *Minzhengbu's* role in hospital provision. Yip does refer to the *Minzhengbu* briefly, but not their hospitals in Ka-che Yip, *Health and National Reconstruction in Nationalist China,* 14–15, as do Carol Benedict, *Bubonic Plague in Nineteenth-Century China* (Stanford, California: Stanford University Press, 1996), 155, Ralph C. Croizier, *Traditional Medicine in Modern China,* 44–45 and S.M. Hillier and J.A Jewell, *Health Care and Traditional Medicine in China, 1800–1982,* 24.
7. See map of Peking in Juliet Bredon, *Peking: A Historical and Intimate Description of Its Chief Places of Interest,* Second ed. (Shanghai: Kelly and Walsh, Limited, 1922), facing page 414.
8. See Carol Benedict, *"Policing the Sick"* 60 and Benedict, *Bubonic Plague,* 154–55.
9. Montague H.T. Bell and H.G.W. Woodhead, *The China Year Book,* 230.
10. Yip, *Health and National Reconstruction,* 15.
11. See Chen Haifeng, *Zhongguo Weisheng Baojian Shi (History of China's Health Care)* (Shanghai: Shanghai kexue jishu chubanshe, 1993), 16–17
12. Zhu Xianhua, "Qingmode Jingchengguan Yiyuan (the Public Hospital in the Capital in the Late Qing Dynasty)," *Zhonghua yishi zazhi* 15, no. 1 (1985). Unfortunately, he does not include his sources.

13. Ibid. 32.
14. John J. Mullowney, "Modern Hospitals for Chinese by Chinese," *CMJ* 26, no. 1 (1912): 39.
15. "Brief Report of the Investigation of Hospitals and Institutions for Defectives Made by a Group of Students Directed by the Y.M.C.A.," (1913), 1.
16. Zhu Xianhua, "Hospital in the Capital," 31–32.
17. Mullowney, "Modern Hospitals for Chinese by Chinese," 38, 40. Zhu expresses it slightly differently: the only patients who paid anything, according to him, were inpatients who paid a fee to cover the cost of food. Zhu Xianhua, "Hospital in the Capital," 31, 32.
18. Zhu Xianhua, "Hospital in the Capital," 31.
19. Isabella Bird, *The Yangtze Valley and Beyond*, 180. N.S. Hopkins and G.D. Lowry, "Hospital Reports: Peking Medical Work," *CMMJ* 20, no. 3 (1906): 148.
20. Mullowney, "Modern Hospitals for Chinese by Chinese," 42.
21. "A Chinese Hospital," *Dianshizhai Huabao* 2 (1885).
22. Trained at the ACM hospital at Anqing in Anhui. Francis W. Peabody and R.S. Greene, "Red Cross Hospital: Kiukiang," (Rockefeller Archive Centre, New York.: 1914), 1.
23. Zhu Xianhua, "Hospital in the Capital," 31. Dr Wu would have been the same one Mullowney met in 1911 who he described as being "of the new school ... [and] trained at the Government medical school at Tientsin, where the teachers are Frenchmen" (that is, the Beiyang Medical School). Mullowney, "Modern Hospitals for Chinese by Chinese," 39.
24. Zhu Xianhua, "Hospital in the Capital," 31.
25. Mullowney was told that originally there had been "four old-school doctors and three new-school doctors in attendance." Mullowney, "Modern Hospitals for Chinese by Chinese," 39. Peabody reported "about five doctors educated in western medicine and ... three doctors of the Chinese school" when he visited. Francis W. Peabody, "Visit to Chinese General Hospital with Dr. Dilley, Peking," (1914), 1 The YMCA students reported five doctors trained in "foreign style (largely Japan) and four Chinese-style doctors "Brief Report," 1.
26. Peabody, "Visit to Chinese General," 1, 2. F. W. Peabody and R. S. Green visited a number of government hospitals on behalf of the China Medical Board, established by the Rockefeller Foundation, in other cities, including Nanchang, Nanking, Kaifeng, see Francis W. Peabody, "Chinese Hospital: Nanking," (1914), Francis W. Peabody, "Police Hospital: Nanchang," (1914), Francis W. Peabody and R.S. Greene, "Government Hospital: Kaifeng," (1914).
27. Zhu Xianhua, "Hospital in the Capital," 31.
28. Ibid. 32.
29. The group of students from the YMCA included both the *Neichengguan yiyuan* and *Waichengguan yiyuan* in their survey of welfare institutions in Beijing. See "Brief Report," J.S. Burgess, "Correspondence from J.S. Burgess, of the Peking Young Men's Christian Association (the Princeton Work in Peking)," (n.d.).

30. From 1903, students studied both Chinese and Western medicine in a four year course run by two departments (medicine and materia medica) at the University. Ma Kanwen, "East-West Medical Exchange and Their Mutual Influence," 171. The situation changed after the end of the Qing but these go beyond the focus of this study.

31. "Chinanfu: Open a Hospital," *North China Herald and S.C. & C. Gazette*, June 26 1903.

32. "Medical Work in Shantung," *CMJ* 26, no. 1 (1912): 112.

33. John Glasgow Kerr, "A Chinese Benevolent Association," *CMMJ* 3, no. 4 (1889): 152. Yu Shenchu lists the Chinese hospitals in Guangzhou, Beijing, Shanghai, Tianjin, Nanjing, Ningbo, Hangzhou, Suzhou, Chengdu, Hangkou, Fuzhou, Xiamen (Amoy) as being set up to vie with the foreigners. Yu Shenchu, *Zhongguo Yixue Jian Shi* (a Brief History of Chinese Medicine) (Fuzhou: Fujian kexue jishu chubanshe, 1983), 374–75.

34. Kerr, "Chinese Benevolent Association (1889)," 154.

35. Ibid. 153–54.

36. E.A. Aldridge, "Report on the Health of Hoihow (Kiungchow) for the Half-Year Ended 31st March 1886," in *Customs Gazette, Medical Reports, No. 31* (Shanghai: Imperial Maritime Customs, 1886), 18.

37. Kerr, "Chinese Benevolent Association (1889)," 154.

38. Ibid. 155.

39. For example, during the plague in Canton in 1894 Mary Niles reported that 296 people had died of plague during the third month in the Fangbian suo. Mary W. Niles, "Plague in Canton," *CMMJ* 8, no. 2 (1894): 119. The *Aiyutang* had supplied 415 coffins to paupers who had died there in 1887. Kerr, "Chinese Benevolent Association (1889)," 153–54

40. John Glasgow Kerr, "Is It an Advance?," *CMMJ* 3, no. 2 (1889): 67.

41. The proportion of men to women admitted to the *Fangbian suo* in 1888 was approximately three to one which compares with the ratio found in mission hospitals between 1904 and 1910. The death-rate among women was slightly less than that of the men: 61.3% to 65.8%. Ibid. See also the discussion of the role of a Chinese institution, established in Hong Kong in 1851, the Kwong Fook I-t'sz (*Guangfu yici* 广副义祠), with similar aims to the *Fangbiansuo*. Elizabeth Sinn, *Power and Charity*, 18–20, 32–5.

42. Kerr, "Chinese Benevolent Association (1889)," 155.

43. Although none had been admitted, the hospital had been built to accommodate 27 inpatients and it was intended that they could choose either to be treated by a staff physician or a private practitioner. Roderick MacDonald, "Report on the Health of Wuchow for the Half-Year Ended 30th September 1898," in *Customs Gazette, Medical Reports, No. 56* (Shanghai: Imperial Maritime Customs, 1898), 25.

44. Aldridge, "Health of Hoihow (Kiungchow) March 1886," 18.

45. Others, like a graduate of the Soochow Hospital, set up in private practice "[and] had two mandarins staying in his house for treatment." "Hospital Reports: Soochow Hospital: October 1st, 1889, to September 30th, 1890," *CMMJ* 5, no. 1 (1891): 18.

46. Thomas Kirkwood, *Report of the London Mission Hospital, Chungking (West China) in Charge of Thomas Kirkwood. M.A. M.B. C.M.* (Chungking: Lungmenhao Press, 1904), 3.

47. *Cixi Xianzhi*, (Shanghai: Zhejiang Renmin chubanshe, 1992), 840

48. "Chinese Medical Enterprises," *CMJ* 31 (1917): 247. The hospital was still in existence in 1987. See *Cixi Xianzhi*, 840.

49. *Cixi Xianzhi*, 12. This hospital's long history has been well documented in Cixi and Ningbo gazetteers: see *Cixi Xianzhi*, 840, 45 and *Ningbo Shizhi*, (Beijing: Zhonghua shuju, 1995). Missionaries were made aware of the enterprise six years after its commencement: see "Chinese Medical Enterprises," 247 and "A Vigorous Chinese Hospital," *CMJ* 32 (1918).

50. "Chinese Medical Enterprises," 247.

51. Jeffrey W. Cody, "Striking a Harmonious Chord."

52. "Chinese Medical Enterprises," 247.

53. Peabody and Greene, "Government Hospital: Kaifeng." This hospital had not begun taking inpatients at the time of their visit.

54. Peabody, "Chinese Hospital: Nanking."

55. Francis W. Peabody, "Visit to Peiyang Hospital for Women and Children: Tientsin," (1914), 2.

56. Called the Red Cross Hospital but apparently with no connection to the National Red Cross Society.

57. Peabody and Greene, "Red Cross Hospital," 2.

58. Francis W. Peabody, "Kung Yee Hospital, Canton," (1914), 1. In 1916 there were five foreign physicians associated with this hospital and medical school and a staff of seventeen Chinese, most of whom were physicians. The hospital would have appeared to cater for a larger proportion of inpatients than other Chinese hospitals: In-patients, 1443 men and 88 women; outpatients 8,425 men and 2,030 women. "Abstract from Chinese Report of the Kwangtung Kung Yee Medical College and Hospital, 1914–1915," *CMMJ* 30, no. 6 (1916).

59. Mullowney, "Modern Hospitals for Chinese by Chinese," 36.

60. Peabody, although he described the "rooms, bed, and patients" as being "in a very dilapidated condition he drew attention to the "attempt at cleanliness and antiseptic" in the surgical dressing room. Peabody, "Visit to Chinese General," 3.

61. Mullowney, "Modern Hospitals for Chinese by Chinese," 38.

62. Wang Zhuqin, December 2001

Bibliography

ARCHIVAL RESOURCES

London Missionary Society Archives, School of Oriental and African Studies, London.

Rockefeller Archive Center, China Medical Board Archives, Record Group 4, Series 1 and 2.

Union Theological College, Burke Library. The Mission Research Library Medical Pamphlet Collection.

CHINESE LANGUAGE PRIMARY MATERIALS

Cixi xianzhi 慈溪县志 Shanghai: Zhejiang Renmin chubanshe 浙江人民出版社, 1992.

Dianshizhai Huabao 点石斋画报 1885–1897 (Shanghai).

Fujian shengzhi-Weisheng zhi 福建省志-卫生志 (Gazetteer of Fujian—Public Health). Zhonghua shuju 中华书局, 1995.

Han Shu 汉书. Ban Gu 班固 (32–92). Beijing: Zhonghua shuju 中华书局, 1975.

Hebei Tong Zhi Gao [Hebei sheng di fang zhi ban gong shi]. Beijing: Beijing Yanshan chu ban she, 1993.

Lau, D. C. and Chen Fangzheng. *Zhouli zhuzi suoyin* 周澧逐字索引 (A Concordance to the Zhouli) Chinese University of Hong Kong Institute of Chinese Studies the ICS Ancient Chinese Texts Concordance Series. Classics: no. 4. Hongkong: The Commercial Press, 1993.

Lau, D. C. *Guanzi Zhuzi Suoyin* 管子逐字索引 (A Concordance to the Guanzi). Edited by D. C. Lau and Zhen Fangzheng, ICS Ancient Chinese Texts Concordance Series: Philosophical Works: No. 37. Hongkong: The Commercial Press, 2001.

Ningbo Shizhi. Beijing: Zhonghua shuju, 中华书, 1995.

Sui Shu 隋书. Wei Zheng 魏徵 (580–643). Beijing: Zhonghua shuju 中华书局 1973.

Yuan shi 元史. Ming Song Lian 明宋濂 (1310–1381). Beijing: Zhonghua shuju 中华书局 1976.

CHINESE LANGUAGE SECONDARY SOURCES

Chen Bangxian. *Zhongguo yixue shi* 中国医学史 (History of Medicine in China). Taipei: Yuandong tushu gongsi 远东图书公司, 1956 (first ed.1919).

Chen Fenglin 陈风林, Liu Shiying 刘士英 and Liang Jun 梁峻. "Beijing daoji yiyuan kaolue 北京道济医院传略 (The Dow Hospital in Beijing)." *Zhonghua yizshi zazhi* 中国医史杂志 28, no. 3 (1998): 141–44.

Chen Haifeng 陈海峰. *Zhongguo weisheng baojian shi* 中国卫生保健史 (History of China's Health Care). Shanghai: Shanghai kexue jishu chubanshe 上海科学技术出版社, 1993.

Gong Chun 龚纯. "Mingdai junyi zuzhide tedian 明代军医组织的特点 (Characteristics of the Military Medical Organization in the Ming Dynasty)." *Zhonghua yizshi zazhi* 中国医史杂志 17, no. 1 (1987): 8–10.

Li Liangsong 李良松. "Luelun zhongguo gudai dui zhuanran bingrende anzhi ji zhuanran bingyuan 略论中国古代对传染病人的安置及传染病院 (A Brief Discussion on Ancient Chinese Infectious Hospital and Setting Down for Patients with Infectious Diseases)." *Zhonghua yizshi zazhi* 27, no. 1 (1997): 32–35.

Ren Yingqiu 任应秋. "Yiyuande jianli—bingfang 医院的建立-病坊 (The Establishment of Hospitals)." *Ming bao yuekan* 明报月刊 57, no. September (1970): 19.

Song Jiong 宋炯. "Liang Song juyang zhidu de fazhan—Songdai guanban cishan shiye chutan 两宋局养制度的发展—宋代官办慈善事业初探 (The Development of the Poorhouse System during the Song Dynasty—Initial discussion of the Song dynasty government-operated charity organization)." *Zhongguoshi yanjiu* 中国史研究, no. 4 (2000): 73–82.

Yu Shenchu 俞慎初. *Zhongguo yixue jian shi* 中国医学简史 (A Brief History of Chinese Medicine). Fuzhou: Fujian kexue jishu chubanshe 福建科学技术出版社, 1983.

Zhen Zhiya 甄志亚 "Zhongguo gudaide yiyuan 中国古代的医院 (Ancient Hospitals in China)." *Beijing zhongyi xueyuan xuebao* 北京中医学院学报 (Journal of Beijing College of Traditional Chinese Medicine) 2 (1980): 55–57.

Zhongguo yixue baikequanshu 中国医学百科全书 Shanghai: Shanghai kexue jishu chubanshe 上海科学技术出版社, 1987.

Zhongguo yixue shi 中国医学史 (History of Chinese Medicine). Shanghai: Beijing zhongyi xueyuan 北京中医学院 (Beijing College of Chinese Medicine): Shanghai kexue zhishu chubanshe 上海科学技术出版社, 1982.

Zhu Deming 朱德明. "Zhejiang guangji yiyuan yu shengliyiyao zhuankexuexiao shilue 浙江广济医院与省立医药传科学校史略 (A Brief History of the Zhejiang Central Hospital and Provincial School of Medicine." *Zhonghua yizshi zazhi* 25, no. 1 (1995): 25–29.

Zhu Xianhua 朱先华. "Qingmode jingchengguan yiyuan 清末的京城官医院 (The Public Hospital in the Capital in the Late Qing Dynasty)." *Zhonghua yishi zazhi* 15, no. 1 (1985): 31–32.

ENGLISH LANGUAGE PRIMARY SOURCES

"Abstract from Chinese Report of the Kwangtung Kung Yee Medical College and Hospital, 1914–1915." *CMMJ* 30, no. 6 (1916): 445–46.

Aldridge, E.A. "Report on the Health of Hoihow (Kiungchow) for the Half-Year Ended 31st March 1886." In *Customs Gazette, Medical Reports, No. 31*, 18–22. Shanghai: Imperial Maritime Customs, 1886.

"Alphabetical List of the Provinces, Departments, and Districts in China, with Their Latitudes and Longitudes." *Chinese Repository* 13, no. 6, 7, 8, 9, 10 (1844): 321–27, 57–69, 418–37, 478–500, 13–34.

"The American Baptist Mission Hospital: Shaohsing, Chekiang." *North China Herald and S.C. & C. Gazette,* March 25 1910, 662.

Anderson, John A. "Medical Work at T'ai Chow-Fu." *CMMJ* 19, no. 5 (1905): 211–13.

Anderson, P. "Foreign Nurses for Chinese Hospitals." *CMMJ* 10, no. 1 (1896): 173.

Annual Report of the Medical Director of Bloomingdale Hospital, White Plains—New York. White Plains, NY, 1925.

Architectural Designs for a Small Hospital. Chicago: The Modern Hospital Publishing Co., 1923.

Arnold, Julean. *China: Commercial and Industrial Handbook, Trade Promotion Series—No. 38.* Washington: Department of Commerce, USA, 1926.

Atterbury, B.C. "Medical Missionary Work in Pekin." *CMMJ* 1, no. 3 (1887): 113–15.

———. "Gratuitous Treatment." *CMMJ* 8, no. 2 (1894): 120–23.

Auburn City Hospital: Thirty-First Annual Report of the Board of Managers (Year Ended September 30, 1910). Auburn, N.Y.: Knapp, Peck & Thomson, Printers, 1910.

Ayers, T.W. "Warren Memorial Hospital, Hwang-Hein, Shantung." *CMMJ* 20, no. 1 (1906): 47–49.

Balme, Harold. "Efficient Mission Hospitals: The Irreducible Minimum." *CMJ* 33, no. 6 (1919): 567–74.

———. *China and Modern Medicine: A Study in Medical Mission Development.* London: United Council for Missionary Education, 1921.

Balme, Harold, and Milton T. Stauffer. "An Enquiry into the Scientific Efficiency of Mission Hospitals in China." Paper presented at the Annual Conference of the China Medical Missionary Association, Peking, February 20–27, 1920.

Barton, H. *Twenty-Ninth Annual Report: C.M.S. Hospital, Ningpo.* Ningpo: C.M.S. Medical Mission, 1915.

Beebe, Robert Case. "Hospital Reports: Philander Smith Memorial Hospital, Nanking." *CMMJ* 1, no. 3 (1887): 177–79.

———. "The Medical Missionary Association of China: List of Members." *CMMJ* 11, no. 2 (1897): 201–4.

———. "Hospitals and Dispensaries." *CMMJ* 15, no. 1 (1901): 6–14.

Bell, E. Hope. "Nursing Requirements in Our Mission Hospitals." *CMJ* 29, no. 3 (1915): 170–77.

Bell, Montague H.T., and H.G.W. Woodhead. *The China Year Book.* London: George Routledge & Sons, Ltd., 1912.

———. *The China Year Book.* London: George Routledge & Sons, Ltd., 1913.

Bercovitz, Nathaniel. "Studies in Sanitation in China: 1 the Disposal of Sewage in Institutions." *CMMJ* 31, no. 5 (1918): 441–44.

Betow, Emma. "Margaret Eliza Nast Memorial Hospital." *CMMJ* 20, no. 4 (1906): 156–57.

Bird, Isabella. *The Yangtze Valley and Beyond: An Account of Journeys in China, Chiefly in the Province of Sze Chuan and among the Man-Tze of the Somo Territory.* London: Virago Press Ltd, 1899. Reprint, 1985.

Bixby, Josephine M. "Kieh-Yang Hospital Report." *CMMJ* 19, no. 6 (1905): 261–63.

Boone, H.W. "How Can the Medical Work Be Made More Helpful to the Cause of the Church in China?" *CMMJ* 8, no. 1 (1894): 13–17.

Bredon, Juliet. *Peking: A Historical and Intimate Description of Its Chief Places of Interest*. Second ed. Shanghai: Kelly and Walsh, Limited, 1922.

"Brief Report of the Investigation of Hospitals and Institutions for Defectives Made by a Group of Students Directed by the Y.M.C.A." 1913. RAC, CMB, Record Group 4, series 2, Box 19, Folder 315.

Broomhall, Marshall, ed. *The Chinese Empire: A General Survey and Missionary Survey*. London: Morgan & Scott, 1907.

Brown, Mary. "The Training of Native Women as Physicians." *CMMJ* 12, no. 4 (1898): 178–82.

Bryson, Mary Isabella. *John Kenneth Mackenzie: Medical Missionary to China*. London: Hodder and Stoughton, 1891.

Burgess, J.S. "Correspondence from J.S. Burgess, of the Peking Young Men's Christian Association (the Princeton Work in Peking)." n.d. RAC, CMB, Record Group 4, series 2, Box 19, Folder 315.

Butchart, James. "Hospital Construction: Paper Read at the Medical Missionary Association, 1901." *CMMJ* 15, no. 2 (1901): 97–102.

Canright, H.L. "Chen-Tu Report." In *Annual Report (1898) of the West China Medical Mission, Methodist Episcopal Church*, 17–21. Shanghai: American Presbyterian Mission Press, 1898.

Cattell, Frances F. "Work in and About Soochow." *CMMJ* 16, no. 2 (1902): 102–4.

Centers of Compassion: Our Hospitals in China. Boston, Mass.: Woman's Foreign Missionary Society, Methodist Episcopal Church, c. 1913.

"Charitable Institutions." *Chinese Repository* 2, no. 8 (1833): 165–66.

Chestnut, Eleanor. "Medical Work in Lien-Chow, Kwangtung." *CMMJ* 14, no. 2 (1900): 123.

"Chinanfu: Open a Hospital." *North China Herald and S.C. & C. Gazette*, June 26 1903, 1253–54.

"Chinese Medical Enterprises." *CMJ* 31 (1917): 247–48.

"A Chinese Hospital." *Dianshizhai Huabao* 2 (1885): 92.

Christie, Dugald. *Thirty Years in the Manchu Capital, 1883–1913. Being the Recollections of Duguld Christie CMG, FRCS, FRCP Edin., Edited by His Wife*. London: Constable and Company, 1915.

Cochran, Samuel. "Hospital Reports: Hwai-Yuen Hospital, An-Hui." *CMMJ* 19, no. 2 (1905): 121–22.

———. "Letter to the Editors: Hospital Plans." *CMMJ* 20, no. 3 (1906): 151.

———. "Fifth Report of the Hwai-Yuen Hospital, September 1, 1905—April 30th, 1906."

CMMJ 21, no. 2 (1907): 98–99.

Cole, A.F. *Twentieth Annual Report: C.M.S. Hospital, Ningpo*. Ningpo: C.M.S. Medical Mission, 1906.

———. *Twenty-Third Annual Report: C.M.S. Hospital, Ningpo*. Ningpo: C.M.S. Medical Mission, 1909.

———. *Twenty-Fourth Annual Report: C.M.S. Hospital, Ningpo*. Ningpo: C.M.S. Medical Mission, 1910.

"The Commercial Value of the Missionary." *North China Herald and S.C. & C. Gazette*, July 10 1901, 55.

"Correspondence from Chinkiang." *CMMJ* 2, no. 1 (1888): 74–5.

Cousland, Philip B. "Medical Training of Native Preachers." *CMMJ* 16, no. 1 (1902): 68–70.

Cox, Geo. A. "Out-Patient Department of Medical Work." *CMMJ* 16, no. 2 (1902): 128–29.

Davenport, Cecil J. "Hospital Reports." *CMMJ* 18, no. 3 (1904): 155–56.

———. "L.M.S. Hospital, Wuchang." *CMMJ* 19, no. 6 (1905): 263–66.

Davidson, Mary J. "Medical Work Amongst Women by Women: Paper Read at the West China Conference, 1899." *CMMJ* 13, no. 3 (1899): 77–83.

Davidson, R.J. "Letter to the Editor." *Chinese Recorder and Missionary Journal* 20, no. 4 (1889): 183–85.

Davis, J.W. "The Opening of the Tooker Memorial Hospital, Soochow." *CMMJ* 14, no. 1 (1900): 58–60.

De Gruche, Kingston. *Doctor Apricot of "Heaven Below": The Story of the Hangchow Medical Mission (C.M.S.)*. Third ed. London & Edinburgh: Marshall Brothers, Ltd., 1910.

"Description of the City of Canton." *Chinese Repository* 2, no. 10 (1833).

Dilley, F.E. "The Hospital Laundry." *CMMJ* 32, no. 5 (1918): 474–77.

"Discussion on Women's Medical Work by Polk." *CMMJ* 15, no. 4 (1901): 299–300.

"Disposal of Patients Dying in Hospital." *CMMJ* 14, no. 3 (1900): 197–98.

Douthwaite, A.W. "China Inland Mission Hospital and Dispensary, Chefoo: 1887 Report." *CMMJ* 1, no. 2 (1887): 82–84.

———. "The C.I.M. Hospital and Dispensary at Chefoo." *CMMJ* 8, no. 2 (1894): 136–37.

"Drs. Ida Kahn and Mary Stone." *CMMJ* 10, no. 4 (1896): 181–84.

Edwards, E.H. "Work among Women." *CMMJ* 1, no. 3 (1887): 167.

Embree, Edwin R. "Letter to R.S. Greene (Rockefeller Foundation) on Behalf of the Building Committee of the Peking Union Medical College." April 3, 1918. RAC, CMB, Record Group 4, Series 1, Box, 32, Folder 660.

"The Emmanuel Movement." *CMJ* 23, no. 2 (1909): 111–14.

"English and Chinese Calendar: 1893." Shanghai: American Presbyterian Mission Press, 1893.

Ennin, and Edwin O. Reischauer. *Diary: The Record of a Pilgrimage to China in Search of the Law*. New York: Ronald Press Co., 1955.

"Entrance to the Anatomy Building." *CMJ* 35, no. 4 (1921): opp. 416.

Fearn, Anne Walter. *My Days of Strength: A Woman Doctor's Forty Years in China*. London: Robert Hale Ltd., 1940.

First Annual Report of the Elliot City Hospital, Keene, N.H. For the Year Ending, December 1, 1893. Keene: City of Keene, New Hampshire, 1894.

Fowler, Henry. "Hiau-Kan L.M.S. Hospital." *CMMJ* 16, no. 3 (1902): 151.

———. "Hiao-Kan Medical Mission: Annual Report." 1905. China India & Local Reports: 1905. SOAS, L.M.S., China India & Local Reports: 1905. London.

———. "L.M.S. Hiau Kan Medical Mission Report for 1902." 1913. China India Local Reports, 1913. SOAS, L.M.S., China India Local Reports, 1913. London.

"General Hospital American Church Mission, Wuchang, Hupeh." *CMMJ* 33, no. 1 (1919): 72–73.

Gibson, Douglas M. "The Old-Time Hospital and Assistants." *CMJ* 33, no. 5 (1919): 475–6.

Gillison, Thomas. "Charging for Drugs." *CMMJ* 16, no. 1 (1902): 20–21.

Gouldy Memorial Hospital, Methodist Episcopal Church, Chungking, West China, 1908. n.p., 1908.

Grant, J.S. "Hua Mei Hospital (Viewed from the River), Ningbo: Built in Stages from 1902." In *Wha Mei Hospital Report for 1913,* frontispiece. Ningpo: American Baptist Foreign Missionary Society, 1914.

———. "Wha Mei Hospital Report for 1915." Ningpo: American Baptist Foreign Missionary Society, 1916.

———. *Wha Mei Hospital Report for 1916 in Connection with the American Baptist Foreign Missionary Society, Ningpo, China.* Shanghai: Presbyterian Mission Press, 1917.

Greene, Roger S. "Letter to Rt Rev. H. L. Roots, Bishop of Hankow." April 29, 1915. RAC, CMB, Record Group 4, Series 1, Box 20, Folder 386.

Hadden, George. "The Registration of out-Patients." *CMMJ* 31, no. 1 (1917): 26–30.

———. "A Standard Clinical Chart." *CMMJ* 32, no. 6 (1918): 576–78.

Harris, Lucy E. "T'ung-Chuan-Fu, Szechuan." *CMMJ* 18, no. 3 (1904): 142.

Haward, Edith J. "Is China Ready for Women Nurses in Men's Hospitals?" *CMMJ* 33, no. 2 (1919): 174–77.

Hedblom, Carl A. "Hospital Efficiency in China." *CMJ* 30, no. 4 (1916): 227–33.

Heimburger, L.F. "The Value of Hospital Records." *CMMJ* 35, no. 3 (1921).

Hertzler, A.E. *The Horse and Buggy Doctor.* New York and London: Harper & Bros., 1938.

Hodge, S. R. "The Church's Duty in Relation to Medical Missions, and the Principles Upon Which Such Missions Should Be Conducted." *CMMJ* 5, no. 3 (1891): 137–44.

Hogg, Alfred. "Letter to the Editor: Wenchow Hospital." *CMMJ* 13, no. 1&2 (1899): 46–48.

Hopkins, N.S., and G.D. Lowry. "Hospital Reports: Peking Medical Work." *CMMJ* 20, no. 3 (1906): 148–49.

"Hospital Reports." *CMMJ* 13, no. 1&2 (1899): 49–54.

"Hospital Reports: Church of Scotland, Ichang." *CMMJ* 20, no. 2 (1906): 97–101.

"Hospital Reports: Fifty-Ninth Annual Report of the Chinese Hospital (Shantung Road) Shanghai, 1905." *CMMJ* 20, no. 5 (1906): 231–32.

"Hospital Reports: London Mission Men's Hospital at Hankow." *CMMJ* 18, no. 3 (1904): 149–50.

"Hospital Reports: Soochow Hospital: October 1st, 1889, to September 30th, 1890." *CMMJ* 5, no. 1 (1891): 38–39.

"Hospital Reports: St. Luke's Hospital for Chinese, Shanghai." *CMMJ* 18, no. 1 (1904): 38–39.

"Hospital Reports: Summary." *CMMJ* 14, no. 3 (1900): 204.

Hospitals in China. Medical Mission Series. Philadelphia, Pa.: The Woman's Foreign Missionary Society of the Presbyterian Church, 1912.

Houston-Patterson, Anne. "Fifty Three Years a Doctor." *Medical Woman's Journal*, no. August (1944): 31–32.

Howie, J. "First Impressions and Experiences in Chang-Poo." *CMMJ* 4, no. 1 (1890): 1–4.

Hume, Edward H. "Opening of the Yale Mission Hospital, Changsha, Hunan." *CMMJ* 22, no. May, No. 3 (1908): 183–85.

———. *Doctors East Doctors West: An American Physician's Life in China*. New York: W.W. Norton and Co., 1946.

———. *Hsiangya Hospital, Changsha, (Hunan)*. New York: W.W. Norton and Co., 1946

Huntley, George A. "Our out-Patient Work." *CMMJ* 16, no. 2 (1902): 111–13.

Hussey, Harry. *My Pleasure and Palaces: An Informal Memoir of Forty Years in Modern China*. 1st ed. New York: Doubleday and Company, 1968.

Jefferys, A.M. "Formal Opening of St. Andrew's Dispensary, Wusieh, Kiangsu." *CMMJ* 22, no. 3 (1908): 185.

Jefferys, W. Hamilton. "Editorial: Chinese Hygiene, by Dr. Arthur Stanley, M.D. Health Officer of Shanghai." *CMMJ* 17, no. 4 (1903): 166–68.

Jefferys, W. Hamilton, and James L. Maxwell. *The Diseases of China*. Philadelphia: P. Blakiston's Son & Co., 1910.

Jex-Blake, Sophia. "Letter to the Editor, Medical Women." *Lancet*, no. 8 November (1873): 688.

Johnson, Charles F. "Hospital Reports: Medical Work at I-Chow-Fu." *CMMJ* 19, no. 5 (1905): 209–11.

Judd, Fred H. "Dieting Patients: Letter to the Editor." *CMMJ* 20, no. 6 (1906): 275.

———. "Enhancing the Value of the Medical Conference: Letter to the Editor" *CMJ* 25, no. 6 (1911): 419–20.

Kahn, Ida. "Self-Supporting Medical Missionary Work." *CMMJ* 19, no. 6 (1905): 223–6.

Kates, George N. *The Years That Were Fat: The Last of Old China*. Cambridge, Mass.: The

M.I.T. Press, 1952. Reprint, 1976.

Kerr, John Glasgow. "The Native Benevolent Institutions of Canton, Part 1." *China Review* 2 (1873): 88–95.

———. "Benevolent Institutions of Canton." *China Review* 3 (1874–1875): 108–14.

———. "Is It an Advance?" *CMMJ* 3, no. 2 (1889): 66–67.

———. "A Chinese Benevolent Association." *CMMJ* 3, no. 4 (1889): 152–55.

———. "The Bubonic Plague." *CMMJ* 8, no. 4 (1894): 178–80.

———. "Self-Support in Mission Hospitals." *CMMJ* 9, no. 3 (1895): 135–37.

———. "History of Medical Missionary Society's Hospital, Canton." *CMMJ* 10, no. 1, 3 (1896): 55–57, 95–98.

Kilborn, Omar L. "Self-Support in Mission Hospitals." *CMMJ* 15, no. 2 (1901): 92–97.

———. *Heal the Sick: An Appeal for Medical Missions in China*. Toronto: Missionary Society of the Methodist Church, 1910.

Kinnear, H.N. *A Year of Waiting: The Thirty-First Annual Report of Ponasang Missionary Hospital for the Year Ending December 1902*. Foochow: American Board of Commissioners for Foreign Missions (A.B.C.F.M.), 1902.

Kirkwood,Thomas. *Report of the London Mission Hospital, Chungking (West China) in Charge of Thomas Kirkwood. M.A. M.B. C.M.* Chungking: Lungmenhao Press, 1904.

Knapp, Ronald G. Personal Communication, November 2002

Kuhne, John E. "The Leper Asylum at Tungkun." *CMMJ* 21, no. 1 (1907): 10–15.

"L.M.H., Hiau-Kan Annual Report." *CMMJ* 17, no. 3 (1903): 124–25.

Lacey Sites, C.M. "The New Methodist Hospital at Yen-Ping, Fuh-Kien." *CMMJ* 20, no. 4 (1906): 211–12.

The Lancaster General Hospital: Thirteenth Annual Report. Lancaster: Press of the New Era Printing Company, 1906.

Latimer James, Mary. "Mary Latimer James, M.D." *Medical Woman's Journal,* no. October (1945): 54–57.

———. "What Is—and What Should Be." In *Our Plan for the Church General Hospital, Wuchang: A Statement of the Most Urgent Needs in the District of Hankow,* 5–8. New York: The Board of Missions, c. 1916.

Lee, Claude M. *Leaves from the Notebook of a Missionary Doctor.* Shanghai: American Church Mission, 1932.

Lennox, William G. "A Self Survey by Mission Hospitals in China." *Chinese Medical Journal* 46 (1932): 484–534.

Lewis, Stephen C. "Opening of the American Presbyterian Hospital at Chenchow, Hunan." *CMMJ* 22, no. 4 (1908): 257–58.

"List of Members of the China Medical Missionary Association." *CMMJ* 15, no. 2 (1901): 167–72.

Lobenstine, E.C. "Letter to the Editor: Relief for Missionary Builders." *Chinese Recorder and Missionary Journal* 46, no. 9 (1915): 578–79.

Lockhart, William. "Report of the Medical Missionary Society's Hospital at Shanghai. From 1st May, 1844, to 30th June, 1845." *Chinese Repository* 15, no. 6 (1846): 281–91.

Logan, O.T. "Westminster Sunday School Hospital, Changteh, Hunan." *CMJ* 30, no. 5 (1916): 353–54.

———. "Five Years' Experience in Aseptic Surgery in an Inland Hospital." *CMJ* 30, no. 1 (1916): 20–26.

Lyall, A. "Swatow Medical Mission." *CMMJ* 4, no. 1 (1890): 24–28.

MacDonald, Roderick. "Wesleyan Missionary Hospital, Fatshan, China, 1893." *CMMJ* 8, no. 2 (1894): 134–35.

———. "Report on the Health of Wuchow for the Half-Year Ended 30th September 1898." In *Customs Gazette, Medical Reports, No. 56,* 16–25. Shanghai: Imperial Maritime Customs, 1898.

Mackenzie, Kenneth J. "The Construction of Hospitals." *CMMJ* 1, no. 2 (1887): 77–78.

Macklin, W.E. "Hwaiyuan Hospital Opening: Letter to the Editor." *CMMJ* 24, no. 5 (1910): 374–5.

Main, D. Duncan. "An Out-Patient Day at the Hangchow Hospital, 12th February, 1889." *CMMJ* 3, no. 4 (1889): 113–18.

———. "Short Sketch of Work in the Hangchow Medical Mission." *CMMJ* 23, no. 1 (1909): 9–14.

Marston, A. "Peking S.P.G. Hospital." *CMMJ* 14, no. 3 (1900): 206.

Masters, Luella M. "The "Pay Doctor" in China." *CMMJ* 16, no. 1 (1902): 1–5.

Maxwell, J. Preston. "Hospital Reports: Eng-Chhun Hospital." *CMMJ* 20, no. 3 (1906): 143–46.

McCartney, J.H. "First (1892) Annual Report: Chungking Hospital, Methodist Episcopal Church, South." *CMMJ* 7, no. 4 (1893): 275–76.

———. *Second (1893) Annual Report: Chungking Hospital of the Methodist Episcopal Church*. Chongqing: Methodist Episcopal Church, 1893.

———. *Sixth (1897) Annual Report of the General Hospital of the Methodist Episcopal Church, Chungking, China:*. Shanghai: American Presbyterian Mission Press, 1898.

———. *Annual Report (1898) of the West China Medical Mission, Methodist Episcopal Church*. Shanghai: American Presbyterian Mission Press, 1899.

———. "Medical Work." *CMMJ* 13, no. 3 (1899): 95–100.

———. *Annual Report (1901) of the General Hospital, Methodist Episcopal Church, Chungking, China*. Chongqing: The West China Missionary News Office, 1901.

———. *12th (1902) Annual Report of Chungking General Hospital of the Methodist Episcopal Church*. Shanghai: American Presbyterian Mission Press, 1903.

———. *15th Annual Report (1905) of the Chungking General Hospital for Men of the Methodist Episcopal Church*. Shanghai: Methodist Publishing House, 1905.

———. *Chungking Men's Hospital (1912), (Gouldy Memorial)*. Shanghai: Methodist Publishing House, 1912.

———. *Report (1911) of the Chungking Men's Hospital, Gouldy Memorial*. Shanghai: Methodist Publishing House, 1912.

McFarlane, Sewell, S. "Opening of the Chi-Chou Mission New Hospital." *CMMJ* 8, no. 4 (1894): 218–21.

"Medical [Mission] Statistics for 1903." *CMMJ* 19, no. 1 (1905): 27–28.

"Medical [Mission] Statistics for 1904." *CMMJ* 19, no. 4 (1905): Endpaper.

"Medical [Mission] Statistics for 1906." *CMJ* 21, no. 3 (1907): Endpaper.

"Medical Mission Statistics, 1905." *CMMJ* 20, no. 6 (1906): Endpapers.

"Medical Mission Statistics, 1907." *CMJ* 22, no. 3 (1908): inserted between 194–95.

"[Medical Mission] Statistics for the Year, 1910." *CMJ* 25, no. 5 (1911): inserted between 338–39.

"The Medical Missionary and the Anti-Foreign Riots in China." *CMMJ* 7, no. 2 (1893): 110–16.

"Medical Work in Shantung." *CMJ* 26, no. 1 (1912): 117–19.

Merrins, E.M. "Foreign Patent Medicines in China—Editorial." *CMMJ* 31, no. 4 (1917): 316–17.

"Methodist New Connection Mission, Laoling." *Chinese Recorder* 1892, 245.

Milne, William C. "Notices of Seven Months' Residence in the City of Ningbo, from December 7th, 1842, to July 7th, 1843." *Chinese Repository* 13, no. 1,2,3,7 (1844): 14–43, 77–98, 127–43, 337–57.

———. "Notices of Seven Months' Residence in the City of Ningbo, Continued." *Chinese Repository* 16, no. 1 (1847): 14–30.

———. *Life in China*. London: Routledge, 1857.

Ministry of the Interior. "Regulations for Dissection in China: Issued by Ministry of the Interior, Nov. 22nd, 1913. Government Gazette 563. Supplementary Regulations Issued April 22, 1914. Order No. 85 of the Board of the Interior." *CMMJ* 30, no. 2 (1916): 126–30.

"Miscellany." *CMMJ* 11, no. 3&4 (1897): 262–65.

"Missionaries and Accuracy." *CMJ* 29, no. 3 (1915): 196–97.

"A Missionary Architectural Firm." *Chinese Recorder and Missionary Journal* 46, no. 11 (1915): 661.

"Missionary News." *Chinese Recorder and Missionary Journal* 22, no. 7 (1891): 338–43.

"Mistakes of Some Missionaries." *North China Herald and S.C. & C. Gazette,* 24 July 1901, 171–72.

Mouat, Frederic J. "On Hospitals: Their Management, Construction, and Arrangements in Relation to the Successful Treatment of Disease." *Lancet* (1881): 3–5; 41–43; 78–79; 125–27; 66–68; 408–10; 580–81.

Mullowney, John J. "Report of the Peking Hospital, October 1910." *CMJ* 25, no. 3 (1911): 206–9.

———. "Modern Hospitals for Chinese by Chinese." *CMJ* 26, no. 1 (1912): 34–43.

Neal, James Boyd. "Diet Lists for Use in the Hospital of the Union Medical College, Tsinan, Shantung." *CMJ* 30, no. 1 (1916): 9–14.

"A New Hospital in Central China, the Hospital of the American Baptist Mission at Hanyang Formally Opened." *CMJ* 21, no. 1 (1907): 123–24.

"News." *CMMJ* 14, no. 1 (1900): 71.

Niles, Mary W. "Native Midwifery in Canton." *CMMJ* 4, no. 2 (1890): 51–55.

———. "Plague in Canton." *CMMJ* 8, no. 2 (1894): 116–19.

"North China Mission American Board: Resolution." *Chinese Recorder* 22, no. 7 (1891): 342.

"Notes and Items: St Luke's Hospital, Shanghai." *CMMJ* 2, no. 3 (1888): 120.

"Notices: Arrivals and Departures." *CMMJ* 1–19 (1887–1905).

Olpp, G. "The Rhenish Mission Hospital, Tungkun." *CMMJ* 23, no. 3 (1909): 172–77.

"The Opening of St James' Hospital, Anking." *CMJ* 22, no. 1 (1908): 116–18.

"Opening of the New Union Medical College Hospital, Tsinanfu." *CMJ* 30, no. 1 (1916): 49–52.

"The Opening of the Pingyin Hospital." *CMMJ* 23, no. 6 (1909): 407–10.

Osgood, Elliott I. "Tisdale Hospital, Chuchow." *CMJ* 25, no. 6 (1911): 413–16.

Park, W.H., and J.A. Snell. "Medical Work: Soochow Hospital Report." Suzhou: Board of Missions of the Methodist Episcopal Church, South, The China Conference, 1914.

Parker, A.P. "Chinese Almanac." *The Chinese Recorder* 19, no. 2 (1888): 61–74.

Pasteur, Louis. "The Germ Theory." *Lancet* (1881): 271–72.

Peabody, Francis W. "Visit to Peiyang Hospital for Women and Children:Tientsin." 1914. RAC, CMB, Record Group 4, Series 1, Box 19, Folder 322.

———. "Chinese Hospital: Nanking." 1914. RAC, C.M.B, Record Group 4, Series 1, Box 21, Folder 412.

———. "Police Hospital: Nanchang." 1914. RAC, CMB, Record Group 4, Series 1, Box 21, Folder 405.

———. "Visit to Chinese General Hospital with Dr. Dilley, Peking." 1914. RAC, CMB, Record Group 4, Series 1, Sub-series 1, Box 19, Folder 316.

———. "Kung Yee Hospital, Canton." 1914. RAC, CMB, Record Group 4, Series 1, Sub-series 1, Box 24, Folder 465.

Peabody, Francis W., and R.S. Greene. "Government Hospital: Kaifeng." 1914. RAC, CMB, Record Group 4, Series 1, Box 20, Folder 356.

———. "Red Cross Hospital: Kiukiang." 1914. CMB, Record Group 4, Series 1, Box, 21, Folder 397. RAC, New York.

Peck, A.P. "Concerning Williams' Hospital, P'ang Chuang Station, in Shantung, of the North China Mission A.B.C.F.M." *CMMJ* 1, no. 1 (1887): 65–67.

———. "The Development of the Medical Department of a Mission Station." *CMMJ* 16, no. 1 (1902): 13–5.

Peill, Arthur D. "Roberts' Memorial Hospital, T'sang-Chou." *CMMJ* 18, no. 2 (1904): 99–100.

———. "Hospital Reports: Roberts' Memorial Hospital, T'sang-Chow." *CMMJ* 20, no. 1 (1906): 44–47.

Peill, Ernest J. "The New Union Medical College in Peking." *CMMJ* 20, no. 1 (1906): 122–25.

"Peking Union Medical College." *CMJ* 35, no. 4 (1921): 457.

Peter, W.W. "The Conference and Dedication at Peking." *CMJ* 35, no. 5 (1921): 486–89.

Phillips, Mildred M. "The Hospital for Women at Soochow." *CMMJ* 3, no. 1 (1889): 30.

Pinel, Phillippe. *The Clinical Training of Doctors: An Essay of 1793. Edited and Translated, with an Introductory Essay by Dora B. Weiner.* Translated by Dora B. Weiner, *The Henry Sigerist Supplement to the Bulletin of the History of Medicine; New Series, No. 3.* Baltimore: The Johns Hopkins University Press, c.1980.

Polk, Margaret H. "Women's Medical Work." *CMMJ* 15, no. 2 (1901): 112–19.

Porter, H.D. "The Medical Arm of the Missionary Society." *CMMJ* 9, no. 4 (1895): 264–68.

Poulter, Mabel C. "Obstetrical Experiences in a Chinese City." *CMJ* 30, no. 2 (1916): 75–89.

Preston, T.J. "The Chinese Benevolent Institutions in Theory and Practice." *Chinese Recorder and Missionary Journal* 28 (1907): 245–53.

R.G.K. "Editorial: Cleanliness." *CMMJ* 15, no. 2 (1901): 156–57.

Randle, Horace A. "How to Encourage the Chinese to Subscribe toward the Support of Medical Missionary Work among Them: Paper Read at the Shantung Medical Missionary Conference, 1898." *CMMJ* 13, no. 1&2 (1899): 13–17.

"Regulations, Etc., of Hall of United Benevolence for the Relief of Widows, the Support of the Aged, Providing of Coffins, Burial-Grounds, Etc." *Chinese Repository* 20, no. 8 (1846): 402–26.

Reid, Gilbert. "Chinese Law on the Ownership of Church Property in the Interior of China: Section I—the General Right Established." *Chinese Recorder and Missionary Journal* 20, no. 9,10 (1889): 420–26.

———. "Chinese Law on the Ownership of Church Property in the Interior of China: Section II—Special Limitations to the General Right." *Chinese Recorder and Missionary Journal* 20, no. 9,10 (1889): 454–60.

Reifsnyder, Elizabeth. "Methods of Dispensary Work." *CMMJ* 1, no. 2 (1887): 67–69.

Report of the Babies' Wards Post-Graduate Hospital. New York: n.p., 1917.

Report of the Board of Managers of the Pennsylvania Hospital Comprising the Report of the Department for the Sick and Wounded and the Departments for the Insane, West Philadelphia. Philadelphia: J.B. Lippincott Company, 1908.

"Report of the Lao-Ling Medical Mission, 1905." *CMMJ* 20, no. 6 (1906): 269–71.

Report of the Soochow Hospital. Soochow: Methodist Episcopal Church (South), 1913–1914.

Rickett, W. Allyn. "Kuan Tzu." In *Early Chinese Texts: A Bibliographic Guide,* edited by Michael Loewe, 244–51. Berkeley: The Society for the Study of Early China and Institute of Asian Studies, University of California, 1993.

———. *Guanzi: Political, Economic, and Philosophical Essays from Early China: A Study and Translation.* 2 vols. Vol. 2. Princeton: Princeton University Press, 1998.

Roots, Logan H. "Letter to Roger S. Greene." June 25, 1915. RAC, CMB, Record Group 4, Series 1, Box 20, Folder 386.

———. *Our Plan for the Church General Hospital, Wuchang: A Statement of the Most Urgent Needs in the District of Hankow, Leaflet 211.* New York: The Board of Missions, c. 1916.

Roys, Charles K. "Some Dispensary Methods." *CMMJ* 21, no. 3 (1907): 110–14.

Ruoff, E.G., ed. *Death Throes of a Dynasty: Letters and Diaries of Charles and Bessie Ewing, Missionaries to China.* Kent, Ohio: The Kent State University Press, 1990.

Saville, Lillie E.V. "Hospital Reports: London Mission Women's Hospital, Peking, Annual Report, 1905." *CMMJ* 20, no. 4 (1906): 188–91.

Seldon, C.C. "Work among the Chinese Insane and Some of Its Results." *CMMJ* 19, no. 1 (1905): 1–17.

Service, C.W. "A Symposium on Methods of Raising Money Amongst the Chinese for Medical Work: Read at the West China Missionary Conference, 1908." *CMJ* 24, no. 1 (1910): 34–42.

Seventeenth Annual Report of the Directors of the Maine General Hospital. Portland: Stephen Berry, 1887.

Shattuck and Hussey Architects. "Letter to Robert H. Kirk (Rockefeller Foundation)." August 9, 1918. RAC, CMB, Record Group 4, Series 1, Box, 32, Folder 660.

———. "Letter to Robert H. Kirk (Rockefeller Foundation)." August 13, 1918. RAC, CMB, Record Group 4, Series 1, Box, 32, Folder 660.

Shin-ping-yuen. "Report of the Public Dispensary Attached to the *Poo-Yuen-Tang* at Shanghai, for the 25th Year of *Taoukwang,* (1845)." *Chinese Repository* 17, no. April (1848): 193–200.

Simpson, James Y. *Anaesthesia, Hospitalism, Hermaphroditism, and a Proposal to Stamp out Smallpox and Other Contagious Diseases.* Edited by W.G. Simpson. New York: D. Appleton, 1872.

Sisters of Mercy. *Annual Report of St John's Hospital and Training School for Nurses: October 1913–September 1914.* St Louis, Missouri, 1915.

Sixth Annual Report of the Highland Hospital, Fall River, Mass. Fall River, Massachusetts, 1915.

Skinner, J.E. "The Alden Speare Memorial Hospital, Yen-Ping, China." *CMMJ* 18, no. 4 (1904): 162–64.

Smith, Arthur Henderson. *Chinese Characteristics*. Shanghai: North China Herald and S.C. & C. Gazette, 1890.

Smith, J. W. "Letter to Weaver (Rockefeller Foundation) Concerning Financial and Contractural Issues." April 27, 1918. RAC, CMB, Record Group 4, Series 1, Box, 32, Folder 660.

Snell, John A. *Report of the Soochow Hospital, Soochow, China*. Shanghai: The Oriental Press, 1917.

———. *Report of the Soochow Hospital, Soochow, China*. Shanghai: The Oriental Press, 1919.

———. "The City Hospital: Paper Read at the Annual Conference of the China Medical Missionary Association, Peking, 1920." *CMMJ: Hospital Supplement* (1921): 41–48.

Somerville, C.W. *Report of the London Mission Men's Hospital, Wuchang*. Shanghai: American Presbyterian Press, 1905.

Soochow Hospital, 1883–1933: Fiftieth Anniversary. Board of Missions of Methodist Episcopal Church, South, 1933.

"Soochow Hospital, Methodist Episcopal Church, South." *CMMJ* 18, no. 2 (1904): 56 ff.

"Soochow Hospital. Southern Methodist Mission." c.1915. RAC, CMB, Record Group 4, Series 1, Box 23, Folder 444.

Speer, Robert E. *"Lu Taifu," Charles Lewis M.D. A Pioneer Surgeon in China*. New York: The Board of Foreign Missions Presbyterian Church in the U.S.A., c.1930.

"St James' Hospital, Ngankin, China." *CMMJ* 18, no. 3 (1904): 133–34.

Stanley, Arthur. "Chinese Hygiene." *CMMJ* 17, no. 1 (1903): 57–63.

"The Statistics Again." *CMJ* 21, no. 6 (1907): 340–42.

Stone, Mary. "Hospital Dietary in China." *CMJ* 26, no. 5 (1912): 298–301.

Stuart, George A. "The Wuhu General Hospital: 1891–1893." *CMMJ* 8, no. 2 (1894): 128–29.

Tallmon, Susan B. *Glimpses of Lintsingchow Hospital: Being an Attempt to Show Briefly What Has Been Done, What We Are Trying to Do, and a Hint of What May Be Done*. Lintsingchow: A.B.C.F.M., 1910.

Tatchell, W. Arthur. "The Training of Male Nurses." *CMJ* 26, no. 5 (1912): 269–73.

Thacker, L.G. "How Best to Obtain and Conserve Results in the Evangelistic Work among Hospital Patients." *CMJ* 26, no. 6 (1912): 339–43.

Thomson, Jos. C. "Medical Missionaries to the Chinese." *CMMJ* 1, no. 2 (1887): 45–59.

———. "Native Practice and Practitioners: Paper Read at Medical Missionary Association Conference, Shanghai May 1890." *CMMJ* 4, no. 3 (1890): 175–96.

———. "Surgery in China: Section I—the History and Present Position of Chinese Native Surgery." *CMMJ* 6, no. 4 (1892): 219–28.

Thomson, Jos.C. "Medical Missionaries to the Chinese." *CMMJ* 4, no. 4 (1890): 231–35.

"Tsing-Kiang-Pu (Qingjiangbu) Hospital." *CMMJ* 19, no. 1 (1905): 32–34.

Tucker, Francis F. "Letter to the Editor: Record Forms." *CMMJ* 18, no. 2 (1904): 94.

Tucker, Francis F., and Emma Boose Tucker. "Williams' Hospital of the American Board." *CMMJ* 19, no. 6 (1905): 257–60.

———. "Letter to the Editor." *CMJ* 22, no. 1 (1908): 69.

Tucker, Francis F., Emma Boose Tucker, and Myra L. Sawyer. *A Chinese Revolution in Physical Well-Being at Pangkiachwang Shantung, China, 1911–1912:* Williams Hospital of the American Board, 1912.

Twenty-Sixth Annual Report: CMS Hospital, Ningbo. Ningpo: C.M.S. Medical Mission, 1912.

"A Vigorous Chinese Hospital." *CMJ* 32 (1918): 484.

"Walks About Canton—Extracts from a Private Journal." *Chinese Repository* 4, no. May (1835): 44–45.

Wang Mien. "Preface to the Report of the Foundling Hospital at Shanghai." *Chinese Repository* 14, no. 4 (1845): 178–80.

Wang Tsinchin. "Report of the Foundling Hospital at Shanghai." *Chinese Repository* 14, no. 4 (1845): 177–95.

Wang Zhuqin. December, 2001.

Wells, Eliza. "London Missionary Society, Report for 1904, Hongkong." 1904. SOAS, L.M.S., South China Reports: 1898–1904; Box 3, Folder 2.

Wenyon, Chas. "Wesleyan Missionary Hospital, Fatshan, South China:Report 1890." *CMMJ* 5, no. 2 (1891): 122–24.

Whitney, H.T. "History of Medical Work in Shaowu." *CMMJ* 2, no. 3 (1888): 121–23.

———. "Medical Missionary Work in Foochow." *CMMJ* 3, no. 3 (1889): 85–90.

———. "Medical Missionary Work in Foochow, II." *CMMJ* 3, no. 4 (1889).

———. "To What Extent Is Charity Incumbent Upon Medical Missionaries?" *CMMJ* 8, no. 4 (1894): 181–87.

———. "The Self-Supporting System in Medical Work." *CMMJ* 8, no. 2 (1894): 93–98.

"Why Medical Missionaries Are in China?" *CMMJ* 14, no. 4 (1900): 278–80.

Williams, S. Wells. *The Middle Kingdom: A Survey of the Geography, Literature, Social Life, Arts and History of the Chinese Empire and Its Inhabitants.* 2 vols. New York: Paragon Book Reprint Corp., 1895. Reprint, 1966.

Wilson, William. "Hospital Reports: Sui-Ting-Fu, Wan Hsien, via Ichang." *CMMJ* 19, no. 2 (1905): 122–25.

Wolfendale, Richard. "An Ideal Medical Missionary Hospital." *CMMJ* 17, no. 1 (1903): 20–23.

Woodhull, Kate. "The Field Women of Foochow." *CMMJ* 16, no. 1 (1902): 44–45.

Woodward, Edmund Lee. "St. James' Hospital, Ngankin, China." *CMMJ* 17, no. 1 (1903): 37.

———. "The Practice of Asepsis in Mission Hospitals in China." *CMMJ* 18, no. 1 (1904): 1–5.

———. "Mission Hospital and Dispensary Construction in China: Paper Read at Medical Missionary Conference at Shanghai, 1907." *CMJ* 21, no. 5 (1907): 252–63.

Wu Lien-teh. "The Central Hospital of Peking." *CMMJ* 31, no. 4 (1917): 271, 352–54.

————. *Plague Fighter; the Autobiography of a Modern Chinese Physician.* Cambridge [Eng.]: W. Heffer, 1959.

Yen, F.C. "An Example of Co-Operation with the Chinese in Medical Education: Paper Read at Biennial Conference of the CMMA, Shanghai, February, 1915." *CMMJ* 31, no. 3 (1917): 218–24.

ENGLISH LANGUAGE SECONDARY SOURCES

Abram, Ruth J. *"Send Us a Lady Physician": Women Doctors in America, 1835–1920.* New York: W.W. Norton & Company, 1985.

Ackerknecht, Erwin H. *Therapeutics: From the Primitives to the 20th Century with an Appendix: History of Dietetics.* New York: Hafner Press, 1973.

Adams, Annmarie. *Architecture in the Family Way: Doctors, Houses, and Women 1870–1900.* Montreal: McGill-Queens University Press, 1996.

Anderson, E.N. "Fishing People's Medicine: Variations on Chinese Themes." Paper presented at the Association of Asian Studies, Pacific Coast Branch, Bellingham, WA 2002.

————. Personal Communication, June 7, 2002

Arnold, David. *Colonizing the Body: State Medicine and Epidemic Diseases in Nineteenth Century India.* Berkeley and Los Angeles, CA.: University of California Press, 1993.

Bak, Sangmee. "McDonald's in Seoul: Food Choices, Identity, and Nationalism." In *Golden Arches East: McDonald's in East Asia,* edited by James L. Watson, 136–60. Stanford, CA.: Stanford University Press, 1997.

Baker, Patricia. "The Roman Military Valetudinaria: Fact or Fiction?" In *The Archeology of Medicine: Proceedings of the Theoretical Archeology Group,* 69–80. Oxford: 2002.

Barr, Pat. *To China with Love.* London: Secker & Warburg, 1972.

Benedict, Carol. "Policing the Sick: Plague and the Origins of State Medicine in Late Imperial China." *Late Imperial China (Ch'ing—Shih Wen-t'i)* 14, no. 2 (1993): 60–77.

————. *Bubonic Plague in Nineteenth-Century China.* Stanford, California: Stanford University Press, 1996.

Bickers, Robert. *Britain in China: Community, Culture and Colonialism 1900–1949.* Edited by John M. MacKenzie, *Studies in Imperialism.* Manchester: Manchester University Press, 1999.

Boltz, William G. "Chou Li." In *Early Chinese Texts: A Bibliographic Guide,* edited by Michael Loewe, 24–32. Berkeley: The Society for the Study of Early China and Institute of Asian Studies, University of California, 1993.

Bonner, Thomas Neville. *The Kansas Doctor: A Century of Pioneering.* Lawrence: University of Kansas Press, 1959.

Bordley, James, and A. McGehee Harvey. *Two Centuries of American Medicine.* Philadelphia: W.B. Saunders Company, 1976.

Bowers, John Z. *When the Twain Meet: The Rise of Western Medicine in Japan.* Baltimore: Johns Hopkins University Press, 1980.

Boyd, Andrew. *Chinese Architecture and Town Planning: 1500 B.C.–A.D. 1911.* London: Alec Tiranti, 1962.

Bray, Francesca. "Chinese Health Beliefs." In *Religion, Health and Suffering*, edited by John R. Hinnells and Roy Porter, 187–211. London and New York: Kegan Paul International, 1999.

Brokaw, Cynthia J. "Commercial Publishing in Late Imperial China: The Zou and Ma Family Businesses of Sibao, Fujian." *Late Imperial China* 17, no. 1 (1996): 49–92.

Bynum, W.F., and Roy Porter, eds. *Companion Encyclopedia of the History of Medicine*. 2 vols. Vol. 1 and 2. London: Routledge, 1993.

Cadbury, William Warder, and Mary Hoxie Jones. *At the Point of a Lancet: One Hundred Years of the Canton Hospital, 1835–1935*. Shanghai: Kelly and Walsh Ltd., 1935.

Carey, John L. "The First National Association." In *The U.S. Accounting Profession in the 1890s and Early 1900s*, edited by Stephen A.Zeff, 373–415. New York: Garland Publishing, Inc., 1988.

Carlin, Martha. "Medieval English Hospitals." In *The Hospital in History*, edited by Lindsay Granshaw and Roy Porter, 21–39. New York: Routledge, 1989.

Chang Che-Chia. "The Therapeutic Tug of War: The Imperial Physician-Patient Relationship in the Era of Empress Dowager Cixi (1874–1908) (Ching-Qing)." PhD, University of Pennsylvania, 1998.

Ch'en, Kenneth S. *Buddhism in China: A Historical Survey*. Princeton: Princeton University Press, 1964.

———. *The Chinese Transformation of Buddhism*. Princeton: Princeton University Press, 1973.

Cherry, Steven. *Medical Services and the Hospitals in Britain 1860–1939*. Edited by Michael Sanderson, *New Studies in Economic and Social History*. Cambridge: Cambridge University Press, 1996.

Cody, Jeffrey W. "Striking a Harmonious Chord: Foreign Missions and Chinese-Style Buildings, 1911–1949." *Architronic* 5, no. 3 (1996). <http://architronic.saed.kent.edu/v5n3/> (December 2002).

———. *Building in China: Henry K. Murphy's "Adaptive Architecture," 1914–1935*. Hong Kong: The Chinese University Press, 2001.

Cohen, Paul A. "Foreword." In *An American Missionary Community in China, 1895–1905*. Cambridge, Mass.: East Asian Research Center, Harvard University, 1971.

———. *Discovering History in China: American Historical Writing on the Recent Chinese Past*. New York: Columbia University Press, 1984.

The Columbia Encyclopedia. Sixth ed. New York: Columbia University Press, 2002.

Conrad, Lawrence I. "Arab-Islamic Medicine." In *Companion Encyclopedia of the History of Medicine*, edited by W. F.Bynum and Roy Porter, 676–727. London: Routledge, 1993.

Cooledge, Harold N. Jr. *Samuel Sloane: Architect of Philadelphia, 1815–1884*. Philadelphia: University of Pennsylvania, 1986.

Couling, Samuel. *The Encyclopaedia Sinica*. Shanghai: Literature House, Ltd., 1917. Reprint, 1964.

Croizier, Ralph C. *Traditional Medicine in Modern China: Science, Nationalism, and the Tensions of Cultural Change, Harvard East Asian Series; 34*. Cambridge: Harvard University Press, 1968.

Cullen, Christopher, Paul Buell, Nathan Sivin, and Philip Cho. "Discussion: Relative Lack of Dissection in China." *EASCI Discussion List* (2000).

Demieville, Paul. *Buddhism and Healing: Demieville's Article "Byo" from Hobogirin.* Translated by Mark Tatz. Lanham, Md.: University Press of America, 1985.

Dols, Michael W. "The Origins of the Islamic Hospital: Myth and Reality." *Bulletin of the History of Medicine* 61 (1987): 365–90.

Dun J. Li. *China in Transition, 1517–1911.* New York: Van Nostrand Reinhold Company, 1969.

Forsythe, Sidney A. *An American Missionary Community in China, 1895–1905.* Cambridge, Mass.: East Asian Research Center, Harvard University, 1971.

Forty, Adrian. "The Modern Hospital in England and France: The Social and Medical Uses of Architecture." In *Buildings and Society: Essays on the Social Development of the Built Environment,* edited by Anthony D. King, 61–93. London: Routledge & Keegan Paul, 1980.

Foucault, Michel. *The Birth of the Clinic: An Archaeology of Medical Perception, 1973.* Translated by A.M. Sheridan. London: Routledge, 1973. Reprint, 1997.

Freidson, Eliot, ed. *The Hospital in Modern Society.* London: Free Press of Glencoe, 1963.

Gernet, Jacques. *China and the Christian Impact: A Conflict of Cultures.* Cambridge: Cambridge University Press, 1985.

———. *A History of Chinese Civilization.* Translated by J.R. Foster. Cambridge: Cambridge University Press, 1985.

Gibbes, R.W. "Regulations for the Medical Department of the Military Forces of South Carolina." (1861). <URL: http://docsouth.unc.edu/gibbes/gibbes.html> (2002).

Giroux, Gary. "Great Events in Business and Accounting History." Available from <http://acct.tamu.edu/giroux/timeline.html> (2002).

Goldschmidt, Asaf. "The Systematization of Public Health Care by Emperor Song Huizong—Benefiting or Policing the Sick." Paper presented at the Tenth International Conference on the History of Science in East Asia, Shanghai, China, October 6, 2002.

Goodall, Norman. *A History of the London Missionary Society, 1895–1945.* Oxford: Oxford University Press, 1954.

Graham, Gael. *Gender, Culture, and Christianity: American Protestant Mission Schools in China, 1880–1930.* New York: Peter Lang Publishing, Inc., 1995.

Granshaw, Lindsay. "The Hospital." In *Companion Encyclopedia of the History of Medicine,* edited by W. F.Bynum and Roy Porter, 1180–203. London: Routledge, 1993.

Granshaw, Lindsay Patricia, and Roy Porter. *The Hospital in History, Wellcome Institute Series in the History of Medicine.* London; New York: Routledge, 1989.

Gulick, Edward. *Peter Parker and the Opening of China.* Cambridge, Mass.: Harvard University Press, 1973.

Guy, William Augustus, and John Harley, eds. *Hooper's Physician's Vade Mecum: A Manual of the Principles and Practice of Physic.* Tenth ed. Vol. 1. New York: William Wood & Company, 1884.

Handlin-Smith, Joanna F. "Benevolent Societies: The Reshaping of Charity During the Late Ming and Early Ch'ing." *The Journal of Asian Studies* 46, no. 2 (1987): 309–37.

Heininger, Janet Elaine. "The American Board in China: The Missionaries' Experiences and Attitudes, 1911–1952." Ph.D., University of Wisconsin—Madison, 1981.

Henderson, John. "The Hospitals of Late-Medieval and Renaissance Florence: A Preliminary Survey." In *The Hospital in History,* edited by Lindsay Granshaw and Roy Porter, 63–92. London: Routledge, 1989.

Hillier, S.M., and J.A Jewell. *Health Care and Traditional Medicine in China, 1800–1982.* London: Routledge & Kegan Paul, 1983.

Hiney, Tom. *On the Missionary Trail: A Journey through Polynesia, Asia, and Africa with the London Missionary Society.* New York: Grove Press, 2000.

Ho, P.Y., and F.P. Lisowski. *A Brief History of Chinese Medicine, 2nd Edition.* Singapore: World Scientific Publishing Co., 1997.

Ho Tak Ming. *Doctors in the East: Where West Meets East.* Subang Jaya, Malaysia: Pelanduk Publications, 2001.

Hoizey, Dominique, and Marie-Joseph. *A History of Chinese Medicine.* Translated by Paul Bailey. Vancouver: UBC Press, 1993.

Horden, Peregrine, and Richard Smith. *The Locus of Care: Families, Communities, Institutions, and the Provision of Welfare since Antiquity, Studies in the Social History of Medicine.* London; New York: Routledge, 1998.

Horner, Charles. "China's Christian History." *First Things* 75, no. August/September (1997): 41–46.

Howard, Paul. "Opium Suppression in Qing China: Responses to a Social Problem, 1729–1906 (Qing Dynasty)." PhD, University of Pennsylvania, 1998.

Huff, Toby E. *The Rise of Early Modern Science: Islam, China, and the West.* Cambridge: Cambridge University Press, 1993.

Hunter, Jane. *The Gospel of Gentility: American Women Missionaries in Turn-of-the-Century China.* New Haven and London: Yale University Press, 1984.

Hyatt, Irwin T. "Protestant Missions in China, 1877–1890: The Institutionalisation of Good Works." In *American Missionaries in China: Papers from Harvard Seminars,* edited by Liu Kwang-Ching, 93–126. Cambridge, Mass.: East Asian Research Center, Harvard University, 1966.

Jing Shao. "'Hospitalizing' Traditional Chinese Medicine: Identity, Knowledge and Reification." PhD, University of Chicago, 1999.

Jones, Colin. *The Charitable Imperative: Hospitals and Nursing in Ancien Regime and Revolutionary France, Wellcome Institute Series in the History of Medicine.* London; New York: Routledge, 1989.

King, Anthony D., ed. *Buildings and Society: Essays on the Social Development of the Built Environment.* London: Routledge & Keegan Paul, 1980.

———*Colonial Urban Development: Culture, Social Power and Environment.* London: Routledge & Kegan Paul, 1976.

Knapp, Ronald G. *China's Vernacular Architecture: House Form and Culture.* Honolulu: University of Hawai'i Press, 1989.

———*China's Old Dwellings.* Honolulu: University of Hawai'i Press, 2000.

Latourette, Kenneth Scott. *A History of Christian Missions in China.* New York: Russell & Russell, 1929.

Leung, Angela Ki Che. "Organized Medicine in Ming-Qing China: State and Private Medical Institutions in the Lower Yangzi Region." *Late Imperial China* 8, no. 1 (1987): 134–66.

———. "Relief Institutions for Children in Nineteenth-Century China." In *Chinese Views of Childhood,* edited by Anne Behnke Kinney, 251–78. Honolulu: University of Hawaii Press, 1995.

Lian Xi. *The Conversion of Missionaries: Liberalism in American Protestant Missions in China, 1907–1932.* University Park, PA: Pennsylvania State University Press, 1997.

Liang Ssu-ch'eng. *A Pictorial History of Chinese Architecture: A Study of the Development of Its Structural System and the Evolution of Its Types.* Cambridge, Massachusetts: M.I.T. Press, 1984.

Lin Yutang. *The Gay Genius: The Life and Times of Su Tungpo.* London: William Heinemann Ltd., 1948.

Ling Oi Ki. *The Changing Role of the British Protestant Missionaries in China, 1945–1952.* London: Associated University Press, 1999.

Loewe, Michael, ed. *Early Chinese Texts: A Bibliographic Guide, Early Chinese Special Monograph Series.* Berkeley: The Society for the Study of Early China and Institute of Asian Studies, University of California, 1993.

Lu Gwei-Djen, and Joseph Needham. "China and the Origin of Examinations in Medicine." *Proceedings of the Royal Society of Medicine* 56, no. February (1963): 63–70.

Lyman, Henry M., Christian Fenger, H. Webster Jones, and W.T. Belfield. *The Practical Home Physician and Encyclopedia of Medicine.* London: World Publishing Co., c.1900.

Ma Kanwen. "East-West Medical Exchange and Their Mutual Influence." In *Knowledge across Cultures-Universities East and West,* edited by Ruth Hayhoe, 154–81. Hubei: OISE Press, 1993.

MacPherson, Kerrie L. *The Wilderness of Marshes: The Origin of Public Health in Shanghai, 1843–1893.* Edited by Wang Gungwu, *East Asian Historical Monographs.* Hong Kong: Oxford University Press, 1987.

Marcus, Karen K. "Twentieth Century Chinese Architecture: Examples and Their Significance in a Modern Tradition." Master of Science in Architecture Studies, Massachusetts Institute of Technology, 1988.

Marrett, Cora Bagley. "On the Evolution of Women's Medical Societies." In *Women and Health in America: Historical Readings,* edited by Judith Walzer Leavitt, 429–37. Madison, Wisconsin: University of Wisconsin Press, 1984.

McEllhenney, John G. "200 Years of United Methodism: An Illustrated History." (1984). <http://www.cros.net/wdrown/archives.htm> (November 2002).

McCool, Audrey C. "The Heritage of Army Dietetics." *Journal of American Dietetic Association* 97, no 10 (1997): 1080–81.

Milburn. "A Comparative Study of Modern English, Continental and American Hospital Construction." *Journal of the Royal Institute of British Architects* 8, no. 3 (1913): 281–301.

Miller, Timothy S. *The Birth of the Hospital in the Byzantine Empire, The Henry E. Sigerist Supplements to the Bulletin of the History of Medicine; New Series, No.10.* Baltimore: Johns Hopkins University Press, 1985.

Minden, Karen. *Bamboo Stone: The Evolution of a Chinese Medical Elite*. Toronto: University of Toronto Press, 1994.

Morantz, Regina Markell, and Sue Zschoche. "Professionalism, Feminism, and Gender Roles: A Comparative Study of Nineteenth-Century Medical Therapeutics." In *Women and Health in America: Historical Readings*, edited by Judith Walzer Leavitt, 406–21. Madison, Wisconsin: University of Wisconsin Press, 1984.

More, Ellen Singer. *Restoring the Balance: Women Physicians and the Profession of Medicine, 1850–1995*. Cambridge, Mass.: Harvard University Press, 1999.

Morozzi, Guido, and A. Piccini. *Il Restauro Dell'ospedale Di Santa Maria Degli Innocenti, 1966–1970*. Firenze: Becocci Editore, 1971.

Murphey, Rhoads. *The Outsiders: The Western Experience in India and China*. Ann Arbor: The University of Michigan Press, 1977.

Murphy, Mary E. "Founding Fathers of the American Accounting Profession." In *The U.S. Accounting Profession in the 1890s and Early 1900s*, edited by Stephen A. Zeff, 339–72. New York: Garland Publishing, Inc., 1988.

Naquin, Susan. "Funerals in North China: Uniformity and Variation." In *Death Ritual in Late Imperial and Modern China*, edited by James L. Watson and Evelyn S. Rawski, 37–70. Berkeley: University of California Press, 1988.

Needham, Joseph. *Science in Traditional China: A Comparative Perspective*. Cambridge, Massachusetts: Harvard University Press, 1981.

———. *Science and Civilization in China: Biology and Biological Technology*. Edited by Nathan Sivin. Vol. 6. Cambridge: Cambridge University Press, 2000.

Opdycke, Sandra. *No One Was Turned Away: The Role of Public Hospitals in New York City since 1900*. Oxford: Oxford University Press, 1999.

Osterhammel, Jurgen. "Semi-Colonialism and Informal Empire in Twentieth-Century China: Towards a Framework for Analysis." In *Imperialism and After: Continuities and Discontinuities*, edited by Wolfgang J. Mommsen and Jurgen Osterhammel, 290–314. London: Allen and Unwin, 1986.

Perkins, Edward Carter. *A Glimpse of the Heart of China*. New York, Chicago: Fleming H. Revell Company, 1911.

Porkert, Manfred, and Dr. Christian Ullmann. *Chinese Medicine*. Translated by Mark Howson. New York: Henry Holt and Company, 1982.

Porter, Andrew. "'Cultural Imperialism' and Protestant Missionary Enterprise, 1780–1914." *Journal of Imperial and Commonwealth History* 25, no. 3 (1997): 367–91.

Porter, Roy. *The Cambridge Illustrated History of Medicine*. Cambridge: Cambridge University Press, 1996.

———. *The Greatest Benefit to Mankind: A Medical History of Humanity from Antiquity to the Present*. London: Harper Collins, 1997.

Purves, Bill. *Barefoot in the Boardroom: Venture and Misadventure in the People's Republic of China*. Sydney: Allen & Unwin, 1991.

Reeves, Carole. *Egyptian Medicine*. Princes Risborough: Shire Publications, 1992.

Reeves, Caroline Beth. "The Power of Mercy: The Chinese Red Cross, 1900–1937." PhD, Harvard University, 1998.

Reeves, William. "Sino-American Cooperation in Medicine: The Origins of Hsiang-Ya (1902–1914)." In *American Missionaries in China: Papers from Harvard*

Seminars, edited by Liu Kwang-Ching, 129–82. Cambridge, Mass.: East Asian Research Center, Harvard University, 1966.

Reischauer, Edwin O. *Ennin's Travels in T'ang China.* New York: Ronald Press, 1955.

Risse, Guenter B. *Mending Bodies, Saving Souls: A History of Hospitals.* New York: Oxford University Press, 1999.

Robert, Dana L. *American Women in Mission: A Social History of Their Thought and Practice.* Edited by Wilbert R. Shenk, *The Modern Mission Era, 1792–1992: An Appraisal.* Macon, Georgia: Mercer University Press, 1997.

Rogaski, Ruth. "From Protecting Life to Defending the Nation: The Emergence of Public Health in Tianjin, 1859–1953." Ph.D., Yale University, 1996.

Rosen, George. "The Hospital: Historical Sociology of a Community Institution." In *The Hospital in Modern Society,* edited by Eliot Freidson, 1–36. London: Free Press of Glencoe, 1963.

Rosenberg, Charles E. *The Care of Strangers: The Rise of America's Hospital System.* New York: Basic Books, 1987.

Royal Commission on the Ancient and Historical Monuments of Scotland, and (RCAHMS). "Pinnata Castra, Roman Legionary Fortress & Marching Camps, Inchtuthill, Tayside." 2004. <http://www.roman-britain.org/places/pinnata_castra.htm and http://www.roman-britain.org/glossary_m.htm> (May, 2004).

Rubin, Miri. "Development and Change in English Hospitals, 1100–1500." In *The Hospital in History,* edited by Lindsay Granshaw and Roy Porter, 41–59. New York: Routledge, 1989.

Rule, Paul. "The Chinese Rites Controversy: A Long Lasting Controversy in Sino-Western Cultural History." *Pacific Rim Report, the Center for the Pacific Rim's occasional papers series,* no. 23 (2004).

Scarborough, John. "Roman Medicine." In *Aspects of Greek and Roman Life,* edited by Scullard. London: Thames and Hudson, 1969.

Schlesinger, Arthur Jr. "The Missionary Enterprise and Theories of Imperialism." In *The Missionary Enterprise in China and America,* edited by John K. Fairbank, 336–73. Cambridge, Mass.: Harvard University Press, 1974.

Scogin, Hugh. "Poor Relief in Northern Sung China." *Oriens Extremus* 25 (1978): 30–46.

Seidler, Eduard. "Medieval Western Hospitals: Social or Health Care Facilities?" In *History of Hospitals—the Evolution of Health Care Facilities. Proceedings of the 11th International Symposium on the Comparative History of Medicine— East and West,* edited by Yosio Kawakita,

Shizu Sakai and Yasuo Otsuka, 5–22. Susano-shi, Shizuoka, Japan: Division of Medical History, The Taniguchi Foundation, 1989.

Shemo, Connie Anne. "An Army of Women: The Medical Ministries of Kang Cheng and Shi Meiyu, 1873–1937 (China)." PhD, State University of New York at Binghamton, 2002.

Sinn, Elizabeth. *Power and Charity: The Early History of the Tung Wah Hospital Hong Kong.* Edited by Wang Gungwu. 1989 ed, *East Asian Historical Monographs.* Hong Kong: Oxford University Press, 1989.

Small, Hugh. *Florence Nightingale, Avenging Angel.* London: Constable, 1999.

Smith, Richard J. *Fortune-Tellers and Philosophers: Divination in Traditional Chinese Society.* Boulder: Westview Press, 1991.

Spence, Jonathon. *To Change China: Western Advisers in China 1620–1960.* London: Penguin Books, 1969.

———. "Ch'ing." In *Food in Chinese Culture: Anthropological and Historical Perspectives,* edited by K.C.Chang and Eugene N. Anderson, 260–94. New Haven: Yale University Press, 1977.

Stanley, Peter. *For Fear of Pain: British Surgery, 1790–1850.* New York: Rodopi, 2003.

Starr, Paul. *The Social Transformation of American Medicine.* New York: Basic Books, Inc., 1982.

Stevens, Rosemary. *In Sickness and in Wealth: American Hospitals in the Twentieth Century.* Baltimore: The Johns Hopkins University Press, 1999.

Su Gin-Djih. *Chinese Architecture: Past and Contemporary.* Hong Kong: The Sin Poh Amalgamated (H.K.) Ltd., 1964.

Swann, Peter C. *Chinese Monumental Art.* London: Thames and Hudson, 1963.

Taylor, Jeremy. *The Architect and the Pavilion Hospital: Dialogue and Design Creativity in England 1850–1914.* London: Leicester University Press, 1997.

Temkin, Owsei. *The Double Face of Janus and Other Essays in the History of Medicine.* Baltimore: Johns Hopkins University Press, 1977.

Thompson, John D., and Grace Goldin. *The Hospital: A Social and Architectural History.* New Haven: Yale University Press, 1975.

Traux, Rhoda. *Joseph Lister: Father of Modern Surgery.* London: George G. Harrap & Co. Ltd, 1947.

Tucker, Sara Waitstill. "The Canton Hospital and Medicine in 19th Century China, 1835–1900." PhD, Indiana University, 1983.

———. "Opportunities for Women: The Development of Professional Women's Medicine at Canton, China, 1879–1901." *Women's Studies International Forum* 13, no. 4 (1990): 357–68.

T'ung-Tsu Ch'u. *Local Government in China under the Qing.* Cambridge, Mass.: Council on East Asian Studies, Harvard University Press, 1988.

Unschuld, Paul U. "The Chinese Reception of Indian Medicine in the First Millenium A.D." *Bulletin of the History of Medicine* 53 (1979): 329–45.

———. *Medicine in China.* Berkeley: University of California Press, 1985.

Varg, Paul A. *Missionaries, Chinese and Diplomats: The American Protestant Missionary Movement in China, 1890–1952.* Princeton, New Jersey: Princeton University Press, 1958.

Veith, Ilsa. "Texts and Documents: Government Control and Medicine in Eleventh Century China." *Bulletin of the History of Medicine* 14, no. 2 (1943): 159–72.

Waley-Cohen, Joanna. *The Sextants of Beijing: Global Currents in Chinese History.* New York: W.W. Norton & Company, 1999.

Walsh, Mary Roth. "Feminist Showplace." In *Women and Health in America: Historical Readings,* edited by Judith Walzer Leavitt, 392–405. Madison, Wisconsin: University of Wisconsin Press, 1984.

Warnek, Gustav. *Outline of a History of Protestant Missions from the Reformation to the Present Time.* Edinburgh and London: Oliphant Anderson & Ferrier, 1901.

Watson, James L. "The Structure of Chinese Funerary Rites: Elementary Forms, Ritual Sequence, and the Primacy of Performance." In *Death Ritual in Late Imperial and Modern China,* edited by James L. Watson and Evelyn S. Rawski, 3–34. Berkeley: University of California Press, 1988.

———. "Funeral Specialists in Cantonese Society: Pollution, Performance, and Social Hierarchy." In *Death Ritual in Late Imperial and Modern China,* edited by James L. Watson and Evelyn S. Rawski, 109–34. Berkeley: University of California Press, 1988.

———, ed. *Golden Arches East: McDonald's in East Asia.* Stanford, CA: Stanford University Press, 1997.

Wei Shang. "Writing, Reading, and Constructing the Everyday World: Studies of Late Ming and Early Qing Reading Materials." (1997). <http://www.aasianst. org/absts/1997abst/China/c153.htm> (October 2002).

Whiffen, Marcus. *American Architecture since 1780: A Guide to the Styles.* Cambridge, Mass.: M.I.T. Press, 1969.

William H. Welch, Photograph Collection. "View of the Peking Union Medical College, Circa 1921." (2000). <http://medicalarchives.jhmi.edu/welch/travelph. htm> (December 2003).

Wong, K C., and Wu Lien-teh. *History of Chinese Medicine: Being a Chronicle of Medical Happenings in China from Ancient Times to the Present Period.* 2nd. ed. Shanghai: National Quarantine Service, 1936.

Wong, K.C. "Chinese Hospitals in Ancient Times." *CMJ* 37, no. 1 (1923): 77–81.

———. "Four Milleniums (Sic) of Chinese Medicine." *The Lancet* (1929): 156–58; 206–8; 60.

Wright, Gwendolyn. *Politics of Design in French Colonial Urbanism.* Chicago: University of Chicago Press, 1991.

Yip, Ka-che. *Health and National Reconstruction in Nationalist China: The Development of Modern Health Services, 1928–1937, Monograph and Occasional Paper Series; No. 50.* Ann Arbor, Michigan: Association for Asian Studies, 1995.

Young, Theron Kue-Hing. "The William Osler Medal Essay: A Conflict of Professions: The Medical Missionary in China, 1835–1890." *Bulletin of the History of Medicine* 47, no. 3 (1973): 250–72.

Yuet-wah Cheung. *Missionary Medicine in China: A Study of Two Canadian Protestant Missions in China before 1937.* Lanham, Md.: University Press of America, 1988.

Zhao Hongjun. "*Jindai Zhongxiyi Lunzheng Shi* (History of the Modern Controversies over Chinese Vs. Western Medicine) Introduction and Summary by Nathan Sivin." *Chinese Science* 10 (1991): 21–37.

Index